D1258756

PRAISE FOR
Paths to Becoming a Midwife

"This book grows out of Midwifery Today's deep commitment to fostering the growth of midwifery as both a profession committed to excellence and a sisterhood in which midwives are mutually respectful of each other, honoring and upholding the value of differences in education and practice styles. It is a must-read for all aspiring midwives, and an invaluable resource for midwifery educators, policy-makers and legislators, social scientists and consumers of midwifery care."

> — Robbie Davis-Floyd, PhD, author of *Birth as an American Rite of Passage* and coeditor of *Childbirth and Authoritative Knowledge: Cross-Cultural Perspectives.*

"*Paths to Becoming a Midwife* is far more than a practical, how-to book, brimming with information. The editors recognize the profoundly political, deeply philosophical and passionately personal issues and questions that underlie midwifery practice, the world of education and learning, and childbirth itself, all of which are represented in this labor of love. They honor, by inclusion, the diverse experience and voices of women who are midwives as well as those who have reflected upon the meaning of midwifery in modern day culture and the political implications for women of how knowledge is acquired, who defines what is legitimate knowledge and what ways of knowing are valued. This book will challenge aspiring midwives to examine their own values and beliefs and the political, communal and spiritual dimensions of the choices they make. This book is a journey, not just a road map, that leads aspiring midwives beyond information and knowledge, to understanding and hopefully the wisdom to choose the path to midwifery that is most suitable for them."

> — Judy Luce, Co-author of *Our Bodies, Ourselves*

For updates to the Directory,
and the latest information on midwifery programs,
visit our Web page at:

http://www.midwiferytoday.com

Dedication

This book is dedicated to
all the midwives
through the centuries,
known and unknown,
who have helped women
bring forth their babes.

There are many paths to becoming a midwife,
and one will be right for you.
This book is for you, searchers who
want to join the loving midwives
who serve mothers and babies
with heart and care.

May your love be strong,
your families happy and supportive,
as you begin the path to
your calling.

Welcome!

ISBN 1-890446-00-9

Copyright © 1998 by Midwifery Today, Inc.

Portions of this book first published in the United States in 1995 by Midwifery Today, Inc.

P.O. Box 2672, Eugene, Oregon 97402

(800) 743-0974 • (541) 344-7438 • Fax: (541) 344-1422 • midwifery@aol.com

Editor-in-Chief, Jan Tritten
Associate Editor, Jill Cohen
Managing Editor, Design, Layout and Cover Design, Joel B. Southern
Content Editor, Jennifer Rosenberg
Proofreading, Editorial Assistance, Cher Mikkola

Special thanks to Robbie Davis-Floyd for reviewing this book, offering sage suggestions regarding its content, and bringing professionalism and balance to our vision.

Cover photo by Harriette Hartigan

PATHS TO BECOMING A MIDWIFE: GETTING AN EDUCATION

A Midwifery Today Book

Second Edition, 1998

MIDWIFERY TODAY, INC.
EUGENE, OREGON

FOREWORD

This book is designed for the aspiring midwife who is searching for an educational focus. Within are descriptions and stories of the many options available for learning the ancient craft of midwifery, be they apprenticeship, formal certified nurse-midwifery or childbirth education.

This book is a guide to the educational programs available for aspiring midwives in the United States and Canada that were known to us at publication. If you are involved in additional programs not listed, or know of other programs we haven't included, please send us information about them so we may continually update the information for future editions.

This book is for those of you who know you are supposed to become a midwife and are now looking for a way to get an education that meets your needs, as well as the needs of your potential clients. Included are articles chosen from past issues of *Midwifery Today* magazine, as well as articles excerpted for or written especially for this publication. They are written by women involved in obtaining their education, written from a student's perspective, or written from the point of view of someone who has designed or created unique programs.

As an aspiring midwife, carefully consider your needs: Do you need to stay close to home to care for your family? Can you spend several years in another location for your education? Have you thought about beginning your study on your own, at home, while you are not able to venture out into the wider community? Have you completed much study and are you searching for an apprenticeship? Is your financial picture relaxed or constrained? Can you/your family easily pay for your education? What kind of environment do you want to work in when your practice begins? Do you need lots of structure in your education, or are you highly self-motivated? Questions such as these may be answered by considering some of the options available to you that we present here.

No matter where you may be on the continuum of aspiring midwives, you will find a way to get your education. Perhaps reading about some of the options presented here will help you clarify your goals and needs. Perhaps the perfect program already exists that meets your needs.

Jump in and see! Contact the programs listed here for information; ask for a list of students who attended. Those students can give you referrals and information about what they liked or didn't like about their education. Begin your path to becoming a midwife!

May your path be challenging and rewarding and may your journey, beginning with your education, be everything you wanted!

CONTENTS

CHAPTER 1
GETTING STARTED

GENERAL:

GUIDANCE:

REALITIES:

CHAPTER 2

POLITICS
&
PHILOSOPHIES

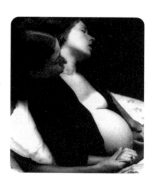

CHAPTER 3

DIRECT-ENTRY
MIDWIFERY

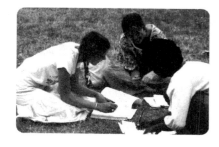

PRACTICE:

EDUCATION:

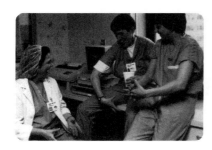

CHAPTER 4

CERTIFIED NURSE-MIDWIFERY

PRACTICE:

CHAPTER 5

CHILDBIRTH EDUCATION, LABOR SUPPORT & POSTPARTUM CARE

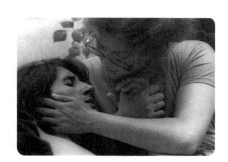

CHAPTER 6

MIDWIFERY
INTO THE FUTURE

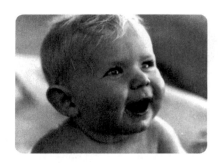

RESOURCES

DIRECTORY OF SCHOOLS AND PROGRAMS

INTRODUCTION

by Jennifer Rosenberg, ICCE, CD(DONA)

At first glance, the number of options available for midwifery education may seem daunting. Or, alternatively, you may feel like there are no options available in your area that fit your needs. This book is designed to help put it all in perspective. There are many options to choose from, but you will find that only a few of them truly fit your goals and priorities. Educational options are frequently limited by geography; you may have to choose between following your "dream path" and finding alternatives based on what is legal in your state and how close you are to the various schools.

Our hope is that with this book you will find the right combination of educational options to help you become the kind of midwife you want to be. We have attempted to cover the gamut of midwifery education, from childbirth education to certified nurse-midwifery, from labor support to certified professional midwifery, from apprenticeships to schools.

If you are just starting out on the path to becoming a midwife, pay careful attention to the first half of this book before you jump into finding a school. Consider all your options. If you are faced with months or more of delay before you can start at an official school of midwifery—nurse or otherwise—there are many things you can do in the meantime to prepare. Many of the stories and articles in this book describe the various options. Do not underestimate the value of life experience, community college work and seemingly unrelated jobs. If you can, volunteer. From public health clinics to NICUs to teen outreach programs, there are real needs for the kinds of nurturing care you long to provide. Consider getting trained in massage, counseling or herbology. Phlebotomy, medical terminology and other technical courses can expand your skills as well. If you keep your mind open, you will find that everyday life has a lot of relevant skills to teach. Read these chapters for more ideas.

One apprentice volunteered at the Midwifery Today office, and although most of her work was routine office work like filing, data entry and envelope stuffing, she said it was a valuable learning experience because it taught her important organizational skills. It also helped her learn to work with a variety of personalities, to adapt to differing expectations, and to take initiative. Though not exciting work, she did not see it as useless. Much of midwifery is waiting, observing, adapting and listening. Take to heart the lessons within these pages, but more importantly, take to heart the lessons within your own life.

Once you have read through the first section of the book, take a close look at the second half. Look at the requirements, expectations and standards of practice for the various national organizations. Compare the different schools. If you can, go on the Internet and look at the Web pages.

Through the course of your education, remember that at the heart of midwifery are the women we serve. Each kind of midwifery is there because a woman needed that kind of midwife. Each path to midwifery is there because a student needed that kind of education. Our goal is to help aspiring midwives find their path, so that women will be able to find the kinds of midwives they need.

SOME TECHNICAL NOTES:

The directory of schools is as complete as we could make it, but because schools are constantly forming, changing, moving or closing, it is impossible to guarantee that any given entry will be correct and complete when you read it. Please contact schools for updated information. If you know of a school which is not listed, encourage them to use the form or a copy of the form on the back page of the book to update their information with us. Updates to the directory will be made available periodically for a small fee.

The political issues in midwifery are in a constant state of flux. Please contact the relevant organizations (see the Resource section) for up-to-date information on policies, certification requirements and legal issues. This book can give you a good foundation for understanding the issues on a national level. It would be impossible for any book to provide a complete picture of the state-by-state legal and political environments for midwifery. Both MANA and ACNM can give you information for your area.

If you want to write for future editions or updates, please send your submission to Midwifery Today, Inc. and note the publication for which it is intended.

You will note that there is a virtual alphabet soup of organizations and certifications in midwifery and midwifery-related professions. Because this is a book of many voices, we have not, in general, arbitrarily changed terminology from that provided by the various authors. Some terms listed:

ACNM: American College of Nurse Midwives

CNM: certified nurse-midwife

CM: certified midwife, direct-entry under the auspices of the ACNM

MANA: Midwives Alliance of North America

NARM: North American Registry of Midwives

CPM: certified professional midwife, direct-entry, specifically refers to a midwife who has met the requirements for NARM certification

TM: traditional midwife, direct-entry, not a certification

DEM: direct-entry midwife. May or may not indicate licensure or certification.

LM: licensed midwife

Lay midwife: Historically refers to non-nurse midwives, but generally refers to a midwife who enters midwifery as a lay person. Many direct-entry midwives still embrace the term lay midwife as a phrase which places the midwife on an equal level with the women she serves, rather than above them. Other direct-entry midwives reject the term lay midwife because it implies a less than professional skill level and training.

TBA: traditional birth attendant, specifically a term used by the World Health Organization to refer to traditional community midwives, usually in Third World countries.

Childbirth Education/Labor Support:

CBE: childbirth educator

CCE: certified childbirth educator

ICEA: International Childbirth Education Association

ASPO/Lamaze: American Society of Psychoprophylaxis in Obstetrics

ACCE/FACCE: CBE certified by ASPO/Lamaze

ICCE: ICEA certified childbirth educator

CPE: certified postpartum educator

ICPE: ICEA certified postpartum educator

CD: certified doula

ICD: ICEA certified doula

DONA: Doulas of North America

CD(DONA): doula certified by DONA

ALACE: Association of Labor Assistants and Childbirth Educators

Terms used to describe various types of labor support:

doula, labor assistant, birth companion, birth assistant, midwife assistant, monitrice

These are not synonyms; they each refer to a slightly different role, training and/or focus on the part of the labor support person. LSP, or labor support person, is a generic term which encompasses any person providing emotional and physical support to the birthing mother, but which generally does not include the person catching the baby.

Again, these lists are not all-inclusive, but will give you a good place to start.

Jennifer Rosenberg is an ICEA certified childbirth educator and a DONA certified doula. She is also a single mom, and works at Midwifery Today.

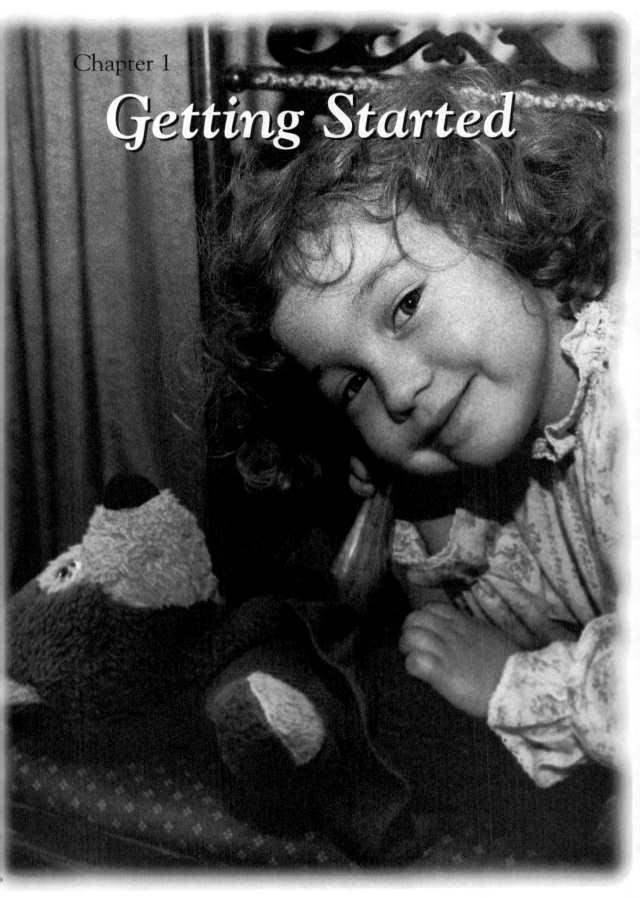

Chapter 1

Getting Started

TO LEARN TO GROW

by Jan Tritten

"The person who seeks an education must involve [her]self in discovering the meaning of [her] own life and the relation between who [she] is and what [she] might become. Without that vision of a personal future and a hard look at the reality of one's own situation, the ultimate purpose of education itself—that is, to grow, to change, to liberate oneself—is almost impossible to achieve."

—Harold Taylor, from Peak Learning by Ronald Gross

Feeding the heart of midwifery through support, good counsel and continuing education has always been the end goal of my efforts at Midwifery Today.

We're realizing some of the dreams we've planned for ourselves. Have you spun a dream of your own lately? Perhaps such a dream would include the investigation of new training or practice options. In this publication, *Paths to Becoming a Midwife*, we'll begin the questioning process with you. We're emphasizing childbirth education and direct-entry programs as well as mapping out certified nurse-midwifery and apprenticeship programs. We contacted many current and former programs by phone and mail; if we missed your training avenue or school, please let us know you're out there and we'll pass the word along.

If you are selecting a new educational route, or modifying your previous training to explore other areas of birth practice, don't just seek a program to glean from. The root of our word *educate* means "to draw out from a dark place."

From the first issue of *Midwifery Today*, I have wanted to create a magazine that would substitute for a good conference, offering practitioners love, support, information and a sharing of ideas and experiences. It's a little ironic, for the magazine still strives to meet these intents, but now I'm looking forward to meeting you in person at one of our Midwifery Today conferences—at our annual domestic conferences, or at one of our international conferences. This is your chance to meet many of your favorite authors and speakers, as well as the chance to learn techniques to enhance your practice, and make new friends. In addition to a wide variety of courses, there will be time to meet a wide variety of birth practitioners, share birth stories, network, and share your tricks of the trade. We're truly eager to meet our readers, and know more about how we can serve your needs. Be sure to call our toll free number (800-743-0974) or access our Web site if you need information about upcoming conferences. We want you to see for yourself—we've planned something just for you.

The task of learning requires humility and attentiveness, and a sometimes painful birthing of our potential. For such a holy event, only an extraordinary teacher will do. Read this book, talk to other midwives, pray and meditate. When you are ready for your educational path to rise up to meet you, the information presented in this book will help open the way.

Jan Tritten became a homebirth midwife in 1976, following the homebirth of her second child. Her first was born in the hospital, and the difference between the two births sent her into her midwifery career. She retired from active midwifery in 1989 in order to devote her time to her work as founder and editor of Midwifery Today and The Birthkit. Changing the way birth is done is her calling.

OBTAINING AN EDUCATION

by Judy Edmunds

Along with all the past and present difficulties midwifery has had to endure, something wonderful is also happening. Educational opportunities are proliferating and improving. There are new, affordable residential schools, at-a-distance didactics, short-term or modular arrangements, supervised preceptorships, and course access via computer. All these opportunities hold great promise for increasing both the availability and caliber of modern midwives.

When I began my practice two decades ago there just weren't many educational choices out there. Those called to midwifery had to be extremely resourceful and persistent in determining their academic needs, doggedly pursuing each bit of available training, and creatively integrating the components. Some midwives were naturally better at this than others, resulting in huge variations in proficiency and practice standards at a time when consumer choice was severely limited. Midwives were often isolated and lacked exposure to other practice styles. Few had any support from or access to resources within the medical community. Thus many, if not most, essentially learned as they went along. Still, since birth usually succeeds on its own, it was not hard to have reasonable outcomes. Challenging situations stimulated the development of new skills. This lack of systematic training, while certainly not ideal, produced important innovations, necessity being the mother of invention. It also bred a generation of fiercely dedicated, independent midwives with hard won and meticulously honed skills coupled with the tenacity required to flourish under adverse conditions. For this, we can be grateful.

My interest in health matters began early, corresponding to personal needs. Because I was in and out of hospitals throughout childhood, illness seemed a constant companion. Despite attentive allopathic treatment, I just kept getting worse. A chance encounter with alternative methods launched my studies in natural health. As I invested in every pertinent workshop, class and book I came across, my accumulation of health and medical texts grew to a sizable library. I tested things out on myself, thrilled with the results. Seeking validation of this knowledge, I eventually earned certificates as a chartered herbalist and registered nutritional consultant from Dominion Herbal College and Donsbach University, respectively. I volunteered in clinics, wherever they would have me (receiving high school credit for some positions). The impetus toward midwifery came when I was eighteen, after I viewed a televised piece about homebirth. The concept made immediate sense, and I enthused to my mother how exciting homebirth was. She cautioned, "perhaps for a second one, but it's best to have the first in the hospital, just in case." (How I've grown to hate that "just in case" line!) Shortly thereafter, I was diagnosed with uterine cancer and endured a series of procedures that ended in hysterectomy. Homebirth would not be something I could personally try out. Still, the spark remained. Having been repeatedly treated with brute, callous disregard or blatant paternalism during my medical adventures, I vowed to help others receive more sensitive, respectful care.

A midwifery intensive was scheduled at a local college. I signed up, not planning to become a midwife (too much responsibility), but to more effectively address the needs of pregnant students attending nutritional and herbal classes I was teaching. The powers-that-be evidently had other plans. In class, we viewed each other's cervices and learned about everything from prenatal care to postpartum hemorrhage. A few months later, I attended my first birth. Now, looking back over almost twenty years of practice and many hundreds of births, certain things stand out as especially useful in learning the art and science of midwifery.

• Organize a midwifery study group and meet regularly to share information and materials, circulate textbooks and journals, review births attended, critique your methods, and learn from each other's mistakes. Invite guest speakers. My group conducted topical research projects and presented reports. A devoted core group kept this up for years.

• Seek formal training for key subjects, such as anatomy and physiology, which is available at most community colleges. Nutrition is the foundation of a healthy pregnancy, so the more you learn the better. Many colleges offer basic nutrition courses that can be supplemented with personal research into women's special needs. Holistic, at-a-distance modules are available and many are quite good, but be cautious of product-oriented programs. Evaluate sample lessons before signing up.

• No matter what you do, document everything. An excellent tool we now have is the North American Registry of Midwives (NARM), and the Certified Professional Midwife (CPM) credentialing process. The CPM credential is being accepted in more and more states as the qualifying standard for direct-entry midwives. Serious students should acquire the application booklet and begin fulfilling the requirements. Besides its utility as a blueprint for obtaining requisite skills and knowledge, the credentialing process provides a convenient means of recording where, when, and how these competencies were achieved. There are forty-nine verification pages, each with about a dozen individual items. By combining a variety of select college courses and workshops, regular conference attendance, an active apprenticeship, volunteer work, and lots of independent study, a motivated student can progress toward primary practice efficiently, even outside a formal program.

• Consider learning in unique ways. Think "outside the box." I took college weight-training classes, which covered weightlifting, applied muscle movement, postural dynamics, diet, metabolism and sports injury rehabilitation. These courses provided a broad understanding of body mechanics and paved the way for the in-depth study required for my massage practitioner license. Because pregnancy changes and challenges a mom's physical structure in profound ways, my broad background has proven very beneficial. Understanding physical discomforts allows me to alleviate many problems and prevent common causes of malpresentations. Alongside structural concepts, I highly recommend studying botanical medicine. Pursued on or off campus, you'll find herbology, homeopathy, and other complementary therapies indispensable. Watch for workshops, conferences, lectures, intensives, and correspondence programs covering areas you're interested in. Different perspectives are

. . . those called to midwifery had to be extremely resourceful and persistent in determining their academic needs, doggedly pursuing each bit of available training, and creatively integrating the components.

refreshing and vital to suitably rigorous thought.

• Subscribe to a variety of journals and newsletters, such as *Midwifery Today, Birth Gazette, Midwifery Matters, The Birthkit, American Journal of Nursing, Mothering, Childbirth Educator, Birth, American Family Physician, Health*, and so on. I cannot overstate the value of this! Share subscriptions with a friend if money is tight, and see what your public library carries. Plan on spending all your extra pennies on pregnancy-related texts. Plan on spending much of your discretionary time reading them. Set goals and read every day. A good midwife must be an avid student, and there is no substitute for accurate, up-to-date information. An appropriate personal library will cost many thousands of dollars, more if you buy all your books new. While this would be difficult to achieve all at once, don't worry. This expense should be spread over many years as you keep building on your resources.

• Learn to respond calmly and efficiently in a crisis. Emergencies are a when, not if, matter, and may define your entire career. Maintain certification in first aid, neonatal resuscitation/ professional rescuer CPR, PALS, ACLS, and other first-responder type programs. Better yet, become an instructor! Vocational colleges offer EMT courses and update modules, which I have found useful. Taking these courses also allows you to meet members of the local emergency response team. Thus, should you call 911, you have an idea of who might come to your aid. Advanced students and practitioners now have the American Academy of Family Physicians' ALSO program available to them. Advanced Life Support in Obstetrics covers a wide variety of perinatal complications and emergency techniques including bleeding in late pregnancy, preterm labor, multiple gestations, medical conditions, birth crisis, breech delivery, shoulder dystocia, postpartum hemorrhage, and much more. Combining prestudy of a thick syllabus, lectures and demonstrations, hands-on workshops, crisis role-play and individual evaluation, this stimulating program is guaranteed to improve your professionalism and self-confidence.

• Investigate nursing training. Even if you decline to take the full program, you can take individual courses in pharmacology, intravenous therapy, phlebotomy, injections, enemas, catheterization, charting, medico-legal issues, infectious disease updates, and so on. Some urban universities, medical centers and research facilities also present classes on a variety of healthcare topics such as sexually transmitted diseases and contraceptive methods. Keep up to date with the latest diagnostic techniques, trends and treatments. I was pleased to find a great program that included many expert lecturers, time in the university's research lab, and a very autonomous clinical rotation through a large hospital's walk-in STD clinic. I highly recommend advanced levels of HIV/AIDS training, including serologic testing certification and partner notification courses. Despite denial and wishful thinking, this matter will eventually come up in every midwife's career, and you have a duty to handle it appropriately.

• Study suturing diligently. Perhaps you might start privately at first, with textbooks and videos. Closely observe experienced practitioners at work. Confer with senior midwives to help you select your equipment. Begin practicing on inanimate matter. Foam models have their place, but repairing living vascular tissue, sensitive to pain, in the confined space of quivering thighs after you've been up all night is much trickier. At least, work on a chunk of fish or chicken flesh since the texture is much more realistic. Then refine your technique at a midwifery school or conference workshop before taking the integrity of someone else's pelvic floor into your hands. (I also worked in a high-volume spay/neuter veterinary clinic where a kind DVM taught me his quick and sturdy stitching style. Think outside the box!)

• Finally, attend as many births as you can because this is where real learning takes place. To students who'd like to be invited more often: Be utterly reliable, helpful, and discreet. If you volunteer to be on call, mean it. This is imperative. I hated it when I was hurrying to load my equipment in the cold, dark, wee hours and paused to phone an apprentice, only to get her answering machine or hear some lame excuse about being too tired, having plans in the morning, no gas in the car, lacking childcare, and so forth. (Please don't even think about bringing your own children.) Once, I foolishly missed the last scheduled ferry, waiting for an apprentice, necessitating an expensive after-hours charter flight. A valued apprentice works hard on her own studies, not expecting to be spoon-fed and led by the hand. She strives to add something unique and worthwhile to the birth team, not just be a spectator. She prepares creatively in advance and brings her own equipment. My favorite helper totes nutritious snacks for herself, the family and me. She asks the family ahead of time which foods they prefer and what she can personally do to make their birth special. She does the dishes, cleans the toilet, starts the laundry, and wipes up puddles without being asked. During a long second stage, she quietly brings everyone juice, attends to the music, rubs backs, and stays optimistic. I don't have to worry about her contradicting me to the family or spreading gossip of the birth to others. I can trust her to keep a confidence. This type of apprentice will have no shortage of opportunities.

So, whatever educational path you choose, remember learning is endless. We are always learning, at each and every birth. Plan on digging deep and offering your best. You will "reap what you sow." To be the best midwife you can, read voraciously, help each other, love birth, and uphold the integrity of midwifery. If this is truly your calling, you will do well.

This article was written especially for this book.

Judy Edmunds has been an active traditional community midwife in northwest Washington since 1981. She is a chartered herbalist, registered nutritional consultant, community health educator and cervical cap fitter. She integrates all her training into whole-woman care. Judy is a contributing editor at Midwifery Today.

PATHS TO MIDWIFERY

by Kate Bowland, CNM

Dear Midwifery Today,

I am writing to ask Midwifery Today readers for advice about midwifery training options. After I decided that I wanted to be a midwife, my sister's homebirth—attended by lay midwives in California—confirmed my decision. However, New York City has no lay midwifery community; therefore, nursing school seemed like the logical first step to take. I don't in the least regret the decision, for I found that I was excited and challenged by most aspects of the profession.

I have recently started working on a high-risk labor and delivery unit, with the intention to get as much experience as possible before I begin my training. Here is my problem: What kind of training will be best for me? The way midwives must practice in the hospital setting, as well as frequent articles in Midwifery Today, have made me question the nursing route. I am attracted to homebirth and envision practicing in a spiritual framework. However, it is not clear that I will leave New York any time soon, and there appears to be no way to train outside the two university programs in the city.

Will training in the medical model, with so much emphasis on technology, enable me to develop my assessment skills? Will I learn what I need to ultimately practice in a more rural setting? Will I become mistrustful of women's ability to give birth naturally? I need advice and welcome input from CNMs and traditional midwives.

> *Merrill Gruver, RN*
> *New York City, NY*

Editor's note: Merrill Gruver's letter is reflective of many of our readers' concerns about educational routes. Kate Bowland, a CNM in Santa Cruz, California, responded.

Dear Merrill,

You want to be a midwife and you ask which path you should take to allow yourself to reach your goal. You are about to make a very personal and political decision. Choosing to be a midwife in the 1990s is choosing the path of the warrior woman.

You will need to carry a machete in one hand, and a shield in the other—a machete to help carve out your space in the medical-industrial-pharmaceutical-insurance complex which runs with the mainstream of unconsciousness in this country. The shield (with a heart on it) you'll need to protect that tender bud of yourself, that spring sprout, new shoot of growth within you, that voice which says birth is a normal natural process to be trusted.

I am a Midwife, BFA, LM, DEM, MOM, ADN, RN, CNM. As you can see, my path was circuitous, with a few detours along the way. I began as an artist, then worked for the San Francisco Chronicle and as a fire lookout. I learned midwifery in an apprenticeship manner, was arrested for the practice of medicine, and went to the California Supreme Court arguing for my right to give birth with whom I choose, and for my right to attend births. I conceived and delivered my two sons at home during the three year long court battle. We lost. The court ruled against us as unlicensed midwives. Charges were dropped against us; they had their test case.

In choosing my battles in the mid-1970s it seemed clear to me that there was a conservative swing in the wind, and that the state would never license midwives under two laws. Lay midwifery was the route of litigious contests, and I wanted to be in the bedroom, not the courtroom.

You ask, "What kind of training is best for me?" You "question" the nursing route, and well you should. Nursing as a profession started off on the wrong foot with Florence Nightingale telling the doctors that she and her nurses would not lift a finger until given doctor's orders. This is not an example of the independent critical thinking and decision making which is necessary in the clinical practice of midwifery. However, the benefit of nursing experience includes learning medical language and working within the hospital system, learning how the team works for birthing mothers and babies. We all know that safe homebirth is dependent upon a good backup hospital and competent doctors and nurses for emergencies.

Personally, I feel the program of physician assistant is a better model for pre-midwifery training than is nursing.

You also ask the important question, "Will I become mistrustful of women's ability to birth naturally?" I ask you, where does your trust lie? In women and nature? Or in test and technology? Are you the same woman coming out of school or after working for a few years than you were when you went into school?

My vision of midwifery training for you would be to teach you the normal first. To begin with, you would work in a low-risk setting, preferably an out-of-hospital setting under the guidance of experienced midwives who know normal. You would be sitting through entire labors without the responsibility or distraction of other patients' needs. You would watch normal birth after normal birth, until normal was ingrained deep in your mind and body. You would have a "feel" for natural, normal, spontaneous birth. You would see only the complications that came up for those women entering labor spontaneously at term. If we look at most homebirth studies that are coming to light from around the world, only about nine to fifteen percent of births need extra help.

Only after you have witnessed the process of progressing labor many times under the guidance of experienced midwives, felt the rhythm of labor with the usual burps and pauses, seen the crowning over the intact perineum, spontaneous expulsions of the placenta and come to know the normal natural way that birth works, only then would you study complications. I believe that the solutions to most complicated births is to recognize problems early and then to imitate nature's usual way.

> I hope you understand that spiritual midwifery is respecting and revering your clients' spiritual belief system.

You ask will training in the medical model with so much emphasis on technology enable you to develop your assessment skills?

As you know, the medical mechanical model of birth came out of the industrial revolution and assembly-line thinking of the last century. We are dealing here as well with the ensuing scientific revolution's persistent influence of ideas which describe the controlling of nature, which value prediction and detection, and which emphasize the rescue of women and babies from the problems that come up in human birth and reproduction. We are dealing with a system of birth care which works within the cultural paradigm of fear.

One ob/gyn resident summed our culture's view of birth when she told me that "birth is a disaster waiting to happen." My experience in a tertiary center was that the students, residents, attending physicians, nurses and midwives in training had no eye for the normal. They were terrified of missing something—particularly something dangerous. There were always stories about sudden disasters and sudden death. If we look to the laws of physics, we are told that to observe something is to change it. I think that if we apply this basic law of physics to birth, I would add that the attending person's feelings change the birth outcome. We have all witnessed how a nervous relative can cause anxiety in the laboring woman. My own observation has been that at birth, fear and anxiety are contagious. Adrenaline seems to flow through the air, and the most normal birth can be turned into an emergency by a fearful attendant. In the hospital, because you have less control over who your attendants are, you are often more vulnerable to the dominant energy becoming fear, rather than faith in the natural birth process.

As to your question, "Can you develop good assessment skills in the high tech world?" my answer is "Yes." And "No."

"No"—if you buy into the fear paradigm of our birth culture.

"Yes"—if you stay in touch with your faith and inner voice. Yes, if you keep notes on your observations and feelings and your perceptions of how things are and how they are going and commit yourself in writing. After the birth, compare your feelings and best guesses to the results of tests and the more objective technology. Compare what your hands felt before the sonogram. You can feel that baby's vitality, integrity, you can feel where its head and feet are, how responsive the baby is to touch and sound. You can carry a fetoscope or Doppler of your own and auscultate the baby's heartbeat. You can do a non-stress test with your hands and your ears first. Sister Angela presented an actual technique for this at a workshop at the California Midwives Association conference in Sacramento. You can feel fluid around a baby in a generous normal amount, or you can feel the shrink-wrapped feeling of the post-dates baby who merits a closer watch in labor. Record your thoughts, diagnoses and predictions for the births you are attending. Afterward, compare your observations with what actually happened. This is a way for you to sharpen your intuition.

You say that you want to practice in a "spiritual framework." Will you lose the spiritual side of your nature if practicing in a medical, technical-hospital based practice? I believe that you are given gifts of the spirit and no one, nothing can take them away. Fire didn't change Joan of Arc's mind. When you go through the valley of the shadow of doubt in nature, please remember that nature doesn't care about individual babies, mothers or midwives, only the overall pattern of reproduction, and the continuing of life, which is overwhelmingly successful.

I hope you understand that spiritual midwifery is respecting and revering your clients' spiritual belief system. That means respecting a Jewish mother's decision to circumcise her son, or a Jehovah's Witness' refusal of blood. It means respecting an atheist's belief in no God, and not imposing your own beliefs on the families you serve. I feel it is not our job to be missionary for our brand of spiritual midwifery.

However, I do not want to negate the value of a midwife's own spiritual practice. I know an African/American CNM who works in an inner city hospital with drug-addicted mothers. She will lay her hands on a woman's belly and baby and bless that baby in her own silent way, and she feels it may be the only blessing that baby will receive. I know a labor and delivery nurse who is a Catholic nun, and she doesn't hesitate to minister with the laying on of hands when a woman is facing a cesarean; she prays silently for a safe vaginal delivery. And I know a midwife who meditates at every birth.

Most midwives espouse the cyclical and flowing model of nature and change. We view the woman's body as normal and healthy in its own right. Our role as midwives is to guard and sanctify the natural process. Birth is viewed as an organic mammal animal sexual act. We believe that a woman's mind talks to her body, and her body talks to her mind, giving her whole being information, stimulating the complex and interrelated flow of hormone and sensations that work together in her opening and birthing.

We are dealing with a culture that believes in a mechanical model of the universe. However, the view from space of Earth as one spaceship, one living organism with complex interrelationships has given rise to global and ecological thinking. I believe this thinking is slowly changing the mechanical model to an ecological cyclical model and that there is hope for natural birth and the midwifery model.

Remember—most of the time, women open, push and deliver healthy babies.

Sincerely,

Kate Bowland, CNM

Santa Cruz, California

CHOOSING YOUR ROUTE

by Diane Barnes, CNM, DEM

Educational opportunities for midwifery have changed considerably throughout my practice. In the old days (twenty years ago), midwives were self-taught, or they were fortunate enough to apprentice with a midwife or at least be mentored by and friends with one. As time passed, more women became interested in the practice of midwifery. Some potential midwives were motivated by their experience in the hospital, both positively and negatively. Some were motivated by the glamour and allure of birth itself.

In the 1960s and 1970s many in the midwifery community thought we didn't need or want regulation. We believed her community would judge the midwife and she wouldn't practice long if she wasn't competent. There were various motivators that changed that scenario. As a community, we became increasingly mobile; our knowledge of our neighbor decreased. Midwives who weren't accepted by their community just moved to another area. Were they competent? Dangerous? We had no way to know. In the 1980s many midwives were searching for ways to increase their knowledge. Independent schools of midwifery opened. Nursing programs expanded their curriculum to include schools of midwifery. These two educational opportunities consisted of very different formats and philosophies.

The Midwives Alliance of North America (MANA) began polling members and opening serious debates regarding regulation and certification and even professionalization. The American College of Nurse Midwives (ACNM) at the same time saw the numbers of non-nurse midwives growing and identified a pool of candidates for their organization. Communication opened between the two and concerns were expressed and similarities identified.

MANA midwives believed that one's home or a birth center is the optimal site for birth. They believed in having good knowledge and skills to attend a birth; however, they did not believe that education had to be university-based.

ACNM believed that women should have midwives attend most births, and because most women deliver in the hospital, effort should be made to get midwives into hospitals. They also believed the education of midwives should be quantified and evaluated, and that midwives should not be accepted without a degree. Concerns were also raised about apprentice midwives being exploited by senior midwives who are put in the position of deciding when the apprentice is trained sufficiently.

The discussions between ACNM and MANA and a consumer consortium led to an agreement that the standards for both organizations match, the ethics statements match, and the basic skills match. MANA decided that the time was right for a sister organization to develop a process to evaluate midwives. The North American Registry of Midwives (NARM) was established first as a registry of midwives who completed an exam of didactic knowledge, and later evolved into a process of complete evaluation including education, knowledge and experience.

Now midwives have two methods of becoming certified: NARM and ACNM. The differences are identified mostly in the remuneration aspects of midwifery. CNMs are accepted in all fifty states. Not all states have hospitals that allow CNMs privileges, however. Nor do all states allow independent practice. Many CNMs work for physicians or are employed directly by them. Many work in public health clinics doing prenatal care only. More regulations are required of CNMs in most states, including insurance requirements to have physician collaboration. Because no home-birth insurance is available, an independent midwifery school education leaves the graduate with limited opportunities in practice. Increasing numbers of states are accepting the certified professional midwife (CPM) certification by NARM, but not all. A CPM's income may be significantly less than that of the CNM, and fewer tuition grants and funds are available.

I began as a physician's assistant in a rural clinic where moms gave birth and went home, and then self-learned the finer points of prenatal and postpartum care, and eventually family planning and general women's health. Then I went to nursing school and became an RN. That helped me put the theory behind my practice. Finally I was accepted to an at-distance program (Educational Programs Associates) in Campbell, California. I completed training and sat for the ACNM exam. My practice hasn't changed much. Although I cover women's general health more, I see a lot more women, and I make a higher income. I am still harassed by the nursing board, and some medical members of the community, but the number of people who appreciate my presence is continuing to grow.

If you are thinking about becoming a midwife, identify your goals.

If you are thinking about becoming a midwife, identify your goals. Do you want to attend homebirth or do you want to make a difference in the hospital? What level of income do you need? What educational opportunities do you have near home? Are you willing to travel? Can you afford the time required of an apprenticeship education and the slower-paced practice, or can you handle the expense of a university-based education? Are you aware of what financial aid is available?

Attending Midwifery Today and MANA conferences as well as ACNM conferences will provide opportunities to interview midwives from all pathways. Understanding the questions and getting answers before you make your decision will lead you to the greatest fulfillment of your dream. Midwifery is my dream fulfilled, and each step on my path has been interesting and rewarding. Each step has increased my ability to serve the women of my community more. Good luck on your path.

This article was written especially for this book.

Diane Barnes, CNM, DEM, has been practicing midwifery in birth centers and in homes for twenty-five years. She operates her own freestanding birthing center in Missouri and attends well over a hundred births a year. She was president of MANA for two terms.

An inspiring excerpt from

Becoming a Midwife

by Carolyn Steiger

Before You Start

Before you are influenced by your teacher, books, experience or other midwives, take a little time to write down your philosophy of childbirth, why you want to be a midwife, and describe what sort of midwife you'd like to be. If you've given birth with a midwife in attendance, what aspects of your midwife's services, personality and attitude were important to you? If you didn't have a midwife or yours didn't meet your needs or expectations, what would you want your ideal midwife to be like? What you'll be describing is an ideal (and perhaps idealistic) picture of a midwife and her connection with birthing women. Look at it from time to time as you are becoming a midwife. You may chuckle at some things you wrote, but other points may re-inspire you and help you remember your greatest dreams.

Life Experience

Birth is not an isolated event, it is part of life. Being an "experienced" midwife includes more than seeing many births. You also need to have experienced a lot of life. You've encountered people of many different cultures, socioeconomic levels and religions. You've been with people under stress, and those who are ill, dying or grieving. You've been in adult relationships, talked with men who have all sorts of attitudes about women. You've felt joy, grief, worry, hope, envy, fear, greed, love, hate—the full range of human emotions—and recognized them in yourself. You may have given birth, raised children, adopted children, taken a child to the hospital for major surgery, or watched a child die. You've nursed your babies and the babies of other women. You've sat and listened to teenage women, old women, women with terrible problems. You've had abrasive or manipulative co-workers. You've been in pain, climbed mountains, taken chances, made a fool of yourself, been humiliated and survived. You've painted your masterpiece, fallen in love, harvested a crop just before the storm. You've watched the moon rise and set, run in a marathon, taken an unpopular stand, bared your soul, and had your heart broken.

Of course, not every midwife has had all of these experiences. But a midwife must have experienced much of life if she is to be non-judgmental, compassionate, and truly able to listen and respond to all types of people.

To feel compassion, to feel "with" a woman, you must see her as your equal—as an equally valuable human being. If you feel superior to women who have less education or money, who aren't as pretty or sophisticated, who are of a different color, religion, ethnic group or culture, who are younger or older, who aren't as healthy as you or as disciplined, you shouldn't be a midwife. If you feel superior to people, you won't serve them, you'll tend to "manage" them and make their decisions for them. If you feel superior to people you will cut yourself off from what they can teach you.

This is not to say you should have low self-esteem. As a midwife you will need to feel good enough about yourself not to need the approval of everyone around you.

You need to have asked questions about who you are, how we all got here and what our place in the Universe is. You must seek Truth and find a rich source of spiritual guidance, comfort and wisdom. You must be a complete person without Birth. Please don't go to births seeking challenges, exciting experiences and a reason to live. The experience of childbirth belongs to that family. It is not yours.

If you are very young or have led a sheltered life, experience more of the world before assuming the role of "wise woman/midwife." Midwifery is a Lifework, not a job to try out for awhile. Some people dread old age. Midwives can look forward to being grannies helping babies they "caught" give birth to their own babies. In many cultures, women only become midwives after menopause. They've raised their own families, and have more time to devote to other families. They have developed character, maturity and wisdom and accumulated years of life experience. The more you prepare, the more you'll have to offer. There's plenty of time.

> To feel compassion, to feel "with" a woman, you must see her as your equal—as an equally valuable human being. If you feel superior to women who have less education or money, who aren't as pretty or sophisticated, who are of a different color, religion, ethnic group or culture, who are younger or older, who aren't as healthy as you or as disciplined, you shouldn't be a midwife.

Excerpted from Becoming a Midwife *by Carolyn Steiger (Hoogan House Publishing, 2915 NE 59th Avenue, Portland, OR 97213, 1987), $24.95, quality paperback.*

Carolyn Steiger has been a licensed midwife in Oregon, speaks regularly at conferences for midwives, and has been involved as a political advocate for midwifery.

WHAT IS THE BEST APPROACH
TO MIDWIFERY EDUCATION?

OPINIONS BY PRACTICING MIDWIVES

CAROLYN STEIGER, A PORTLAND, OREGON MIDWIFE, IS THE AUTHOR OF THE PRACTICAL AND INSPIRING BOOK, *BECOMING A MIDWIFE*.

There are several legitimate ways to train midwives. The traditional method is through apprenticeship: An experienced midwife passes on her knowledge to another woman, shares her insights and gives the student the opportunity to learn from pregnant and laboring women and from birth itself. If we can strengthen and support the concept of apprenticeship we will strengthen midwifery itself and ensure its survival and autonomy.

Through the use of apprenticeship, we retain control over midwifery education. Schools which are answerable to the state are all too often dictated to by the state, which in turn looks to the medical community for direction. Of course, there are schools which provide training similar in nature to an apprenticeship. But those which are patterned after medical schools will only produce mini-doctors or practitioners who must spend years deprogramming themselves if they are to rediscover the strength of women, the beauty of birth, and the wisdom of the midwifery model.

For many, apprenticeship is the most accessible form of education in terms of distance, time and cost. Young people may be able to leave home to travel to distant schools, but women who have acquired wisdom over a lifetime of rich and varied experiences, who may indeed make the finest midwives, may also have families who depend on them and babies to breastfeed. Apprenticeship offers hometown training to these women.

Midwives are likely to serve many low-income women. If our training is costly, we will incur debts that prohibit us from serving everyone who needs us. Women with families may not have the financial resources to pay tuition and to support their families as well. Apprenticeship is generally much less costly.

Apprenticeship can be interwoven with the rest of daily life and is not as disruptive as having mom leave home for her training.

The way we teach midwifery should reflect our ideals. We should use the art and spirit of midwifery to teach the art and spirit of midwifery.

Midwifery requires the development of many intangible qualities. We believe, for example, that humility, compassion and honesty are as essential as technical ability. Even if the student can perform skills, pass tests, accumulate experience and graduate from a school, it doesn't mean she should be a midwife nor does it guarantee that she will be a good one. Intangible qualities are best evaluated in a one-to-one relationship by someone who also has developed these qualities. For example, assessing a student's intuitive response to labor can be done only by someone sharing the experience with her and responding intuitively herself.

Self-examination is an important part of midwifery education. The student must search her heart, confront her fears and prejudices, and seek her own healing first. Nurturing this personal growth is easiest in the intimate, non-competitive setting of the one teacher-one student relationship. A competitive spirit has no place in midwifery.

In an apprenticeship, skills, experience and study are blended perfectly with the spirit of midwifery. Proper performance of skills requires more than efficiency and technical ability. The teacher passes on, by example, the ability to approach each woman with a respectful and loving touch. Through frequent contact with her teacher, close relationships with birthing women, and many hours of labor-sitting, the apprentice has the opportunity to acquire highly developed observational skills. She learns to use her hands, her senses, her intellect and intuition.

Through apprenticeship, experience is gained in a traditional manner: The apprentice "studies" the birth process in its natural setting, the home. She is then able to evaluate the dramatic impact of intervention, environment and procedures on the birth process more clearly than can hospital personnel. Apprenticeship usually limits the number of births each month to those the teacher attends. This establishes a certain pace which in itself affects one's attitude toward birth. The apprentice isn't in a hurry to "get the baby out." She can be more "process-oriented." She is more likely to see each birth as special. She is able to become close to each woman and therefore can sense which techniques will "work" for that woman. She is able to see the entire labor and birth and gain a better perspective on what is happening.

Well-designed apprenticeships can provide a solid foundation of skills in the study of women's health, pregnancy, childbirth and newborn care. The apprentice must learn to make critical evaluations from a midwifery perspective because most textbooks are based on a male, medical perception of women giving birth at the hospital. In an apprenticeship, the student adapts what she reads to the needs of her community and her study is guided by a teacher who has her own philosophy of midwifery and style of practice. This is how we retain a rich tradition, distilled through the centuries and gleaned from diverse cultural and ethnic backgrounds.

Too many of us are trying to invent apprenticeship as we go along; many problems have arisen. We must become as dedicated to apprenticeship as we are to midwifery. If we direct as much energy toward its design and are as devoted to its growth it will, in turn, revitalize midwifery and nurture the blossoming of a new generation of powerful, wise, and compassionate women to carry on our dreams.

JULIE LITWIN IS A PHYSICIAN'S ASSISTANT WHO PRACTICES IN SANTA CRUZ, CALIFORNIA.

I trained to be a midwife in 1979, and practiced with partners in California for several years. Because we were harassed for being unlicensed, a partner and I decided to return to school so that we could practice legally. We elected to become physician assistants instead of nurses because we could learn a lot more about primary healthcare in a shorter amount of time.

There are a number of physician assistant programs around the country which differ a lot in terms of length, emphasis and curriculum. The program that we chose, at Stanford University in California, was fifteen months long. It was designed to train practitioners to provide primary healthcare for people in medically underserved areas. The classes were held at Stanford and a clinical preceptorship offered in one's own community. The program required a number of prerequisite classes and previous medical experience for which midwifery counts.

A physician assistant can specialize in many different areas after graduating if one so chooses. I specialized in women's healthcare and midwifery. The only program I found at the time was located in Campbell, California, through Education Program Associates. The program is equivalent to nurse-midwifery training but is implemented in a self-paced format to enable the student to work at other jobs while completing the program. It took me a little over one year to finish.

> A physician assistant is actually able to practice midwifery without going through specialty training if the doctor who supervises her/him allows it.

A physician assistant is actually able to practice midwifery without going through specialty training if the doctor who supervises her/him allows it. The specialty training provides another piece of paper that says you know what you are doing.

The laws regulating PAs are different in each state, so I'm not sure whether what is true in California is true elsewhere. In my state, the basic difference between practicing as a PA and practicing as a nurse is that the physician supervision requirement is a little different. PAs are more restricted.

A PA works under specific protocols and the doctor has to sign a certain number of her/his charts. This has created some difficulty in securing doctor backup. Furthermore, in California no malpractice insurance that covers doctors will also cover me while doing homebirths. [Ed. note: The political climate for midwifery in California changes rapidly, and at this writing, malpractice coverage may not be as difficult to obtain.]

I'm not sure what the ideal form of midwifery education is. I think the more practical experience one can get from working in different places and with various midwives who have individual styles, philosophies and practices, the better. I certainly don't think that one has to be a nurse or a PA to be a midwife, although that kind of training does add other dimensions to a practice.

SHERRY WILLIS, A FLINT HILL, VIRGINIA MIDWIFE, IS CO-FOUNDER OF THE COMMONWEALTH MIDWIVES' ALLIANCE AND HAS SERVED AS VIRGINIA REPRESENTATIVE FOR THE MIDWIVES ALLIANCE OF NORTH AMERICA (MANA).

In order to acknowledge the uniqueness of each woman seeking her station as midwife, we must think in terms of multiplicity of answers to midwifery education. I view midwifery as an art rather than vocation, and when creatively expressed, as multifarious by nature. My ideal would be, whether by way of apprenticeship or formal schooling, that all education be founded upon fundamental precepts that would afford greater freedoms in methods of practice than currently available. While I practice in the Wise Woman Tradition and respect all ways of education and practice, I strongly feel that no course of study should hinder midwives from using methods that respect the unique experience of each family served and the individual family's beliefs and needs.

More specifically, the greatest portion of any midwifery education should be experiential in nature, with midwives teaching midwifery, not obstetrical technology. Aspiring midwives would ultimately apprentice to birth, respecting women as the true experts in giving birth, and babies in being born. Women and their babies would be regarded as the primary teachers of birthing.

The following is an exploration of some of the precepts I refer to as the foundation for ideal midwifery education:

(1) A much broader definition of normalcy during the childbearing year than our contemporary narrow and rigid view.

(2) A redefinition of commonly accepted childbearing complications to that of normal variations in the process.

(3) Development of a greater sensitivity to the interferences with normalcy in childbearing (physical, cultural, emotional), the subtle as well as obvious, with special emphasis on those created by midwives themselves.

(4) Specific instruction about the ecosystem created by mother and child, the natural laws governing it, and the responding sense of natural timing that nature maintains as an instrument for success.

(5) Instruction in developing a criteria for practice that will make homebirth accessible to a greater number of women. Of critical concern to me is that the popularly accepted midwife criteria creates an elitist group of women "acceptable" to birth at home and excludes many women who could safely choose homebirth as an option.

(6) Exploration of our own fears surrounding childbearing and how they alienate us from the women we attend, and their experience.

(7) Development of intuition as a rational and intellectual skill.

(8) Facilitation of personal empowerment in becoming a midwife—only through our own empowerment can we enable another. Specific issues would be fostering internal validation of ourselves as midwives, and validation from the communities we serve in order to balance our obsession with external validation (licensing, certification and so forth). Throughout this process we would be encouraged to creatively express our individuality and uniqueness.

I assert that midwifery education faces powerful and beautiful transformation. We need to serve consciously and with great discretion as we follow the path of change. Our education, or re-education, can recreate the reality of childbearing in this country only by helping women reclaim their inherent right to normal birthing practices. My ideal vision is that through midwifery education we will creatively construct and implement numerous avenues to realize the station as midwife. Our safest passageway is unity through diversity.

IDA LASERSON, CNM, PRACTICES IN EUGENE, OREGON.

Slogans to the contrary, midwifery is not "just catching." There is a large body of basic knowledge requisite to safe entry into the practice of midwifery, and that knowledge and experience can best be gained through formal education in a post-RN accredited school of nurse-midwifery. The prerequisite education grounds the student in the basic sciences of normal anatomy, physiology and microbiology. Nursing skills and procedures are gained through classroom study and the all-important clinical practicum under the guidance of experienced teachers. Additionally, many certified nurse-midwife programs require the entering student to have had at least one year's experience as a labor/delivery RN.

CNM programs offer an organized, systematic curriculum which covers all the basic areas of experience. Periodic written and clinical testing verifies the student's mastery of the material. In order to exercise her skills during normal labor and delivery, the CNM must be able to recognize and respond appropriately to the abnormal. Student nurse-midwives gain all or part of their clinical education in hospitals where they are exposed to complicated labors and births as well as to the normal. This exposure is extremely valuable as the student can learn to handle emergencies in the relatively sheltered environment of a well-supervised clinical setting. The student gains knowledge; the birthing mother is protected.

The CNM can be legally licensed to practice in all fifty states. Licensure grants credibility and the power to work for change in prenatal and birthing care from within the system. The current trend toward family-centered, gentle, non-interventionist hospital births is largely due to the example set by nurse-midwives and the pressures they and the families they serve apply to these large institutions.

As more CNMs demonstrate safe care in homes and birth centers, these kinds of out-of-hospital births will become more accepted by the mainstream. Consequently, more birthing options will then be available with the assurance of competent medical backup for complications. Indeed, CNMs who now attend out-of-hospital births can obtain hospital privileges in order to give continuity of care to those laboring women who must be transported due to complications.

Grounded in the basic midwifery knowledge gained through formal education, CNMs can and do look to other resources such as naturopathy, acupuncture, herbal medicine, massage, psychology and direct-entry midwifery for a variety of "born again" old approaches and innovative and creative new approaches to perinatal care. Incorporating non-medical methods and practices into the core foundation of CNM education produces a well-rounded midwife who has a versatile repertoire of skills to offer birthing families—a midwife whose skills are embroidered upon her firm foundation in the science of midwifery.

STANDARDIZED EDUCATION:

DOES IT PREPARE BETTER MIDWIVES AND BIRTH EDUCATORS?
WHAT ARE THE SHORTCOMINGS AND STRENGTHS OF YOUR OWN PREPARATION?

A collection of responses from practicing midwives

ALISON OSBORN IS A MIDWIFE IN GRASS VALLEY, CALIFORNIA.

Obviously midwives need to learn bottom lines, parameters of standards of care, ethics and what constitutes normalcy in birth. We need to know how to recognize when things aren't within normal limits and what to do about it.

Rather than ask if standardized education prepares better midwives, the question should be "How can we make available the true scope of midwifery practice in standardized form?"

When the focus is on the jillion little things that can possibly go wrong, we teach fear and distrust of the body's innate ability to do its work. We need to stay in the norm and cushion students in their first year of education—with normal birth. We need to remain within the circumference of "nutrition-plus-exercise-plus-relaxation-equals-outcome" model. If we try to teach the medical model—and especially if we teach this initially—we cannot hope to prepare midwives to advocate and facilitate normal birth.

In our attempts to get one hundred thousand midwives working by 2050, we will need to standardize programs. I personally am unable to teach all that I know to an apprentice in less than three years, and I can only teach one at a time. We'll never train enough midwives to serve the demand by the apprenticeship method alone.

As to the shortcomings and strengths of my own education, my training took over ten years. The desire to become a midwife started five years before that, and I attended college, taking anatomy, physiology, microbiology plus all the standard classes. I also went to births—around ten per year for ten years—and looked up in reference texts what I had seen at these births. I had the great advantage of working with a collective, and we had chart review weekly.

This training was wonderful in several ways: I learned my skill while being a single mom—I didn't have to separate my life or leave my girls; I learned very thoroughly, one birth at a time (one birth per month is much easier to absorb, in terms of psychosocial dynamics than three births in ten hours). Most of the women I served I knew as friends before they became pregnant, and these are friendships we've maintained, so I experienced pregnancy and birth to be truly an event in the continuum of life. And perhaps not the least beneficial is the amount of time I gave to the pursuit: As years passed, I matured.

The negative aspects to this approach to training are that not many women can train in this manner—there aren't enough births; as well, it is necessary to have an income while you learn (I was on welfare), and it is not the way to gain exposure to the variety and variance which occurs even within the range of normal—you just don't see a lot of what can happen, and if you haven't seen it, chances are you are left with a gap in your training.

I addressed this concern with a three month internship at Casa de Nacimiento in El Paso. I attended more births in three months than in the preceding ten years! A good deal of what I saw was on the outside fringe of normal; as a result, I got a great education and went on to start making my living as a midwife.

Liz Esty is a new age midwife, partner and mother in Oregon.

How did I become a midwife? How could I stop it? I had a homebirth, everyone heard, and they all wanted me at their births. I couldn't stop it. My training? I learned by doing. After a few years, there were so many of us that we would gather together in study groups. It's not the most formal way to begin, but that's how it happened.

In the 1970s there was a renaissance in midwifery. The rebellion of the 1960s had defined a group of people who felt they had the right to choose their place to birth. Women who had their children at home found themselves called upon by their families, friends and neighbors to attend their homebirths. These women had no formal training, and had to be motivated to find ways to further their education.

Time has passed, and the renaissance has ebbed. The 1990s have brought in a new group of midwives—women who are called to midwifery by their hearts rather than their neighbors. These women have more choices in their learning process; today there are schools, homestudy programs and apprenticeships. But these women are not always called by their community and therefore, they are left to make their own way.

They may have to travel hours, even days to attend classes and conferences. They may leave their families for months to obtain training. Then they have to make their own way into the midwifery community.

These women are often ostracized by their peer midwives. "You left your families," or "You didn't learn by apprenticeship" are criticisms one often hears directed toward the new midwife. The community close at hand is often closed when they return home; competitive feelings surface: "You are taking a piece of the pie"; "Your education is not sufficient [like mine]"; "How great that you're a midwife—just be sure to practice somewhere else." After years of professional wasteland, where there were so few options available, now it seems unbelievable—some states are now setting up training programs for midwives in the interest of promoting midwifery, while the regional midwifery organizations may greet a newcomer's expressed interest in relocation with, "Sorry, there is no room at the inn." It is simply devastating to return home after pursuing one's desire with all one's being, only to be treated with such an attitude of indifference.

The New Age midwife's blend of academics and experience also seems to threaten some established practitioners. What if she has really learned quite a lot? What if her experience covers a wider spectrum than that of the practitioners? What if she sets up practice in their back yard? What if pregnant women are drawn to her personality and choose her to attend their births?

In this "new age" of midwifery, those midwives who are choosing to combine the old with the new may feel as if they are scaling a sheer cliff. They hear about sisterhood. They hear about expanding midwifery care. They know that there are thousands of women who are unable to obtain adequate prenatal care; finding a way to bloom, to set up practice, to serve women, to continue their "becoming"—this may be an excruciating uphill climb.

As midwives, we preach our grandiose wisdom. "We are sisters on a journey." "We need to expand midwifery care and services." "Every woman has the right to choose how and with whom she births." But the New Age midwives often feel little or no support from their sister midwives. Alone, on their own, they often seek other New Age midwives who remind them to persevere in their uphill climb and to trust that they will become.

Is it any wonder that we are in a state of persecution? Is it any wonder that there are vast numbers of women who receive no prenatal care at all? Are we sisters on a journey, or are we our own worst enemy? The time has come to stretch and mature, and to live up to what we say we believe. The only way we will ever see midwifery grow is to truly support each other on our road to becoming— regardless of the educational pathway chosen. "Does standardized education prepare better midwives?" It will hardly matter how well prepared the new practitioner is if she has no acceptance from the community of her peers. It seems clear that we need to give up the "piece-of-the-pie-that's-mine" attitude, for with each new midwife who takes her training to the service of empowering women to birth where and with whom they choose, many more families will be attracted to midwifery care.

If on the other hand, we refuse the challenge to humble ourselves, to accept and to welcome our sisters in their beginnings, then midwifery will remain a dying art, available to a precious, persistent few. I ask each of you to open your hearts, and to live what you profess. Please remember—we are always becoming.

AT THE HEART OF BIRTHING EDUCATION

by Elizabeth Davis, CPM

Passion for the subject, and passion for sharing what we know—most educators agree that these qualities keep our teaching fresh and vital. In my growth as a teacher, I have acquired yet another sense of the importance of passion, and it is this: It is paramount to acknowledge my students' passion as a key to their success.

From adult education theory, we know that mature learners will only accept that which incorporates their already established sense of self. I worked from this premise in my childbirth preparation series, and I also emphasized this established sense of self with student coaches, guiding them in finding their best avenue of communication—physical, verbal, or empathetic—and showing them how to use it as a focal point in birth assisting. In curriculum development, I encouraged students to identify which aspect of childbirth preparation excited them most, whether a particular subject or learning activity; I recommended they build their first class firmly around this interest, as a springboard.

Even while stressing personal enthusiasm, I did not neglect certain "bottom-line" information. This closely parallels what we know in midwifery practice as "maintaining the boundaries of safe care." In fact, the art of blending the highly personal with the starkly objective is not only relevant to the learning experience of individual adult students. I believe it is also of significance to the larger scope of midwifery education.

As we move to retain the apprenticeship model of midwifery training, we find we must articulate competencies as well as curriculum—both what a midwife needs to be able to do, and what she must study and experience to learn this. Thus far, we have focused primarily on technical abilities, and to some extent, the more elusive caregiving techniques. But what of the more fundamental capacities? For example, how do we teach a midwife to "conduct deliveries on her own responsibility?" How do we teach her to empower women and their families to take responsibility for themselves? And in the highly individualized course and process of birth, where variables are at once standard and changing minute-to-minute, how do we teach a composite view of "maintaining the boundaries of safe care?" A seldom-discussed but highly relevant attribute in this regard is common sense—and how may this be taught, or evoked?

The ACNM's ad hoc committee on homebirth may soon begin to formulate curriculum for nurse-midwives who wish to practice out-of-hospital. This prospect underscores the need for training which blends both affective and cognitive learning styles. In addition to skills essential for an expanded scope of practice, what else might nurse-midwives need to know? How is caregiving different when one enters someone else's environment as a guest, particularly when one's hostess/host are well educated about this experience to be shared with them, and especially if they have definite ideas of their own about the tone and measure of its unfolding? *[Ed. note: The ACNM has since published a guidebook for CNMs on homebirth practice.]*

Curriculum for practitioners in this field must have a major component of self-assessment. This would not be a separate segment or module, but would be an overall learning objective interwoven within all areas of study and preparation. This can be accomplished in many ways. My midwifery students use journal work to help discover their emotional reactions to class material and activities, which we further debrief with discussion. Having students identify personal agendas, expectations and limits in general as well as in birth-related situations is critical. We also work extensively with the role-playing of psychologically challenging situations. To learn to be a team player, to give and take constructive feedback, to know when to ask for help, and to be able to do so when necessary—these are all affective abilities which can be valued, cultivated, taught and tested. In doing so, we come close to the heart of an optimal standard of care.

A program which emphasizes self-assessment teaches students to stay in touch with their personal passion. And a teacher who is acquainted with the effectual blending of personal and objective learning will seize the moment when passion runs high, and temper it with hard, pertinent facts. Without this passion, where will practitioners find courage, vitality and staying power in the demanding birthing professions? And without self-awareness and ongoing self-assessment, how can we hope to be truly responsible practitioners?

A critical formulation of the Inter-Organizational Work Group/Carnegie meetings is that educational methods cannot be separated from the way we define practice. To shape our models for the future, we need only reflect on what sort of care provider a particular avenue of training will generate. We can place the student in a context which intimidates and usurps personal power and passion. Or we can choose an educational model that "midwifes" the student, with all the care for the wholeness of her learning that we would devote to any birth.

This article originally appeared in Midwifery Today Issue No. 20.

A renowned expert on women's issues, Elizabeth Davis, CPM, has been a midwife, women's healthcare specialist, educator and consultant for the past twenty years. She has served as a representative to the Midwives Alliance of North America for five years, and president of the Midwifery Education Accreditation Council for the United States. She is co-founder of the Midwifery Institute of California, a three-year, apprenticeship-based midwifery program. She holds a degree in Holistic Maternity Care from Antioch University, and is certified by the North American Registry of Midwives. She is the author of four other books, including Women, Sex & Desire, and The Women's Wheel of Life: Thirteen Archetypes of Woman at Her Fullest Power (with co-author Carol Leonard). Elizabeth lives in Windsor, California, and is the mother of three children.

FACING REALITY:

HOW TO BEGIN YOUR MIDWIFERY CAREER

by Karen Parker, CNM

I t's two o'clock in the morning. You have been soundly asleep for three hours when the telephone rings. It takes a while to register in your dreams but it clicks and you jump to quiet the offending noise. It's time. Your good friend is in active labor and you have been invited to participate both as a support person and helper to the midwife attending. As you hang up the phone you notice you have a good case of the "shakes" and you hurry to find your robe in hopes the warmth will calm your excited psyche. This is your fifth birth, and each one so far has been an exhilarating and beautiful pleasure. Your love of birth has become apparent within your circle of friends and you have felt honored to be asked to attend.

Once dressed, you feel compelled to kiss your sleeping children, and your mate only opens one groggy eye as he wishes you love and good luck. As you hurry to the car the autumn air welcomes you, causing you to slow your step to look at the moon, so still and majestic in the solitude of these wee hours. You wonder if other women are gazing at its strength right now as they also embark on a similar adventure. You shiver, and hop into the car thinking haste is in order here.

It's early yet as you observe your friend in her labor. Her mate envelops her body with strong, supportive arms as they lie together in gentle breathing. You busy your-self, quietly assisting the midwife as she prepares for her work. And with God's speed the passage draws near; the wet smells, now familiar, signal the approach of this new and precious life. Your body sweats yet your hands feel cold as you watch the midwife deftly slip the cord over the baby's head. She then hands the little, wet, wiggling Being into the loving embrace of her mother and father. Your tears are silent as you remember your own birthings and the special emotion felt when you first met your children. You feel the great privilege and the blessing of childbirth. Your heart is stirred. You wish it for yourself again and always and forever.

INITIAL DECISIONS

Deep emotion usually motivates the initial decision to pursue a career in mid-wifery. Each of us is different but the decision-making process still requires great for-titude and soul searching. A number of issues present themselves as decisions, often at the most inopportune moments. Some are but a nuance at the time, only to man-ifest with volcanic force at a much later date. The most obvious considerations con-cern your family, the type of training most suitable for you, personal sacrifice, and your level of commitment. Some feel they can sidestep these decisions by allowing birth to just come their way. However, the personal demands in this profession are tremendous, requiring constant reevaluation of goals. It is beneficial if one begins with a clear idea of personal direction.

Family Considerations

Most of us become interested in midwifery through our own birthing experiences. You hold the memories close, feeling a sense of accomplishment, self worth. However, a strong fresh memory of your birth usually indicates that your children are still very young. This means that often you feel bound to the priority of caring for your young family. Thoughts of pursuing a career are viewed as a luxury rather than a serious step. We have all experienced becoming deeply absorbed in an exciting new book or article only to have to halt our train of thought to kiss yet another "owee." So your heart yearns in one direction while your soul reminds you of your existing commitments. Sound familiar? Part of this struggle is a result of our cultural upbringing. Our mothers, guided by their mothers, believed that keeping a home and raising a family were the all-encompassing role of woman.

There are no magic words out there in the universe that can help you with that struggle. It depends upon your own sense of timing. Only you can determine the course of your unfolding. The answer lies within.

It is likely that your mate is a major influence in the decision-making process. If you were to choose to begin your career what would this mean to him? More work, more money, more sacrifices from him, more, more, more? Certainly it challenges his present lifestyle which may be quite comfortable the way it is. You can determine his true feelings by using gentle encouragement, and quiet his fears as well. After all, you are not replacing your marriage with a career, only complementing it. It is sad that our society continually places women in a position in which they must validate their right to happy and fulfilling work. For those considering a change, an encouraging partner is valued beyond gold. Generally, men tend toward one of three reactions when informed of their mate's desire to begin a career in midwifery: He will wait it out patiently until she "changes her mind when things get rough"; he will use guilt to make things as tough as possible; or with love and support, he will take pride in the growth and fulfillment she is experiencing.

Every relationship has weaknesses which can become more troublesome with change. You can prepare yourself by strengthening your commitment both to your partner and to your career. Make it clear that anyone who continually argues your limitations or makes life difficult during your work hours is not using acceptable behavior. Your happiness is your right and personal responsibility. Gold stars to the loving supportive mate who thrills at your joys and can be your spine when yours can't hold you up anymore. Blessed be the mate who can listen to his partner's desire to challenge herself outside the home and supports her in word and deed. This precious man is worth all the juicing up you can provide along with constant acknowledgment of his output and personal sacrifice.

But what about all your children, your babies? (No matter what their age, they are still your babies.) It is true that they will also learn the concept of "letting you go." The birthday party you prepared for, then missed, is not easily reconciled with a four-year-old. Midwifery is often a very impromptu work, full of juggling where time is concerned. One of the things your children will come to learn is "wait." Your end of this deal is to be impeccable in your follow-up of "wait." Focusing on quality time is also imperative. Your children will need the same juicing and acknowledging as your mate. There is no limit on ways to say thank you. Be creative in ways that include your children in your career. When I have arranged a film night or public event it is a special time for my family. We present ourselves as a unit to the public and have good fun at the same time. We prepare snacks together and the children like to set them up and serve. I find that this contributes to the picture that they have in their mind's eye of what goes on in their mom's life when we're apart.

SELF-SACRIFICE

Perhaps you have already come across areas in your life you must relinquish in order to pursue midwifery. Maybe there is no more time for your exercise class, or the garden just went to weeds for lack of attention. And what about those special walks at sunset? Suddenly there just isn't time. Fortunately for most aspiring midwives the reverent pleasure of attending is an equal trade-off for these personal forfeitures. However, I do not intend to prepare you for a no-fun existence. In fact, midwives need to play more than anybody because their work is so stressful. It is necessary to get involved in a recreation unrelated to the career side of your life. All throughout my apprenticeship I maintained an avid rock climbing career. I did find that after a while I absolutely preferred to be birthing and that my work had become, in fact, my play. I so enjoyed my midwifing that I didn't mind at all being called away to deliver instead of going off-call and trekking into the mountains. This ultimately created resentment within my family, most especially with my mate, and took lots of work to undo. Elizabeth Davis says it best in her book *Heart and Hands, A Guide to Midwifery:* "It is the power derived from increasing clarity that leads a midwife beyond her capacity." This concept of total immersion in one's work will take you to great heights, yes. But the price is often too great to bear.

> Fortunately for most aspiring midwives the reverent pleasure of attending is an equal trade-off for personal forfeitures.

COMMITMENT

So, you have looked deeply and closely at these decisions. You have concluded that the time is right to take steps toward learning this exciting and fulfilling work. Your family will love you through it and you have juggled everything in your mind so you can be available to study and attend with a minimum of hassle. And yet it still seems an insurmountable task to put everything in order enough to allow yourself the time for study, prenatals, births, postpartum follow-ups, classes, public events and on and on!

It all boils down to personal commitment. Remember when your heart stirred? Remember the blessing of being present as new life emerged? When was the last time you were so thoroughly inspired? How many times in your life have you fallen in love, completely, forever . . . over and over and over again? (Oh, those sweet little babies!) Commitment. How deep does yours go? How willing are you to examine the reaches of your own courage and ability to love? How dedicated have you become to safe and loving passage? Commitment—it is the foundation of a caring midwife's career.

Once you realize you are truly committed and wish to pursue this profession, you will be faced with the choice of training methods. There are basically two kinds of midwives in America: certified nurse midwives (CNMs) and direct-entry midwives (DEM or lay midwives). For those deciding how to obtain their midwifery education, choosing the correct direction can be difficult and time consuming.

TRAINING

These choices may be limited for you in your locale. For some, apprenticeship in lay training is the only available course. Others may have college programs available to them in certified nurse-midwifery. This involves years of classroom study. It also means becoming a nurse first and then going on to a midwifery degree. It means three to four years of nursing school, then another year to get your nurse-midwifery degree. Of course those years give you orientation within the high-tech medical world. Even after years of effort to secure the degree, some areas are still politically hostile to any homebirth (or alternative birth) care provider. Depending on locale, your license could be threatened or revoked or hospital privilege denied. This is terribly unfortunate and is something we can all work to change within our own states. There is a place for each of us and certified nurse-midwives are an important complement to each community.

For those women who choose not to become a nurse there are special considerations. Do you view midwifery as a separate profession from nursing? It is essential that you do if you choose to take the training via apprenticeship. Can you accept no diploma on your wall after a long and in-depth study process? Diplomas don't insure competency but neither does a lack of one! Can you deal with a medical world which may constantly ignore you for lack of credential? Will the pleasure of successfully going about your work be enough or do you need the status of letters after your name? And those letters mean more than status. They mean prescription privileges, hospital privileges, instant (sometimes) credibility, more ease in obtaining doctor backup (sometimes), and on and on. Can you accept that your only insurance policy is TOTAL honesty and your credential, experience? If you can, then apprenticeship with a practicing midwife could be your most suitable answer. One common fallacy is that apprenticeship is an "easier" way to learn the art. I don't agree. If anything, there is greater challenge. You assume responsibility for your own knowledge and ability to absorb information. You must also develop strong skills in transforming your observations into clinical information on the spot. No grades are issued but being asked to step into the role of primary assistant far surpasses any "A" you'll ever receive!

One established midwife, Christine, points out, "For me, convincing people that I was serious about my work seemed most difficult. Because my apprenticeship ended with no resulting diploma, I encountered much resistance in the medical world. It took years of effort within my community before practitioners would listen to me in a credible way. Unfortunately, the hardship seemed to extend to my clients. I would be persistent and thorough in my endeavors to secure information or care that I needed for them. But if there was a transport to the hospital, especially a time-crucial emergency, I sometimes had difficulty getting everyone to listen to me concerning what was needed, past events and so forth. After a few years in the community, this lessened but I was concerned about the compromise in care my clients might have to face because of my lack of standard credentials."

Christine lives in an area where lay midwives are the only care providers for homebirth couples. Even so, it is a graphic portrayal of what can be encountered and it is only with diligent and careful persistence that she came to be viewed as an intelligent and capable midwife.

It may be helpful to keep the possibility of nursing credential in mind during your apprenticeship. You can always change your direction. We are as free as we deem ourselves to be.

IN CONCLUSION

Certainly, your acceptance as a midwife within your community varies with the legal status of each state. How you go about securing your training is a matter of personal choice. Making the initial decisions is tough to say the least. A woman's family must be supportive and loving even though it will be very demanding at times. Their payoff is simply to see her happily working at her contribution to the universe. Her personal happiness could also vastly improve her ability to contribute to the relationships within her family. Self-sacrifice is balanced by personal gain as one achieves a long sought-after dream. All of it comes full cycle to how committed you are to accomplishing your goal. If you can encounter each obstacle as a way of solidifying your commitment to becoming a conscious, competent midwife, you will arrive there with a firm belief in your own purpose.

This article originally appeared in Midwifery Today Issue No. 4.

Karen Parker, CNM, began attending births in 1976 as an apprentice, is a certified midwife in Oregon with a nursing degree and a CNM degree. She is now in private, independent practice with three ob/gyn physicians at Providence Hospital in Portland, Oregon. She loves her practice which includes complete care of women: providing lactation consultation as well as midwifing women through menopause.

MIDWIFERY EDUCATION:
A GLOBAL PERSPECTIVE

by Vicki Penwell

In a home in the Philippines, a new mother scoops up her newborn daughter, still attached by the pulsing umbilical cord, and hugs her to her breast.

A Lahu tribeswoman in northern Thailand squats beside a fire to cook rice, her baby strapped to her back with a bright length of cloth.

In a hospital in the war-ravaged country of Laos, a young woman strains stoically, soon to deliver her third child.

What makes these women different from their American and European sisters? The fact that over one million of them will die this year while trying to bring forth new life.

The developing world accounts for 99 percent of all maternal mortality—an average of three thousand women each day die of pregnancy related causes. For mothers in developing countries, the risk of dying is 50 to 200 times higher than that of a woman in a developed nation. A typical woman in Africa or South Asia faces a lifetime chance of one in 20 of dying while pregnant or in childbirth.

The World Health Organization (WHO) has been tracking the problem of maternal death, looking for solutions. Data points to the need for more trained midwives. In the WHO publication, *Safe Motherhood*, a recent article carried the headlines "Midwifery Education: A Life Saving Solution."

Could it be that midwifery education can really save lives, and on such a large scale? The answer is a resounding yes, according to Dr. Barbara Kwast, midwife and scientist with WHO's Safe Motherhood program and a former lecturer in community obstetrics in Ethiopia. "Midwives could safely handle 70 to 80 percent of deliveries and more if they were adequately trained," Dr. Kwast says. "They are also able to fill the gap in health services between the village and the district hospital."

Dr. Mark Belsey, Chief of WHO's program called Maternal and Child Health, told a recent conference in Geneva, Switzerland, "The number of nurses and midwives is falling, and mid-level care—where the midwife should be—is disappearing." The meeting called particular attention to the need for effective training initiatives to combat the increasing global shortage of midwives.

The world is in need of midwives, ones who know how to work outside of hospitals. Over 70 percent of mothers in the developing world give birth with no trained assistant, with 85 percent receiving no prenatal care at all. The prediction is that without a reordering of priorities, the annual number of deaths from reproductive causes will double by the end of this century, reaching at least two million.

There are many problems related to training midwives for effective service in the underdeveloped world that must be overcome. It is vital that the midwife be trained to recognize and understand the traditional beliefs and traditional practices of the population she is caring for. She develops strategies to close the cultural gaps between the midwife and the community. The midwife must present health education to communities within the context of that culture (often through skits or storytelling), teaching the preventable factors that lead to maternal death. And she must be competent in skills to identify and successfully manage the five major causes of maternal death—hemorrhage, illicit induced abortion, sepsis, obstructed labor and eclampsia.

One of the problems of midwifery education was summed up in an article in *Midwifery: An International Journal*, by Barbara Kwast. Author Kwast wrote, "Unfortunately too few midwife teachers have relevant experience in rural areas and have little practical appreciation of the problems. . . . Teachers have little contact with midwives practicing outside hospitals, and that is where most midwives should be working, if lives are to be saved."

I have seen the women of the Third World. I was there when the Philippine woman gave birth. I cared for the Lahu mother's baby when he was sick. I received the little Lao baby into my hands, in that dirty, forsaken hospital in the capital city of Laos.

The other side of the world is not so far away. Are we willing to share? What resources, what knowledge, what hope?

This article originally appeared in Midwifery Today Issue No. 20.

Vicki Penwell has been a licensed midwife since 1983 in both New Mexico and Alaska. She is married and has three sons. Since 1990 Vicki has traveled widely, teaching midwifery and primary healthcare for women and children in the underdeveloped world. She has set up and currently oversees birth centers and clinics in the Philippines and Mexico among the poorest of the poor. In her duel role as mission pastor for the Vineyard Christian Fellowship, Vicki teaches midwifery in the context of church-based missions and community development.

References

World Watch Institute Report, June 1991.

"Postpartum Haemorrhage: Its Contribution To Maternal Mortality," Kwast, Barbara, in *Midwifery: An International Journal*, Vol 7, No. 2, 1991.

"Preventing The Tragedy of Maternal Deaths," Starrs, Ann, 1987. A report on the International Safe Motherhood Conference held in Nairobi, Kenya.

"Challenge for the Nineties," Starrs, Ann with Diana Measham, 1990. Proceedings of a Safe Motherhood South Asia Conference held in Lahore, Pakistan, 1990.

"Midwifery Education: Action for Safe Motherhood." Report of a collaborative ICM/WHO/UNICEF pre-congress workshop, International Confederation of Midwives Conference, October 1990, Kobe, Japan.

"Woman's Health and the Midwife: A Global Perspective." Report of a collaborative pre-congress workshop, International Confederation of Midwives Conference, August 1987, The Hague, Netherlands.

Chapter 2

Politics
&
Philosophies

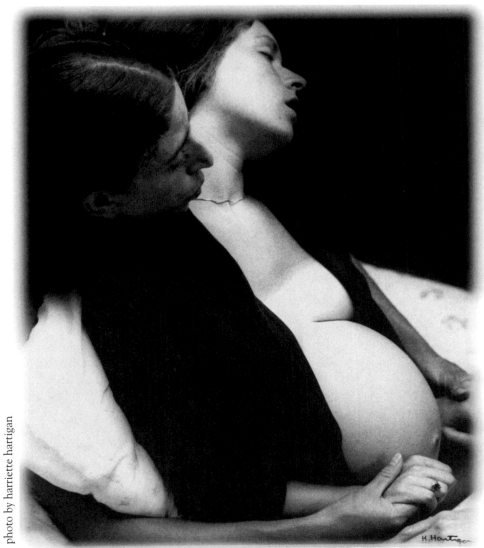

POLITICS: AN INTRODUCTION

by Jennifer Rosenberg, ICCE, CD(DONA)

There is a tremendous debate right now among midwives, and there are gravitational forces at work. On the one hand, the explosion of philosophical differences in what midwives should be, how midwives should be educated, who should certify midwives and who should control them threatens to destroy the community, and will at the very least reshape it into something completely new. On the other hand, the strong desire for unity and common ground pulls us back together.

In this section you will read a number of strong opinions, arguments and philosophies. Midwifery Today has for many years attempted to walk a tightrope between science and art, medicine and normalcy, intuition and deduction. We've worked hard to show that midwifery is not an either-or proposition. Thus, despite the strong biases and views of each of the authors in the section, you will see that each of them acknowledges that there is room for other kinds of midwifery, other kinds of midwives.

We have compiled this chapter not to air midwifery's dirty laundry, but because it will help you, the aspiring midwife, understand why each side feels so strongly. You will read these articles and see commonalities between your own heart and one or another of the views expressed herein. This is a valuable aid to you to determine what kind of midwifery you will ultimately be most comfortable in. Do you feel strongly about being able to work in a hospital environment, or with higher risk women? Would you rather change the system from within than without? Or is your heart in homebirth, and do you feel that to be true to yourself you must serve women in the environment you feel is the most normal? These are important points to recognize, and the debate in this section will bring up many more issues for you to consider when making your choice.

We at Midwifery Today hope you will view this chapter as an opportunity to see both sides of the story, to understand the whole debate before stepping into the profession. There is a middle road. Many midwives, of all backgrounds, yearn for unity. Not uniformity, but simply cooperation and the understanding that there are many kinds of midwives and many kinds of education, and that this is a good thing. This is why there are certified nurse-midwives in MANA, and why apprentice-trained homebirth midwives become CNMs. If Midwifery Today can be said to take a side, it is this middle road that we land on. Our goal is to promote midwifery care. Not just hospital-based midwifery care. Not just homebirth midwifery care. Not just certified nurse-midwifery care. And not just traditional midwifery care. We advocate for all of them. There is a need for each of them. Whatever road you land on, our hope is that you end up being a good midwife and serving women well.

Jennifer Rosenberg is an ICEA certified childbirth educator and a DONA certified doula. She is also a single mom, and works at Midwifery Today.

A BALANCED MIDWIFERY EDUCATION
IS A WORTHWHILE GOAL

by Jan Tritten

The giving of love is an education in itself.

How do we best educate midwives? Does a system like the American College of Nurse Midwives (ACNM) provide the best education in order to achieve the midwifery model? The ACNM method may yield technical competence, but at what cost? Can the "soft" aspects of midwifery be retained, even nurtured, in an environment where the technical aspects are emphasized? Conscious synthesis of right brain (sensitive/esthetic) capacities and left brain (rational) makes the best midwife. If the balanced teaching technique of woman helping woman is de-emphasized, then we slip too far into the medical model.

The current, sad trend is to require higher and higher degrees in order for an aspiring midwife to gain entry to midwifery school, even though there is no proof that such degrees correlate with better outcomes. It limits competition and drives the price of midwifery services up. This is far from the ideal of "with woman." Instead, we need good programs for entry-level midwifery. The ACNM looked at the issue of direct-entry schools, but as you will see in later articles, the results of that effort have been mixed, with some unfortunate and unexpected consequences for direct-entry midwives.

Just as a baby needs a mother for guidance, so a mother needs a midwife.

Potential midwives are often called to the profession after their children are born. One option for the aspiring midwife is to practice at the direct-entry level, although it is illegal in many states. Another option involves the aspiring midwife who perhaps has a degree in counseling or biology. She may have to move to a state which offers a program such as Yale's where nursing is picked up with midwifery in a three-year stint. Or, a woman may first become a nurse, gain experience in obstetrics and go through midwifery school, all of which takes about the same amount of time it would have to become a doctor. Most young mothers can choose neither of the last two options due to potential cost both in money and family hardship.

We as a profession must consider alternative methods in order for aspiring midwives to gain an appropriate education. Many good ones are emerging, and apprenticeship is an excellent example.

In January 1994, the Midwifery Certification Task Force endorsed standard qualifications for national certification of midwives. The qualifications represent hands-on skills proven by a specific amount of experience in certain areas of prenatal, intrapartum and postpartum care, as well as successful completion of the North American Registry of Midwives (NARM) exam. This standardization of skills gives apprentices (and the public) the opportunity to evaluate their midwifery abilities.

A college-based program would provide better access to the hospital learning experience, but unfortunately, midwifery training would again be fit into the medical model and would be difficult for midwives to control.

Direct-entry midwifery education provides a good alternative to the present nursing system because it keeps midwifery a calling rather than merely a career. In that midwifery education is locked into nursing with so few midwifery schools in operation, it limits who can attend. And there is no good reason why a midwife must first be a nurse. This mode of education has kept midwifery from being an autonomous profession by molding it to the authoritarian medical model. (In England, both educational systems exist.) Moreover, midwifery is one of the only fields where you must train into one profession before you can pursue the one you have truly chosen. By using the teaching model, in four to five years a student midwife can gain a bachelor's degree and a midwifery education concurrently. Requiring preliminary work in childbirth education or a brief apprenticeship in home or clinic births with practicing midwives would ensure that the normalcy and beauty of birth would be emphasized as a prelude to the more technical instruction which must follow.

It takes about three years to learn midwifery, more for some, a bit less for others, depending on the intensity of the program. In most situations, midwifery is 90 percent spirit and 10 percent scientific/technical. Because that 10 percent saves lives, it must make up 90 percent of our education. In practice, however, we can assume that each woman's birth will be normal. Yet, we must always use our skill in technical evaluation in case it isn't. As midwives, it is our job to help women have normal births by using all our resources and good counsel.

The challenge to the profession still remains: to make midwifery education attainable all across the United States. We need to maintain alternative routes of entry into the field through apprenticeships, correspondence, direct-entry and nurse-midwifery schools. The different kinds of practitioners make a great checks and balances system and serve our diverse culture well. Above all we must increase the number of midwife-attended births to 75 percent or more of the country's births.

Every birthing woman needs a midwife—to guard the sanctity of her birth and act as her caregiver and advocate. Just as a baby needs a mother for guidance, so a mother needs a midwife.

This article originally appeared in Midwifery Today Issue No. 4.

Jan Tritten became a homebirth midwife in 1976, following the homebirth of her second child. Her first was born in the hospital, and the difference between the two births sent her into her midwifery career. She retired from active midwifery in 1989 in order to devote her time to her work as founder and editor of Midwifery Today and The Birthkit. Changing the way birth is done is her calling.

UNDECIDED? BECOME A CNM!

by Judith Rooks, CNM, MPH, FACNM

In advising a young woman considering the different paths to becoming a midwife, I would question her about why she wants to be a midwife, her circumstances and what kind of life she wants to lead. Although my response would depend upon her answers, in most cases I would probably advise her to become a CNM. This article lays out the reasoning for that advice and provides a summary of some of the relevant history of both nurse-midwifery and direct-entry midwifery in this country. Anyone who wants to be a midwife should know this history.

Although I am a CNM, I am not in practice—most of my career has been in public health (in this country) and in international maternal and child health and family planning—mainly as an epidemiologist, consultant, teacher and writer. I tend to view midwifery in the context of my public health concerns. However, I have also been active in nurse-midwifery, including serving as president of the American College of Nurse-Midwives from 1983–1985. I have spent much of the past several years researching, writing and dealing with the aftereffects of having published a comprehensive book, *Midwifery and Childbirth in America*. Although I was well steeped in nurse-midwifery and childbirth, honoring a commitment to write a book explaining midwifery in America required me to learn much more about direct-entry midwives. I did this through the extreme generosity of many wonderful direct-entry midwives and their supporters.

Having entered midwifery from public health, I developed respect and affection for midwives in general. From my experience as a nurse-midwifery student at Johns Hopkins from 1972–1974, from research I have conducted on nurse-midwifery and birth centers, from teaching in CNEP,[1] and from my experiences as a member and leader of the ACNM, I have great respect for nurse-midwives. I have also developed increasing respect for direct-entry midwives and have real affection for the free-spirited lay midwifery movement that played such a significant role in the 1970s and 1980s. I am especially respectful of direct-entry midwives' steadfast commitment to the essential qualities of midwifery and birth, and their arduous struggle to preserve those qualities in the face of long-standing barriers and opposition. Both arms of the profession have fascinating histories, have made important contributions to individual women and to the development of midwifery in the United States (and the world), and both are relatively powerful and effective forces in our society. Their goals for women are the same, but their major contributions, role and place in society are different. With some exceptions, CNMs and direct-entry midwives lead very different lives.

DIFFERENCES IN HISTORY

Profound differences in the culture of nurse-midwifery and direct-entry midwifery have resulted from their histories. Nurse-midwifery was brought to the United States when Mary Breckinridge founded the Frontier Nursing Service in Kentucky in 1925 amidst a long, successful medical campaign to defame and eliminate midwives. The medical community at that time insisted that midwives were untrained and incompetent.

Mary Breckinridge was an extraordinary woman from a prominent family. Her grandfather had been vice president of the United States and her father was an American ambassador to Russia. She was well educated and spent much of her youth traveling and living in Europe. She married, was widowed, remarried and had two children, both of whom died at young ages in rapid succession. She then divorced and determined to use the rest of her life to improve the lives of children. She became trained in public health nursing, and at the end of the first World War went with the Red Cross to France, where she imported goats to supply milk for starving babies and created the first French Child Hygiene Visiting Nurse Service. Although impressed by French midwives, she thought it odd they had no background in nursing—just the opposite of America, where nurses had no training in midwifery. Then she encountered British nurse-midwives who had the combination of training she thought was needed to help the children of impoverished families in the mountains of Kentucky, where she was from and the part of the world she knew best.

Mary Breckinridge established the Frontier Nursing Service—the first American nurse-midwifery service—in a remote, doctorless county in the Kentucky mountains. She and the FNS established many of the basic principles and assumptions that have guided nurse-midwifery.

Figure 1: Principles and Assumptions Established by the FNS:

- Formal training in nursing and midwifery
- Providing care to women who lack access to medical care
- Collaboration with physicians
- Nurse-midwifery as a tool of public health
- Meticulous record keeping with analysis of data on outcomes

---

Already a nurse, she prepared herself by obtaining formal midwifery training in Britain. For staff, she recruited British midwives, sent American public health nurses to Britain for training, then started a formal nurse-midwifery school at FNS.

She brought nurse-midwifery to America to provide care to families who lacked access to medical care. Yet she knew that midwives and their patients also need physicians. As soon as she arrived in Kentucky, she recruited a medical director and developed protocols defining the clinical relationship between the FNS nurse-midwives and physicians.

Breckinridge saw nurse-midwifery as a tool of public health, worked in close collaboration with state and local health departments and sought and received financial and other support based on the public health benefits of providing nurse-midwifery care to a needy population. The Frontier Nursing Service kept meticulous records and thus could assess the results of the care it provided, including remarkable reductions in both maternal and infant mortality.

The second nurse-midwifery service was started by a New York City women's club to provide care to impoverished inner-city women and their babies. The third was started with government funds to serve poor black women in rural Alabama. The fourth was started by a Catholic missionary group concerned about Hispanic women in New Mexico. Every new service needed help from the few existing services and schools—a close-knit conspiracy of evangelical public health nurses cum midwives nurturing a nascent profession in pockets of poverty and rural isolation that were not served by physicians.

> Both arms of the profession have fascinating histories, have made important contributions to individual women and to the development of midwifery in the United States (and the world), and both are relatively powerful and effective forces in our society.

Although every service had a training program, only a few of the midwives trained in those programs practiced midwifery in the United States. It was very hard to start a service, in part because midwifery was not legal in most states. By the early 1960s—nearly forty years after the FNS was started—fewer than forty nurse-midwives were in practice in this country. Most of those few worked in Kentucky, New Mexico or New York City, the only three jurisdictions in which their practice was explicitly legal. A few worked under granny midwife laws in other southern states; some worked as missionaries in developing countries. Many of the early nurse-midwives taught nursing or worked in public health. Nurse-midwives introduced the concept of family-centered maternity care into American nursing education, played a significant role in the development of childbirth education, demonstrated the radical concept of mother-baby rooming in, and urged mothers to breastfeed at a time when most hospitals were teaching women how to make formula and sterilize bottles.

The few nurse-midwives who were practicing midwifery did only homebirths until the mid-1950s, when they were invited into Johns Hopkins and several other teaching hospitals to help obstetricians cope with the post-war "baby boom." They proved that they could assist the poor and improve the quality of care in those hospitals. Obstetric leaders speaking at a 1968 conference described the "shameful and humiliating circumstances" experienced by poor, black women in "our great public hospital clinics . . . conditions and attitudes of callousness" that "almost defy description." An obstetric department chairman who had worked with nurse-midwives during his residency at Hopkins described the interest, competence and dedication they brought to their work and the need to introduce those attitudes into charity-hospital obstetric services in order to "produce a more humanitarian quality of service."

But everyone at the meeting agreed that nurse-midwives should be restricted to caring for the poor. The nurse-midwives did not complain. Many were Catholic nuns (or would have been nuns except that they were Protestants) and most came from public health nursing. They knew the problems of poor mothers and babies, and had become midwives to improve the care of women who were poor. In order to serve women who had little money and many health problems, they needed an institutional base and the involvement and support of physicians. Nurse-midwives did not venture from care of the poor for almost fifty years because their hands were full with the needs of the women they were serving and because they could not do so and retain their institutional and medical support.

With time more women, physicians, and health service administrators saw the advantages of midwifery, and the nurse-midwives' role began to broaden. By the 1970s they were filling substantial roles in the military services, in the Indian Health Service and in programs established after enactment of Medicaid and federal support for family planning. Health maintenance organizations in the West began to use CNMs—at first because they were short of obstetricians, then for financial reasons and finally, because some of their subscribers wanted and demanded midwives. CNMs began to enter private practice, mainly as employees but, in some cases, as partners of physicians. But most practiced in collaboration with obstetric faculty and residents in busy tertiary hospitals, where they were taught and expected to use the obstetric interventions practiced in all academic obstetric departments.

While many nurse-midwives adapted their practice to complement the predominant medical model, the desire to avoid routine use of medical interventions played an important role in motivating midwives to develop birth centers as places designed for the midwifery model of care. CNMs were the major force in the development of freestanding birth centers.

DIRECT-ENTRY MIDWIFERY

Direct-entry midwifery arose from lay midwifery, which was opposite from nurse-midwifery in virtually every way. Lay midwifery arose as part of the free-spirited, anti-authoritarian, anti-bureaucratic movement of the 1960s and 1970s, and consisted mostly of young, mainly middle-class college students and graduates with the nerve and verve to buck the medical paradigm. They initially took care mainly of women like themselves. Focusing on homebirths, lay midwifery developed purposefully outside the matrix of mainstream medical institutions and authority. They did not need or want institutional support. Some acquired training and backup from individual physicians, but those who didn't were willing to work without it. Many practiced illegally, and thus clandestinely; most simply worked without reference to the law. They were of great interest and very attractive to the women's movement and the press. They ignored the concept of midwifery as care only for the poor, and were reviled by obstetric leaders. Members of local medical associations encouraged police to arrest them. Entering the "system" was not even a consideration for most of them for many years. Although a few schools were developed, most were short-lived, and there were no widely accepted educational standards.

The 1980s were the beginning of a new era for lay and direct-entry midwives in that it saw the development of a national organization, passage of laws that sanction and regulate their practice in an increasing number of states, new schools and intense discussion about the pros, cons and process of evolving into a profession. The Midwives Alliance of North America (MANA) was founded in 1982 and welcomed all kinds of midwives with a vision of unity. Although some of its members are CNMs, MANA focuses on direct-entry midwives. During its first fifteen years, MANA created an organizational structure; developed written statements of midwifery ethics and values, standards, and core competencies; and launched separate organizations to develop processes to accredit direct-entry midwifery educational programs and examine and certify direct-entry midwives. Progress was slowed by internal disagreement about the desirability of national standards, as well as concern that accreditation and certification processes would discriminate against apprentice-trained midwives. Direct-entry midwifery developed outside the system, and some midwives want to keep it that way. They feel that nurse-midwifery has compromised too much in order to enter and survive in the system and fear that setting standards will lead to "professionalization," creating artificial distances between women and their midwives.

Four states have passed laws that require at least three years of midwifery education (the standard called for by the International Confederation of Midwives and the World Health Organization) or a bachelor's or higher degree.[2] Thirteen states license direct-entry midwives but do not require extensive formal midwifery education. The law passed in New York in 1992 was the first intended to cover CNMs and licensed direct-entry midwives under the same set of regulations. (See Robbie Davis-Floyd's article, "The Ups, Downs and Interlinkages of Nurse- and Direct-entry Midwifery: Status, Practice and Education.")

Given great variation in direct-entry midwives' practice, the anti-authoritarian culture of the lay midwifery movement, hostility from the medical profession, paranoia based on the history of midwives being arrested and jailed, and the fact that many direct-entry midwives had been in practice for many years and had become knowledgeable and competent while having had no formal midwifery education—for all these reasons it was difficult for this group of maverick midwives to agree among themselves to establish national standards regarding the necessity of formal education, or to consider it substandard or unethical for a midwife to practice without a working relationship with a physician.

Nevertheless, part of this group has always had long-term goals of achieving full professional status and standards for direct-entry midwifery and integrating midwife-attended homebirths into the mainstream healthcare system. With time, this faction and this goal have become predominant, and they have made substantial progress.

Despite much progress, direct-entry midwives account for only five percent of all births attended by midwives in this country. Nurse-midwives account for 95 percent. Although the proportion of all United States births attended by midwives is low—about six percent in 1995—it is increasing every year, as shown in Figure 2:

Figure 2:

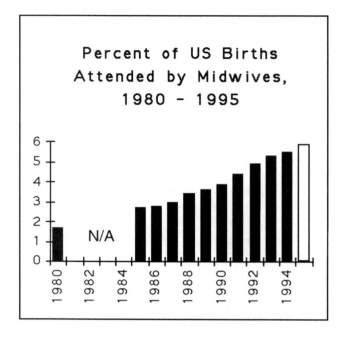

All this increase has come from births attended by CNMs in hospitals. National data on births come from birth certificates. Based on that source of data, direct-entry midwives attended between 11,500 and 12,500 births each year between 1989 and 1995. That amounted to 0.3 percent of all births in the United States during each of those years. (See figure 3.) There is some under-reporting of births attended by both CNMs and direct-entry midwives. Under-reporting of births attended by direct-entry midwives is probably greater, so the numbers for them are low. The true percentage is a little higher but is not likely to be more than one half of one percent.

Direct-entry midwives have a stable niche, though one that is not growing. Women who choose homebirths do so for many reasons, and most are very committed to their choice. But it is not the choice of many women. In fact, there has been an overall decline in the proportion of births in homes and birth centers since 1989. Homebirths declined from 0.67 percent of all births in 1989 to 0.62 percent in 1995. Birth centers accounted for 0.36 percent in 1989, but only 0.27 percent in 1995. Most of the reduction is due to physicians withdrawing from out-of-hospital birth.

The idea of normal birthing was in the air in the 1970s. Women inhaled it, took childbirth education seriously, and some sought the care of midwives. Out-of-hospital births peaked at 1.5 percent in 1977. The proportion quickly fell back to one percent, where it remained throughout the 1980s and 1990s to date. The 1970s image of a homebirth with a lay midwife was romantic and vivid, and it is still attractive. Many women are attracted to homebirths, but they're afraid it isn't safe and they're afraid of pain.

Figure 3: Percent of U.S. Births Attended by Midwives, 1989–1995

Year	All Midwives	CNMs	Direct-Entry Midwives		
	As % of all U.S. Births	As % of all U.S. Births	Number (Based on Birth Certificates)	As % of all U.S. Births	As % of all U.S. Births Attended by Midwives
1989	3.6	3.3	12,400	0.3	8.5
1990	3.9	3.6	11,575	0.3	7.1
1991	4.4	4.1	12,085	0.3	6.6
1992	4.9	4.6	11,767	0.3	5.9
1993	5.3	5.0	12,281	0.3	5.4
1994	5.5	5.2	11,396	0.3	5.0
1995	5.9	5.6	11,396	0.3	5.0

Nevertheless, there is evidence of a much greater demand for homebirth where appropriate standards are in place, such as in Washington state, where licensed direct-entry midwives are moving ahead. The Midwifery Act passed in Washington in 1981 requires licensure based on three years of formal midwifery education and passing a state examination. The Seattle Midwifery School offers a three year program that was based on the curriculum used in the Netherlands. It has been in operation for twenty years. In 1995 the Group Health Cooperative of Washington, an HMO that has one-third of the healthcare market in that state, surveyed its members to determine how many might consider having their next baby at home with a midwife if that service was covered by the HMO. Eight percent of the women said they might use such a service if the Co-op offered the same benefits for a homebirth that it provides for a birth in a Group Health hospital!

Because of these findings, homebirths attended by licensed direct-entry midwives became available to members of the Group Health Cooperative of Washington in January 1996. Each regional unit of the Co-op agreed to develop contracts with some direct-entry midwives in its geographic area. To be eligible for a contract, a midwife must be licensed by the state and have professional liability insurance. Insurance is available through a joint underwriting agreement that all liability insurance companies operating in Washington have to participate in. The state organized the joint underwriting agreement. Midwives covered by the insurance policy must participate in a program of quality assurance that includes a practice review and continuing education. The obstetrics department of local Group Health hospitals provide medical backup.

This kind of progress requires high educational standards. It cannot be extrapolated to other states or the nation as a whole until the direct-entry midwifery community is willing to accept and demand strong mandatory national educational and certification standards that invoke confidence and are easily understood. Direct-entry midwives also need to develop stronger working relationships with physicians and backup hospitals and conduct rigorous, objective studies to measure the safety and effectiveness of the care they provide. Although I support the NARM certification process as an important move in the right direction, it does not require completion of a formal midwifery education program, and CPM certification is voluntary. MANA has never been willing to support mandatory certification as a requirement for the legal right to practice as a direct-entry midwife.

When I last examined the situation, thirteen states were licensing direct-entry midwives without requiring substantial formal education in midwifery. The state of Oregon licenses direct-entry midwives but does not require a midwife to be licensed in order to practice,[3] and does not require any kind of formal midwifery education as a requirement for licensure, although the midwife has to pass a test.

The significance of the "CNM" title, however, is very specific. A person authorized to refer to herself as a CNM has met clearly defined educational and competency standards. In addition, the term "CNM" and "nurse-midwife" are virtually interchangeable. In common and legal usage, a person who says she is a nurse-midwife is representing herself as a CNM. In contrast, the term "direct-entry midwife" does not denote a person who has met any specific set of standards. "Licensed midwife" is also amorphous, because the qualifications vary greatly from state to state. Implementation of the NARM certification process, leading to the credential of certified professional midwife, or CPM, provides a title with clear meaning and standards. However, it doesn't solve the problem, because MANA has taken the position that NARM certification is voluntary. As a consequence, "midwife" and "direct-entry midwife" continue to refer to people with a wide spectrum of qualifications. In my opinion, voluntary certification cannot take direct-entry midwifery where it needs to go. Without a clear, uniform way to identify who is and who is not qualified to practice midwifery and refer to themselves as midwives, we can't even count noses. Currently no one knows how many direct-entry midwives are practicing or how many births they attend.

In addition, the International Definition of a Midwife calls for formal midwifery education, and the standard length for direct-entry midwifery education in Europe is three years. The standard for the education of direct-entry midwives in the United States should be similar to the standard in Europe. The history of direct-entry midwifery in this country has created a unique situation that calls for tolerance of variation from this standard during a period of transition. That tolerance should be temporary.

ADVANTAGES OF BECOMING A CNM

Nurse-midwives have spent nearly three-quarters of a century trying to build a place for midwifery within the American healthcare system, demonstrating the midwifery model of care within the system and trying to change the system from within.

There are pros and cons to being in the system. I am going to focus on the advantages. I will not go into the advantages of being a direct-entry midwife instead of a CNM or the disadvantages of being a CNM, although there are some of both. Nor do I address differences in the quality and completeness of the educational preparation of CNMs as compared to direct-entry midwives. The educational preparation of CNMs varies but has a very definite floor; all programs must provide experiences sufficient to develop the core competencies of a certified nurse-midwife as defined by the ACNM. In addition, no nurse-midwifery program graduate is allowed to take the certification examination until the director of her program signs a document stating her belief that the person applying to take the exam is capable of safe beginning-level nurse-midwifery practice. The educational experiences of direct-entry midwives are so diverse that I would not attempt to compare them to those of CNMs. Some direct-entry programs may not be adequate; some are probably excellent. But there is no clearly defined floor. That difference alone would make me choose to be a CNM. The following are advantages of that choice. They include advantages to the CNM as a person and as a practitioner, and advantages to the CNM's clients. They are presented more or less in that order.

1. Any CNM is qualified to become licensed to practice legally in all but a few states.[4] A CNM with a master's degree in nursing is qualified to practice legally in every state. Americans are a mobile people. It is difficult to foretell when, where and how many times you will want or need to move.

2. The perks to being in the system—reasonable middle-class salaries, paid vacations, retirement programs, healthcare insurance and so forth—are important. Nurse-midwives can support themselves and their families on their own, if necessary.

3. Being a nurse as well as a midwife gives you flexibility. In today's society, job market and healthcare system, flexibility is valuable. Life may lead you down paths that are impossible to predict. If there are no jobs for midwives in your community, your nursing credential will help open other jobs to you. In addition, nursing education is valuable for what is learned. Much of the knowledge and clinical experience from mental health, public health, pediatrics, medical/surgical nursing and pharmacology are relevant to midwifery, as are general principles and practices related to infection control.

4. Receiving widely accepted credit for your education, including a college degree and a higher degree if possible, will open doors to opportunities and challenges that you may not know or care about now. As your life continues and you grow and learn, your interests may change and compound. You may want to teach, to do research, to become involved in health-service administration or the development of healthcare policies at the state or federal level, or to work in another country. Having university degrees and a widely accepted credential and being part of a well-known, respected profession will give you the qualifications to follow new interests as they evolve.

5. You will become familiar with the healthcare system, how it works and how to work within it. Your professional organization, the ACNM, has a distinctive, respected place and voice within the American healthcare system.

6. You will have greater and easier access to the legal right to administer and prescribe necessary medications.

7. With only a few exceptions (midwives who attend homebirths in some states), you will be able to obtain insurance against claims of damage from malpractice. Unless you are self-employed, you may be covered by an insurance policy purchased by your employer. If you are ever sued (it can happen to anyone, even if you make no mistakes, and everyone makes some mistakes), you will most likely be assisted and supported by your colleagues and the institution that employs you. The good record and reputation of nurse-midwives will help support you; no one can argue successfully that you were wrong simply because you are a midwife and not a physician.

8. You will have more opportunities and easier access to more resources for continuing education.

9. Being in the system will allow you to provide care to a larger number and variety of women. Nurse-midwives have always played a significant role in the care of women who are at higher than average risk of poor pregnancy outcomes because of adverse social and economic conditions, lack of information, and unhealthful practices. The problems confronting these women and their children are among the most important challenges facing our country. Providing effective care to these women gives CNMs an opportunity to make personal, creative contributions to solving one of our society's gravest problems. This is challenging work; nurse-midwives are proud of their accomplishments in this arena, and they have earned high respect for them.

10. You will be able to attend births in all settings, although you may need additional mentoring to prepare you to attend homebirths. But you will be fully qualified to practice in hospitals, which is where 99 percent of American mothers give birth. Many women feel that a homebirth is too risky but want the care of a midwife during prenatal and postnatal care, as well as during labor and birth. CNMs who attend births in hospitals generally provide supportive, respectful, empowering midwifery care—care that can make a significant difference for both the physiological and psychological outcomes. Most women who give birth in American hospitals are attached to electronic fetal monitoring equipment, have an epidural and are given a remote control for the in-room television set and a button to call a nurse. No one needs a midwife more than women who are giving birth in hospitals!

11. Your potential scope of practice will be much broader because of your own knowledge and skills and because of your ability to work collaboratively with doctors. As a result, you can provide care to a greater proportion of pregnant women, you can meet a greater range of your clients' needs for healthcare during pregnancy and you can extend your care to women before and after, as well as during their pregnancies.

12. You can offer your clients a fuller range of therapeutic options, by providing them yourself or by accessing the services of other professionals on behalf of a client. Women will not have to accept that if they choose you as their maternity-care

provider, they are simultaneously limiting the therapeutic modalities that will be accessible to them within their primary maternity-care relationship. This can be important. Many women would like to go through labor with midwifery support and no unnecessary use of interventions, but are unwilling to foreclose the option of pharmacologic pain relief before they have even started labor.

13. The quality of a woman's experience during pregnancy, birth and motherhood is heavily weighted by whether or not she wanted to become pregnant, and nearly half of all pregnancies in the United States are unintended. Family planning can be an important and satisfying part of midwifery care, and you will be able to offer clients a variety of effective contraception methods. Overall, a CNM has more respect and power, greater options and therefore greater choice.

There is also an obvious underside to being a CNM. The perks of the system are important, but there are wonderful attributes to not being in the system. Being a nurse gives you flexibility and a useful background, but in the long run, I want midwifery to be a freestanding profession, true to its ancient origins and the international definition of a midwife. College degrees are necessary door openers in our society, but that does not mean that the education provided in universities is necessarily superior to learning in other ways and in other environments. Universities have some particular shortcomings when it comes to educating practitioners. Being in the system will allow you to provide care to a larger number of women, but being in some managed healthcare settings may force you to accept responsibility for the care of more women than you can provide good midwifery care to within the available time. Being able to provide or access labor and delivery interventions may lead to their overuse. There are no simple, black and white answers. No one way is best for everyone.

A different set of issues present themselves when comparing nurse-midwifery with direct-entry midwifery from the perspective of the health and vigor of the midwifery profession as a whole. Whatever form it may take, midwifery is good for women and babies and society and should be the standard of care in the United States; it should be broadly available and used by most women as it is in Western Europe. Nurse-midwifery is growing and has great potential within the healthcare system and within universities, which have significant influence and special access to many important resources. Nurse-midwifery also has a strong, widely respected quality assurance system. Nurse-midwifery care has been closely scrutinized and studied, showing high quality and excellent outcomes. Direct-entry midwifery is far behind in these areas but is developing in other important ways. Nevertheless, MANA and the direct-entry midwifery community have made important contributions. Every phenomenon is seen more accurately and more richly if looked at from more than one perspective. Midwifery will be stronger if we can preserve this diversity. In addition, some important things that need to be accomplished can be done more effectively if both groups work together. I value direct-entry midwives and want them to succeed—to change in some ways, but to succeed. But for the present, the advantages of nurse-midwifery education are clear—more flexibility, more choice, better perks and a wider scope of practice.

But I am talking about choice. I am not categorically against any kind of obstetric intervention. All of them have a place; all of them are of distinct benefit to women and their babies when used appropriately. This is even true of epidural anesthesia, in my opinion. My complaint with the usual care provided to American women during labor and birth is that it fails to provide the benefits of midwifery care, and it overuses many painful, invasive, ineffectual and/or dangerous obstetric interventions. But you do not diminish the advantage of providing midwifery care simply because the midwife is able to use or access medical interventions that might be needed. If you become a CNM, you can choose to limit yourself to homebirths and to limit yourself to the more narrow range of methods common to direct-entry midwives. You would still have that choice, although you might need to seek additional experience with homebirths, in which case you could choose to also become credentialed as a certified professional midwife (CPM). If you become a CNM, you will have to make choices constantly. For example, you can refuse to accept positions in which you are expected to overuse obstetric interventions.

Just as I am sure there are CNMs who overuse some medical interventions, I am sure some direct-entry midwifery clients are denied timely access to interventions they need because their midwife is unable to use it, and that some clients are not offered methods that they ultimately would have wanted to use. Of course we have to depend on midwives to make good choices, but it is better to have more options and more tools at your disposal.

Direct-entry midwifery is not currently growing. Even in Washington state, where all pieces of the essential structure are in place and most barriers have been removed, licensed direct-entry midwives complain of lack of demand for their services. I want homebirth to survive, though not many women choose it. If I had a dozen eggs to invest, I would put some of them in the direct-entry basket, because I think it is important. But I wouldn't put them all in the basket that isn't growing. Since you have just one life, I would invest my education in the career path that offers the most choices. Then work with the rest of us to keep all those choices available for women. The best of all worlds is a situation which provides the most advantages to the most birthing moms.

---

1. CNEP is the Community-based Nurse-midwifery Education Program, a nationwide distance-learning program operated by the Frontier School of Midwifery and Family Nursing, part of the Frontier Nursing Service based in Hyden, Kentucky.

2. Washington, Florida, New York and California.

3. Based on an attorney general's decision that midwifery is not the practice of medicine and thus cannot be prohibited under the state's medical practice act.

4. As of January 1998, Alabama, Louisiana, Montana, Oregon, South Carolina and Washington state also require a master's degree in nursing or a health-related field. Tennessee and Wisconsin require a master's degree for prescriptive authority, but not for basic licensure as a nurse-midwife. Idaho, Mississippi and New York required baccalaureate degrees.

I want to acknowledge the assistance of Robbie Davis-Floyd, who reviewed a draft of the article and gave me extremely helpful comments and suggestions.

References:

American College of Nurse-Midwives. (1998). Quick Reference Tables, table 5, Jurisdictions that require educational degree preparation for nurse-midwifery practice. ACNM, Washington, DC.

Rooks, J.B., Fischman, S., Lescyznski, P., Kaplan E., Morgan, G., & Witek, J. (1978). *Nurse Midwifery in the United States: 1976-1977.* American College of Nurse-Midwives, Washington, DC.

Rooks, J.P. (1997). *Midwifery and Childbirth in America.* Temple University Press, Philadelphia.

Rooks, J.P., Weatherby, N.L., Ernst, E.K., Stapelton, S., Rosen, D. & Rosenfield, A. (1989). "Outcomes of care in birth centers: The national birth center study." *New England Journal of Medicine.* 321:1804-1811.

This article was written especially for this book.

Judith Rooks is a nurse-midwife and epidemiologist with a long career in public health. She has taught in a school of nursing, a school of medicine and a school of midwifery (CNEP). She has worked at the U.S. Centers for Disease Control, in the Office of the Surgeon General, and for the U.S. Agency for International Development. She has authored more than fifty scientific and professional publications, including the National Birth Center Study, which was published in the New England Journal of Medicine in 1989, and a comprehensive book entitled Midwifery & Childbirth in America, published by Temple University Press in 1997. Judith served as president of the ACNM in the mid-1980s and is currently on the editorial bodies of both Birth and the Journal of Nurse-Midwifery. In 1993 she received the American Public Health Association's Martha May Eliot Award for exceptional service to mothers and children. She is married and lives in Portland, Oregon.

THE DAUGHTERS OF TIME
ON THE PATHS TO MIDWIFERY

by Barbara Katz Rothman, PhD

Direct-entry to what? A path to where? What is it that we are entering, and where is it we are going? Much as I would like it to be, "midwife" is not a self-evident, all inclusive term. A midwife is, like everything else in this world, very much in the eye of the beholder.

Having studied midwifery issues for nearly twenty-five years now, I have quite the collection of midwifery T-shirts, including one from the first MANA meeting, from organizations long defunct, shirts with women and babies and moons and stars. But my favorite is the first one I ever got. Between the words "The Midwives" on top, and "Daughters of Time" on the bottom, is a drawing of two women, clearly intended to be midwives, striding forth. One is from the 1800s, wearing a shawl, long skirt and high button shoes, hair knotted back. The other, younger and taller, has long loose hair, an open-necked shirt with rolled-up sleeves, a wristwatch, sandals and bell bottoms. Midwives of the 1970s are now as much a part of our history as are midwives of the 1870s.

What is the continuity between these two midwives, and the midwife just starting to stride forth on her path today? All are daughters of time, speaking to the continuity of midwifery across time, just as each is also a daughter of her own time, speaking to the different kinds of midwifery that different moments of time call forth.

The midwife of the 1970s was aspiring toward her midwifery: it was a goal, an ideal. She could not, as her sister/foremother of the 1800s could, take midwifery for granted. For an earlier midwife, the practice of midwifery was important, valued and respected, but also a part of ordinary life. Of course there were midwives and of course what midwives did was practice midwifery. The work needed to be done, and someone would have to do it, like for instance cobblers, the people who made shoes. It is not to say that the work wasn't much appreciated, and not to say that better cobblers weren't much in demand, but one wouldn't think to venerate grand cobblers or hold up the ideals of cobblery.

Because midwifery has been deeply damaged, so all but completely destroyed in the years that separate the two midwives on my T-shirt, it can no longer be taken for granted. Midwifery came to be something more than the people who practice it—it came to be something of an ideal, a goal, a model to which one could aspire. The distinction arose between midwifery as an occupation or a practice, as something one does, and midwifery as a model. I am the person who first wrote about the distinction between a "medical model" and a "midwifery model" of pregnancy and childbirth. When Marsden Wagner pointed out to me that I was the first person who made this distinction, I was surprised—hadn't we always known this?

I had a homebirth in 1974 with the assistance of a feminist obstetrician, someone who understood and agreed in principle with my right to birth as I saw fit, in the location of my choosing. In fact, she was clueless. When the baby was born and I was reaching up to take him, the doctor passed the child back over her shoulder to where she presumably expected a nurse to materialize. My mother—standing in the right place—was the first to hold my newly born son.

Homebirth, I saw, was real different than hospital birth, not only for the birthing woman but also for the women attending. I chose this topic to research for my dissertation as a graduate student in sociology. Living in New York City, I tracked down and interviewed all the people I could find who were attending homebirths. All were nurse-midwives. Some had gone through regular nurse training and then moved on to hospital-based midwifery before doing homebirths; some had been trained and worked as midwives before becoming nurse-midwives.

I observed a few births, but it was less what the midwives were doing that interested me, and more how they were thinking about what they were doing. Their knowledge, their understanding, their way of thinking about birth intrigued me. How do people know what they know? That's a basic question in sociology, and it was the one that captured my attention.

My key insight was seeing that there are different models underlying practice, different ways of thinking about birth that resulted in different ways of practicing. Ways of thinking, ideology and concepts underlie ways of practicing, of behaving and doing. I read the obstetrics literature and I read the literature of the developing homebirth movement—newsletters, conference reports, Ina May's *Spiritual Midwifery*—what little there was out there on homebirth. I started comparing the way people think about birth at home and the way they think about it in the hospital. It was the difference between the two places that first caught my attention.

Most of the midwives I was interviewing were in a way just like the feminist obstetrician who delivered my baby. They had the best of intentions, but they were really out of their element in the home. They didn't know what to think much of the time. They were confused about what they were doing and seeing. I worked with a study group at the time in which we read each others' dissertation work. Continually talking about these different midwifery paths, I had a hard time articulating the differences between home and hospital birth.

One day my friend and colleague Eileen Moran came back to my house the day after a study group meeting. She sat down with me in my office and drew two circles on a piece of paper. The one on the left, she said, is the way doctors think about birth—the way midwives are taught about birth in their hospital training. The circle on the other side of the paper, the homebirth approach, represents the lay midwives in California and what *Spiritual Midwifery* is about. And here in the middle, trying to find their way, are these midwives you're interviewing.

That was exactly right. Those were the midwives, as I quickly came to call them, "in transition," that most painful, intense, hardest part of labor right before you make clear and obvious progress. Those midwives were right there, that part where you don't know if you'll ever pull through, that part where you are vulnerable and scared and working very, very hard.

It wasn't really about "home" or "hospital." A midwife could bring the hospital way of thinking into the home with her. And a midwife could bring the home way of thinking into the hospital. Many of those midwives would tell me stories of doing homebirths one day and then doing hospital births the next, trying to take what they had learned at home and apply it in the hospital. "Midwifery" was a way of thinking to which most of these nurse-midwives were aspiring. I started to call these different approaches "medical" and "midwifery," rather than hospital and home.

Like many graduate students of the time, I was heavily influenced by the work Thomas Kuhn had done in his book *The Structure of Scientific Revolutions*, in which he introduced the idea of a paradigm shift. Science, Kuhn pointed out, doesn't proceed at an even pace. Data is collected and analyzed and collected and analyzed. And then there comes a moment when the data no longer seems to fit the old analysis, and a "scientific revolution," a paradigm shift, lurches the science ahead to a new place.

Kuhn gave a simple example from a psychology experiment. Subjects were asked to identify playing cards flashed on a screen. Most were from a standard deck, but some were made anomalous—a red six of spades or a black four of hearts. Something interesting happens when you show people these cards: At first, they "normalize them." They identify a black heart as a regular red heart, or see it as a spade. After a while, though, subjects begin to hesitate. More and more hesitation is shown, until they switch over and come to see a black heart as a black heart, and a red spade as a red spade. Kuhn said science works like that too. "Novelty emerges only with difficulty, manifested by resistance against a background provided by expectation."

But medicine and midwifery aren't sciences. They are clinical practices. Science has as its goal the production of knowledge. Medicine and midwifery are geared to the provision of services, to the improvement of outcome. It is the nature of scientific work to expose inconsistencies, to show the flaws in the old paradigm. Clinical practice, on the other hand, is not about generating data; it's about treating people. There are no control groups in clinical practice; once something is accepted as a treatment, it is offered. It works or it doesn't work, but the situations in which treatments are offered—the real world—are far too complex for us to consistently learn anything about the treatment. Maybe the condition would have cleared up without the treatment, maybe it only cleared up in spite of the treatment, maybe it wasn't the condition diagnosed anyway. Maybe the patient never really followed the treatment. Who knows?

Not only is clinical work not organized to produce new knowledge, but one could argue that it is really designed to avoid the production of knowledge. If the data you see—what is actually happening in the patient before your eyes—does not conform to the model of the illness, the practitioner is expected to reconsider the patient. For example, medical texts offer both the theoretical effectiveness of a contraceptive, how it is supposed to work, and also its "use-effectiveness"—how well it actually works in practice. If a contraceptive doesn't work the way it is supposed to, the problem lies with the user.

While I found the story Kuhn was telling extraordinarily useful, I didn't want to adopt his vocabulary. If science works with paradigms, what could I say clinical practice works with? "Models" are what I came up with. Models serve much the same purpose for the clinical practitioner as paradigms serve for the scientist: they attract groups of adherents, they become focal points for social organization as well as the organization of knowledge. And while paradigms are open-ended enough to leave all sorts of problems for the scientist to solve, models are useful to provide guidelines for practice. Both make work possible. Kuhn looked at paradigm shifts and scientific revolutions; I saw shifts in models and clinical revolutions.

What makes a clinical revolution? If, unlike science, clinical practice is not designed to produce new knowledge, where does new knowledge come from?

Where does knowledge come from in the first place? We learn from each other. We are taught to think from one another. Models or paradigms or whatever you want to call them give us the picture we have in our heads, against which we look at the world. We hold up what we know to be true and judge what is before us against that. If the model tells me what a normal labor is like, then what is this labor I am seeing when compared to that? Longer? Shorter? Stronger? Weaker? Or take something very simple: We have learned what a newborn baby should look like. There is a model, an ideal type—not ideal in the sense of being the "Gerber baby," but ideal as in paradigmatic, the essence of new babyhood—having the necessary and essential characteristics that mark it as a new baby. Given that model, we can look at any new baby and ask if it varies, and how. In the direction of pathology? Is the head too big? Too small? Are the limbs proportional? How is the muscle tone? Compared to what? Compared to what you know is "normal," compared to the model you have in your head of what a baby's muscle tone should be at birth.

So where do models come from and how are they developed? We are accustomed to thinking that we know what we know from what we have observed, but it is just as true that how we practice sets up what we can observe—what is observable in the first place. If every new baby you ever saw was born from a deeply anesthetized mother, what would you know about normal muscle tone in a newborn?

That was the type of problem, if less dramatic, that was confronting the midwives in transition—these hospital trained nurse-midwives doing homebirths for the first time. Their models did not apply. So how could they know what was normal? Clinical practice in hospitals was structured to avoid the production of just the knowledge they now needed. Want to know how long a placenta can take to separate from the uterine wall and still be healthy? You will never find out if all placentas are removed within fifteen minutes of the birth, as is done in hospital delivery rooms. Want to know if you are looking at a "second stage arrest," a pathological condition, or a normal "rest period" for a woman who has had a difficult labor, before she begins the work of pushing forth the baby? If you always and immediately treat any cessation of contractions after full dilation as second stage arrest and rush to pull the baby out, as they do in hospitals, you will never observe the rest period or its resolution.

Examples like these flowed forth in those early years as midwives confronted the limits of hospital-based knowledge for home-based practice.

Setting—place, location—counts. The difference between medical and midwifery models of birth are not just about attitudes, not even just a set of guidelines for practice. Different bodies of knowledge are produced in different settings.

Education is about the passing on of knowledge. It would be very difficult to teach obstetrics at homebirths. It is no less difficult to teach the midwifery model of birth in the hospital. Because nurse-midwifery has come through the hospital, it has been very hard to become a midwife, to develop a midwife's body of knowledge, in that medically dominated setting. I have brought midwives I respect and admire to tears by saying this. Get angry, hate me if you will, but a midwifery model does not develop under medical domination. And hospitals are places where medicine sets the rules.

> . . . a midwifery model does not develop under medical domination. And hospitals are places where medicine sets the rules.

On the other hand, it is hard to reach women who most need midwifery care without going through medically based certification. It is hard enough then. Nurse-midwifery—medically based midwifery— needs home-based midwifery to produce and maintain the midwifery base of knowledge, which some midwives bring into hospital settings. That is the problem confronting the midwife just starting to stride forth on her path today. Unlike the midwife of the 1800s for whom midwifery was a self-evident destination, today's midwife-to-be faces different paths leading to different places.

It is tempting to talk only about how we all share a concern for birthing women, how all kinds of midwives and mothers need each other and how women need all kinds of midwives in all kinds of circumstances. But this focus alone does a disservice to the serious attempt to achieve an alternative body of knowledge, a disservice to midwifery not just as a practice but as a goal, as a model, to minimalize the differences between midwifery as it is developed and practiced in different places.

We're used to thinking about how home-based and apprenticeship midwives need hospital-based midwives—to accept the transfers, to work with the women who "risk out" of homebirth, to work with the women who have learned to fear birth. But hospital-based, medically entrenched midwives need the outsider's view of the other midwives just as much or even more if they are to retain sight of midwifery as a goal.

If I were to design a new T-shirt now, I'd show the Daughters of the Millennium, striding forth, seeking their own paths, recreating midwifery for their own time.

References

Kuhn, Thomas. (1970). *The Structure of Scientific Revolutions*. University of Chicago Press.

Rothman, Barbara Katz. (1979). *Two Models of Maternity Care: Defining and Negotiating Reality*. New York University. Also published in *In Labor: Women and Power in the Birthplace*. (1993). W.W. Norton.

This article was written especially for this book.

Barbara Katz Rothman, PhD, is a professor of sociology at the City University of New York.

Excerpted from

RECREATING MOTHERHOOD: IDEOLOGY AND TECHNOLOGY IN A PATRIARCHAL SOCIETY

THE MEDICAL AND MIDWIFERY MODELS

by Barbara Katz Rothman, PhD

MIDWIFERY AS FEMINIST PRAXIS

Long before obstetricians arrived on the scene, there was a practice and a tradition of midwifery. And that tradition continues today: with full professional autonomy (that is, the right to control itself as an occupation) in some states, and underground, even illegally, in other states. I am speaking here of woman-taught and woman-controlled midwifery, and not the medically, obstetrically trained nurse-specialist programs which have incorporated the word "midwife." Some women trained as nurse-midwives are, and some are not, part of the midwifery tradition, but it is that alternative tradition, that non-medical model of procreation, which I address.

Midwifery is, I believe, feminist praxis. Marx used the word praxis to mean conscious physical labor directed toward transforming the material world so it will satisfy human needs. Midwifery works with the labor of women to transform, to create, the birth experience to meet the needs of women. It is a social, political activity, dialectically linking biology and society, the physical and the social experience of motherhood. The very word midwife means with the woman. That is more than a physical location: it is an ideological and political stance. Midwifery represents a rejection of the artificial dualisms of patriarchal and technological ideologies. The midwifery model of pregnancy rejects technological mind-body dualism as it rejects the patriarchal alienation of the woman from her fetus. That of course is too negative, and too self-conscious a way of putting it. Rather than rejecting dualisms, midwifery continues to see unity.

The political agenda for feminism is quite clear: we must empower the midwives, enable them to practice midwifery as a fully autonomous profession, not subject to the control of physicians.

It is very difficult, in this society at this time, to even think of pregnancy, and especially childbirth, in non-medical terms, to imagine that midwives are doing anything other than being maybe "nicer," "kinder," or more "sensitive" than obstetricians. But it is not just warmth or empathy that midwives have to offer: there are some lovely obstetricians around too. And it's not just their gender that distinguishes midwives, especially as more and more women enter obstetrics. What midwives offer us is an alternative ideological base, and consequently the potential for developing an alternative body of knowledge about procreation. The medical model sees a vulnerable fetus caught in a woman's body (the child of man held by woman) and a woman, although stronger than the fetus, also made vulnerable by its intrusion (weakened by what the man has "done to her," what he has growing in her). The job of the obstetrician is to help effect the separation of the two, so they can "recover," so that the woman can "return to normal," and the baby can be "managed" separately. The ideologies of technology and patriarchy focus the vision and the work of obstetrics.

In such a model, the development of the hospitalization for childbirth made sense, and the increasing regionalization of maternity services (locating "high-risk" services in a central large teaching hospital) is perfectly rational, even imperative. One would not expect, after all, to do the best job of auto repair in the driveway, or even in the local gas station; the most well-equipped garage is the place for the best repairs. The workman is only as good as his tools. Birth is best done, as are auto repairs, where the access to tools is best.

But there are inherent problems in limiting our vision of childbirth to its technical, medical dimension. That vision of childbirth enables us to think only in terms of morbidity and mortality rates, and not the often wrenching social and personal implications involved in childbirth management programs and technology.

Compare this situation with a very different example of technological progress, that which has occurred in transportation with the introduction of automobiles. What if we approached the history of transportation with the same narrow focus with which we approach childbirth, defining it entirely in terms of life and limb, morbidity and mortality rates, as they vary with different modes of transportation? It is obvious that the shift over time from a horse-based to an engine-based transportation system has had effects on the morbidity and mortality rates associated with transportation. We might try to figure out the effects in terms of lives lost each year in transportation accidents, or in the more sophisticated comparison of lives lost per mile traveled in each system. It would be an interesting and valuable history of transportation to consider. But would anyone claim it is *the* history of transportation, that this is the most salient, most far-reaching effect of new modes of transportation in our lives?

The introduction of new technology in transportation has had a fundamental impact on American life. it has influenced family organization, our perceptions of time and space, our vision of the world in which we live. There is a context, a social context, in which we see the meaning of technology in transportation. A medical history of transportation is interesting and important, but it is only one (rather narrow) facet of the story. And so it is with childbirth.

The medical monopoly on childbirth, its control by physicians, has meant defining birth in medical terms, and thus narrowing our scope of perception. The other equally salient, humanly meaningful aspects of childbirth are lost to us, outside our narrow range of vision. This narrowed vision has given us detailed knowledge of some of the physiology of pregnancy, childbirth and newborns, but without context. The woman whose pregnant uterus we think we understand is located three bus fares away from the facility we have designed for her care. The newborn whose blood is so finely analyzed is placed at a distance that must be measured in more miles from the family on which she will ultimately depend.

What midwifery offers us is not just tossing in a few social or psychological variables, but a reconceptualization of the "facts" of procreation. A professional controls not only people—as doctors control nurses who "follow orders," the patients who "comply"—more important, a profession controls the development of knowledge. In regard to birth, the profession of medicine determines not only who may attend a birth, or what birth attendants may do, but it controls also what we know of birth itself.

> The midwifery model of pregnancy rejects techno-logical mind-body dualism as it rejects the patri-archal alienation of the woman from her fetus.

In its control over practice, the profession of medicine maintains control over research—research in its broadest sense. Data are collected, both formally and informally, to support and develop the medical body of knowledge. But the data are themselves generated by the medical practices. The methods of observation in medicine have often been criticized as not being "scientific" enough, but the more fundamental flaw is in not recognizing the social processes involved in the generation of the data, of that which is there to be observed. So it develops that in our society the obstetrical perspective on pregnancy and birth is not considered just one way of looking at it, but rather the truth, the facts, science; others may have beliefs about pregnancy, but we believe medicine has the facts. However, obstetrical knowledge, like all knowledge, comes from somewhere: it has a social, historical and political context. Medicine does not exist as something "pure," free of culture or free of ideology. The context in which medical knowledge develops and is used shapes that knowledge. In particular, the setting of practice is an important part of the generation of the data on which the knowledge is based.

To begin to make this point clear, I am going to draw examples from two very different worlds, different "settings of practice." I am going to contrast medical obstetrical knowledge with the knowledge of a lay midwife practicing outside of medical settings. The same physiological event, the birth of a baby, can occur in many places—women labor and babies are born in a variety of settings. But the social definitions, our ideas about what is happening, are vastly different in different settings, and these differences create new social realities. In turn, these new realities, or definitions of the situation, create new physiological reality, as the birth process itself is shaped by the settings in which it occurs. Let us begin with a simple, everyday event.

Situation 1: A woman comes to the maternity floor of a large hospital. She is upset, almost crying, holding her huge belly and leaning against her husband, who seems nearly as upset as she is. "My wife's in labor," he states, and hands over a scrap of paper with times marked off—the seven- to twelve-minute intervals they have timed between contractions. The woman is ushered into a cubicle and examined. The examination might be repeated an hour later. "No," the doctor tells her, "you're not in labor yet. You have not yet begun to dilate. This is just a false alarm, a false labor. You can go home and come back when you really are in labor."

Here we have a physiological event—the painful contractions of the uterus—defined in two different ways, as labor and as not-labor. The woman and her husband are basing their definition on her feelings, the sensations she is experiencing as she has been taught to measure them—in minutes, for example. The doctor is basing his or her definition on what he or she feels as an examiner, the degree of dilation—how much the cervix has dilated. Each definition of the situation carries with it a way of acting, a set of behavioral expectations for the people involved. As not-labor, the doctor is finished with the woman and can turn his or her attention elsewhere. The woman is to go home and stay simply pregnant a while longer. Defined as labor, however, the situation is very different. The woman changes from her status of pregnant woman to the new status of laboring woman. She will put on the appropriate costume (change from "maternity clothes" to a "hospital gown") and become a patient. The doctor will be expected to provide examination and treatment, to begin managing her condition. Only in labor will she become the doctor's responsibility.

> **Situation 2:** Cara (an empirical midwife): I got a call that Roberta was having heavy rushes but wasn't dilating and was having a hard time. I wanted to go see her and help. When I got there, Roberta was writhing with each rush and shaking. She just didn't have any idea how to handle the energy. Joel was sitting beside her looking worried. The whole scene was a bit grim for a baby-having. I got them kissing, hugging and had Roberta really grab onto Joel and squeeze him. Joel is a big, strong, heavy-duty man. He and I rubbed Roberta continuously and steered in the direction of relaxed. I let her know that she was having good, strong rushes and that if she'd relax and experience it and let it happen, her rushes would accomplish a lot and open her up. She gradually accepted the fact that there was no getting out of this except to let it happen and quit fighting it.

Here we have the same physiological event, a woman experiencing the same sensations and the same lack of dilation, defined along yet other lines. First note the difference in the language being used. The empirical midwife describing this situation is not talking about "contractions," the medical word for what the uterine muscle is doing, but "rushes." This midwife lives and works on the Farm, the Tennessee commune that published *Spiritual Midwifery*. The midwives explain their language:

> On the Farm we've come to call these contractions of the uterine muscle "rushes" because the main sensation that happens when these muscles contract is exactly the same as the sensations of rushing while coming on to a heavy psychedelic, which feels like a whole lot of energy flowing up your back and into your head. It leaves you feeling expansive and stoned if you don't fight it.

This language relies on internal or subjective cues, sensations the woman herself experiences. The medical language, in contrast, relies on external or "objective" cues, information available to the examiner—how much the woman has dilated. Thus when the subjective and objective cues are at variance, in the medical situation the subjective cues are discounted. The woman's sensations of labor are "false" and the doctor's examination is "true." In the midwifery situation, the woman's experienced reality of the rushes is acknowledged. The "problem," the variance between subjective and objective measures, is here defined as the woman's inability to cope effectively, to "let it happen." This definition, of course, also carries with it consequences for the people involved: the midwife and the husband are expected to help her cope, relax, let it happen. For the woman, one of the negative consequences of this definition of the situation is that it tells her that it is in some way her own fault that she is having a hard time. In that way the midwives are doing the same thing as the doctors: imposing their definition of the situation on the laboring woman. The doctor's responsibility is very narrowly defined: to manage only "real" labor. The midwife's responsibility, in contrast, is defined more broadly, to include "helping" or "managing"—controlling the emotional as well as the physical situation.

Thus each of these alternative definitions carries with it quite different consequences, consequences that will shape the experience of all those involved, but most dramatically of the pregnant woman. It is one thing to be a pregnant woman, and quite another to be "in labor." And it is one thing to be told that the labor you are experiencing is "false" and yet another to be told that the rushes are real and you have to learn how to relax and stop fighting them. The meaning given the particular uterine contractions of any particular woman becomes the basis for the way the event, and thus the woman, is treated.

These scenarios, and their implications, explain why it matters, even to those of us who are not midwives, that midwives come to have professional autonomy. With professional autonomy comes the power to control the setting of birth, and ultimately to control the birthing woman. As someone who is not a midwife, I prefer midwifery control to obstetrical control because obstetrical control, the "objective" medical reality if you will, diminishes the birthing woman. It makes her an object upon whom the art and science of obstetrics are practiced. The underlying ideology is that of technology, the body as machine. This depersonalizes the birthing woman, making her a suitable candidate for being hooked up to yet other machines.

The organization of the hospital maternity floor influences this mechanistic vision of the woman. Labor rooms look more like regular nursing care rooms; delivery rooms more like operating rooms. As the woman is transferred from one to another, there is basis for more and more narrowly defining the relevant parts of her, as she first loses full personhood to become a patient, and then in the delivery room, where all the doctor sees of the woman is the exposed perineum centered in draped linen, becomes simply a pelvis from which a fetus is removed. The alternative birth settings—homes, "birthing rooms," and the like—provide a contrasting image, in which the mother is not lying flat, and is surrounded by friends and family, tied to a full social world. Such a setting may very well encourage the awareness of the social and emotional factors in the birth. Thus "contractions" may be the salient feature when palpating the abdomen of a semiconscious woman, but "rush" may seem more appropriate when talking to a woman who is experiencing one.

Is the woman I described "really" in labor when she experiences contractions with "no progress"? Who defines? Who sets the policy about whether such a woman could or should be admitted to a particular hospital? If midwife and physician disagree, upon whose judgment will the insurance company's decision to pay for the day of hospitalization rely? And so how will we learn from which definitions of the situation results in the better outcome for mother and baby? Unless and until midwifery achieves professional status, it controls neither the birthing woman nor the development of an alternative body of knowledge.

In sum, for midwifery to develop an alternative body of knowledge, to reach new understandings about what is happening in birth, midwives must have control over the setting of birth. I have come to see that it is not that birth is "managed" the way it is because of what we know about birth. Rather, what we know about birth has been determined by the way it is managed. And the way childbirth has been managed has been based on the underlying assumptions, beliefs and ideologies that inform medicine as a profession.

WILL THE CIRCLE BE UNBROKEN?

Childbirth is managed within the guidelines established in accordance with "obstetrical facts," but those facts themselves have grown out of the setting of practice established by medicine. The circle is tight, and usually closed. When it is broken, startling things happen.

I have made a study of the breaking of that circle of knowledge. I have studied nurse-midwives, trained within medical settings, who began doing homebirths. For a nurse-midwife with standard hospital-based training (that is, someone who began her career as a nurse, and then entered a postgraduate hospital-based program in midwifery), doing homebirths is a radicalizing experience. It makes her think hard about her work and its meaning. In this new setting, she has to question many of the taken-for-granted assumptions of the medical setting and medical model. And she finds herself constructing a new model, a new way of explaining what she sees. This is the process of reconceptualization, taking something you've confronted maybe a hundred times, and suddenly seeing it as something else entirely.

For the nurse-midwife making the transition from the hospital to homebirths, many anomalies present themselves. The nausea she was taught was part of normal labor may not be there. She may begin to see that in the hospital this discomfort was caused by not letting the woman eat or drink anything during labor. The amount of time something takes, such as expelling the placenta, may begin to look, in this new setting, very different from the way it did in the hospital delivery room. At first she will try to apply the medical knowledge in this new setting, attempt to utilize the knowledge gained in the hospital for what she is seeing in the home. That won't always work for her. When she is faced with an anomaly in the medical model that she cannot ignore or "normalize," she has a radicalizing experience: she rejects at least part of the medical model. She may share that experience with other nurse-midwives, and many such stories are told. Hearing the resolutions achieved by others supports and furthers her own radicalization. What were perceived as facts come to be seen as artifacts: obstetrical constructions, artifacts of the medical setting.

Let me review a small sample of these questioned "facts":

1. Vomiting and nausea are a common part of labor.

Working outside of medical control, midwives who have not denied food and drink to laboring women have observed that nausea is uncommon. The question: is nausea caused by labor, or by lack of food?

2. Infection is likely to occur if much time passes after the rupture of the membranes and before birth.

Careful and frequent vaginal examinations were standard practice in the hospital to assess progress of dilation once the membranes ruptured (the "waters broke"). Midwives working outside of medically controlled settings, faced with a natural rupture of membranes at term (when the woman is due) but before labor began, have on occasion avoided the examinations, fearing that they may be a source of infection. The question: how likely is infection, and at what interval after the membranes have ruptured, if hospitalization and vaginal examinations do not take place?

3. Milk does not come in for three days after birth.

Working against what had been standard medical practice, women (inside hospitals as well as outside) demanded their babies be brought to them earlier and more often. The new knowledge, now no longer even a question, is that milk comes in more commonly within twenty-four to forty-eight hours after birth when mother and baby have unrestricted access to each other. A corollary of this is that the time required for the infant to regain birthweight has been adjusted downward.

4. Once full dilation is reached, second stage (pushing the baby out) begins. If it does not, the condition, called second-stage arrest, is a sign of pathology.

Working outside of medically controlled settings, midwives sometimes observed a woman who, on reaching full dilation, rolled over, exhausted, and fell asleep. That is not something one would often see on a delivery table. After a nap, the labor resumed, with a healthy baby and mother. The question: what is pathological second-stage arrest and what is a naturally occurring rest period?

The examples abound. Some of the most interesting, like most of these examples, have to do with medical timetables, with how long the various stages of pregnancy, labor and the postpartum period are claimed to take. Other questions have arisen about the distinctions between voluntary and involuntary control—just how much of the birth process can and does the mother control?

Where does midwifery stand amidst these questions? Can we turn to midwives to learn answers?

The answer: only to the extent that midwifery emerges as a full profession.

The implications of allowing medicine the monopoly on childbirth management thus go beyond the relatively simple question of the infringement of other occupations' right to practice. What I am arguing is that our usual assumptions need to be turned on their head. As a society we claim that medicine has the monopoly because childbirth is more than anything else a medical event. The truth might more nearly be stated that childbirth is a medical event because medicine holds the monopoly on management.

If birth were moved out of the hands of medicine, if birth were denied in other than medical terms, the implications would be far-reaching indeed. Some of the "facts" about birth, as I have shown, would be seen to be "artifacts" of medical management. But it is not just that a new, more lenient and more individually varied set of timetables would be developed to replace the obstetrical timetables. As important as this would be, the effects of demedicalizing childbirth would go beyond even this evaluation. Demedicalizing childbirth would allow us to perceive the experience in new ways.

Such demedicalization would open up the possibility of new outcome measurements for birth. If birth were defined in other than medical terms, other outcome measures would be perceived as equally appropriate. As things stand now, if two approaches to childbirth result in equal mortality and morbidity rates, the two approaches are perceived as being roughly equivalent. Thus homebirth is demonstrated to be at least as safe as hospital birth because mortality rates are equal and morbidity rates are lower.

But birth is also an event in the lives of families, and if perceived as such, outcome measures based on familial experience would also be considered appropriate, along with infection rates or other measures of physiological morbidity. To take extremes, childbirth management that routinely leaves older siblings with nightmares and separation anxiety as the mother is removed from the household to return days later engulfed in the care of the new infant is not the same as a birth that leaves older siblings strongly attached to the newcomer, unshaken in their own secure position within the family—even if the rate of morbidity is the same. A birth management that leaves wives angry at husbands, and husbands feeling that they have failed their wives, is not the same as a birth that draws the two closer together. A birth experience that leaves the woman unsure of her mothering abilities and unable to comfort a crying new baby is not the same as a birth experience that leaves the woman feeling confident and competent. And a birth experience that excludes the father, or whomever the woman is planning on raising that child with, is not the same as a birth experience that leaves the co-parent intensely attached to the child and feeling his or her own parenting competence grow.

Childbirth is also a learning experience for women. Perceived in those terms, birth outcome can also be measured in terms of the woman's knowledge about her body, her baby and her birth. With demedicalization, teaching skills, long valued in midwifery and largely ignored in medicine, would be considered important. A pregnancy and childbirth experience, again looking at the extremes, that leaves the woman fearful of her bodily function, unsure of just what was cut "down there" or why, is not the same as a birth that leaves the woman feeling strong and positive about herself, more rather than less comfortable with her body.

In sum, the medical monopoly on childbirth management has meant defining birth in medical terms, and thus narrowing our scope of perception. A birth management that routinely leaves psychological and social trauma in its wake for the members of families, using this narrow definition, is measured as perfectly successful, unless the trauma is severe enough to be measured in appropriately "medical" terms—that is, infant weight gain or some such crude measure.

Because I challenge the usefulness and the validity of such measures, I thus challenge the medical monopoly on childbirth. The policy implications that follow from this challenge are admittedly radical. If childbirth is redefined in other than strictly medical terms, medicine as a profession loses its long-standing monopoly on childbirth management in the United States. The demand by midwives to practice their profession is not an attempt by a less qualified group to engage in the practice of medicine, as it has most often been seen, but rather the claim of a more qualified group to practice midwifery. The state, as granter of professional licensing, remains in a position to license—or to refuse to license—individual midwives or classes of midwives. But redefining birth in non-medical terms means that it will be midwives and not physicians who determine appropriate midwifery qualifications, who set the standards for midwifery practice, and who advise the state on the licensing of midwives.

If childbirth is not merely a medical event, then physicians are simply one profession with relevant expertise. That expertise will continue to be used, as birthing women and midwives will continue to call on physicians for their skills. But breaking the circle of medical dominance would mean that medical practice would not determine women's experience of birth: women's experience of birth would determine medical practice.

— Excerpted from Recreating Motherhood: Ideology and Technology in a Patriarchal Society, by Barbara Katz Rothman. 1989. W.W. Norton & Co. New York. London. Pg. 169+

Barbara Katz Rothman, PhD, is a professor of sociology at the City University of New York.

THE UPS, DOWNS AND INTERLINKAGES OF NURSE- AND DIRECT-ENTRY MIDWIFERY:
STATUS, PRACTICE AND EDUCATION

by Robbie Davis-Floyd, PhD

In this article and the one that follows, I seek to provide an anthropological overview of both the upside and the downside of recent transformations in the status, education and practice of nurse- and direct-entry midwives. My motivation for writing stems from the many inquiries I receive from student midwives, or those thinking about becoming student midwives, concerning my opinion about which educational path they should follow and what kind of midwife they should become. For the past several years, through interviews and participant-observation, I have been studying the development of two new direct-entry certifications by members of the Midwives' Alliance of North America (MANA) and the American College of Nurse-Midwives (ACNM), and the differing educational philosophies these two certifications represent. As a result, students often ask me to explain what I have learned about the divergence between ACNM and MANA over the issues of scope of practice and appropriate educational routes. This and the following article are my attempts to make my understandings about both nurse- and direct-entry midwifery more available to such students, as well as to midwifery educators, practicing midwives, consumers and social scientists interested in these issues.

In the course of carrying out this research, I have interviewed approximately thirty direct-entry midwifery students and thirty nurse-midwifery students about their motivations for becoming midwives and their educational experiences. In addition, I have conducted over one hundred interviews with experienced nurse-and direct-entry midwives on a variety of topics, from their training to the nature of their practices to their motivations for developing direct-entry certification. At present, I am still actively conducting research and many of my interview tapes have not yet been transcribed. Since I have been asked to write this article before my research is complete, I have relied heavily on editorial assistance from a number of prominent nurse- and direct-entry midwives, all of whom are listed in the acknowledgments.

During this editorial process, it often became apparent that midwives in both organizations are extremely concerned about how they will be represented in print. It seems that both nurse- and direct-entry midwives want me to represent them as they would like to be, not necessarily as they are. The passion both groups put into their critiques of my portrayal of the downsides shows very clearly the depth of their desire to be the best midwives, the best educators, the best caregivers they can be, according to their respective values and beliefs. They want their ideal image to be presented in print, *because they strive to live up to that ideal,* and are concerned about printing anything that might threaten a profession that is still at a fragile evolutionary stage.

But I see midwifery as increasingly strong—strong in practitioner-client relationship, strong in safety, strong in evidence-based care. During my interviews with midwifery students, I was struck by the fact that almost all the students I spoke with, direct-entry and nurse-midwifery alike, felt spiritually called to practice midwifery. I take this fact as another indication of midwifery's strength—it is an ancient profession with powerful appeal to new generations. It is clear that no matter what the individual drawbacks in their training and practice styles, midwives are the best care providers for the vast majority of mothers and babies. The benefits of midwifery care have been well and thoroughly described by numerous authors (see for example Rothman 1982, Goer 1995, Arms 1997). Most recently Judith Rooks has provided thorough summaries of nearly every study done on the outcomes of midwifery care in her comprehensive *Midwifery and Childbirth in America* (1997; see also MacDorman and Singh 1998). I do not need to recapitulate these findings here. Suffice it to say that midwives' nurturant, woman-centered, evidence-based care produces excellent outcomes, generally with lower rates of intervention and lower costs than births attended by physicians.

Nevertheless, the medical monopoly in the United States is still firmly in control of birth: obstetricians and family practitioners attend 94 percent of American births. Most American women think only of calling an obstetrician when they become pregnant; many people are unfamiliar with the benefits of midwifery practice and do not know that midwives are available in almost every city. The 8,700 or so midwives who attend 6 percent of American births[1] are culturally marginal in relation to the 35,619 obstetricians (and other doctors) who attend all the rest. Much work needs to be done to educate the public about the benefits of midwifery care. I am a firm believer that midwives themselves are the most effective public educators because they often speak out about who they are and what they do. This country needs many thousands more midwives than it has. Students are the key to midwifery's future; it is in the interests of helping them make informed choices about how to become midwives that I offer the following assessments. In these assessments, I include both the upside and the downside as I see them, so that the students for whom I write will be as informed as possible and, whichever route they take, will understand the benefits to seek and the risks to guard against.

In what follows, I first present a general overview of the ups and downs of nurse- and direct-entry midwifery. I then describe the historical reasons for the present tensions between the ACNM and MANA, the professionalization of "lay" midwifery, the development of two new direct-entry certifications by members of these two national midwifery organizations, and the tensions generated by the exclusive establishment of one of these certifications in the state of New York. I consider the potential role of each of these new certifications in keeping open the full spectrum of midwifery care, including homebirth. And I offer an evaluation of the stylistic and philosophical differences between experiential and didactic models of midwifery training, describing the trend toward the incorporation of both models in all current versions of midwifery education. In the concluding sections, I venture to express my own vision of a midwifery future in which harmony between the two national organizations prevails and unity in diversity is the dominant theme.

Please note the following sections refer *only* to members of ACNM and MANA. I have not studied and cannot speak about midwives not affiliated with either organization.

THE UPS AND DOWNS OF NURSE-MIDWIFERY

Nurse-midwifery has strong roots in homebirth practice and the home care of the poor during the 1920s and 1930s, when Mary Breckenridge adapted the British combination of nursing and midwifery to serve the rural poor of Appalachia through the Frontier Nursing Service, which she founded in 1925. Today nurse-midwives practice in many settings, but mostly in the hospitals where 99 percent of American women give birth. Ninety-six percent of births that CNMs attend take place in hospitals (Rooks 1997). They made and have stuck with a decision that the best place for midwifery is inside the healthcare system. They got in by being trained as nurses, which meant that midwifery could be construed as an advanced form of nursing, which put it solidly inside medicine (Roberts 1995: 121; Rooks 1997:40).[2] At the time, this was a very strategic move: the nurse-midwives who founded the ACNM in 1955 were (and still are, to a lesser degree) trying to legitimize midwifery in the face of powerful medical opposition and a long and relentless medical campaign to convince the public that midwives were unsafe practitioners (Donegan 1978, Donnison 1977, Leavitt 1986, Wertz and Wertz 1989). Training midwives as nurses not only made sense in terms of the increased range of care they could offer, but also in terms of (1) convincing the public that they constituted a legitimate and trustworthy profession; and (2) convincing physicians that they should be part of the American system of obstetrical care.

Now that the members of ACNM are expanding into "direct-entry" midwifery education and certification (see box 1), they are doing so in careful alignment with nurse-midwifery. Nursing was their ticket to entry and legitimacy; although they are willing to drop a nursing degree as a requirement, they will keep all other aspects of their educational standards by creating ACNM's version of direct-entry midwifery in the image of nurse-midwifery. To succeed within medicine, as they are doing, they must mirror the standardized education of all medical professions. Their leadership believes that success within the technocracy[3] requires a college degree, and that it is disempowering to women to require them to obtain an education worthy of a college degree without also requiring them to obtain the degree. That is why, starting in 1999, the ACNM will require that all CNMs obtain a baccalaureate degree (in any field) either before, during, or upon completion of their midwifery education.[4] Presently there are no undergraduate nurse-midwifery programs leading to a baccalaureate degree; thus in effect, for the immediate future, the baccalaureate will be a requirement for entry into all such programs. (Some nurse-midwifery certificate programs, which at present lead to an associate degree, will become post-baccalaureate programs; others may investigate mechanisms for offering the baccalaureate.[5]) Some in the ACNM strongly advocate that the master's degree should be required for certification, but the ACNM Board of Directors has recently reaffirmed that the master's is not a requirement. Seventy percent of nurse-midwives already do have a master's degree.

Box 1

THE USE OF THE TERM "DIRECT-ENTRY" IN THE U.S.

I must stop here to explain the complexities of the term "direct-entry," which in its simplest form means that one enters directly into midwifery education, instead of first passing through the discipline of nursing. This is the definition utilized by most non-nurse midwives, many of whom chose as early as the mid-1980s to replace the term "lay" with "direct-entry"—a term already well-known in Europe—because it conveys their strong sense of themselves as professionals and carries the definite if subtle implication that nursing is at best a roundabout way to enter midwifery. Direct-entry midwifery is the norm in Europe, where most midwives do not become nurses, but rather attend formal three-year midwifery training programs in post-secondary educational programs or universities.

There appears to be some disagreement within the American nurse-midwifery community over the proper meaning of the term "direct-entry." Some nurse-midwives favor the broad definition (entering directly into any type of midwifery education). Others point to the European use of the term to mean government-accredited formal education. Still others seek to limit the use of the term in the United States to mean very specifically that one enters midwifery education not through nursing but through an ACNM-accredited university-affiliated midwifery training program (which will require completion of basic science prerequisites and a university degree). Many "direct-entry" midwives see this as a costly and indirect route.

It is essential to understand that we are dealing with two radically different educational paradigms, even though they are called the same thing. There are important ramifications of this semantic confusion: because both groups are using the same label, some members of each feel that the other is co-opting their process, not to mention their terminology.

Another problem that confounds the use of the term "direct-entry" is the fact that some ACNM members believe that all who call themselves direct-entry midwives should at a minimum meet the criteria laid out in the international definition of a midwife (see box 2); many direct-entry midwives do not meet these criteria. A few in the ACNM have attempted to resolve this problem by suggesting that all American midwives who do not meet the international definition should be called TBAs (traditional birth attendants)—an idea that MANA midwives find not only inaccurate but also insulting in the extreme. In developing countries, generally speaking, TBAs, while often highly respected in their own communities, have far less formal Western-style training and lower overall social status than "midwives" who meet the international definition. The evidence-based knowledge and skills of NARM-certified CPMs (see below), including those who are apprentice-trained, are very different from those of most traditional midwives; to lump them together in the same category would be extremely misleading. In addition, most MANA midwives believe that even TBAs shouldn't be called TBAs, as this is a somewhat derogatory label that often obscures their locally valued roles as community midwives.

What nurse-midwives have gained from these strategies is multiple: legal status in all fifty states (and the District of Columbia), insurance reimbursement and malpractice coverage, participation in some managed care programs, a degree of respect within the medical community and in the wider society, the ability to offer the benefits of midwifery care in hospitals where the vast majority of women give birth, and the credentials and skills to carry out and publish much-needed research on midwifery practice. Because they are integrated into the healthcare system, CNMs can find employment throughout that system. Most are employed by hospitals, physicians, or HMOs; some choose to enter midwife-run private practices. CNMs in private practice tend to know all the women in their practices and derive a great deal of satisfaction from their work, but often suffer from burnout and find it difficult to also "have a life." At such a point they can fluidly choose to enter larger practices where they may have less patient involvement but more time for themselves and their families (Cecilia Wachdorf, personal communication). In between these two extremes are many nurse-midwives working in large practices who struggle to maintain a balance between the risk of burnout and their desire to offer personalized care with some degree of continuity (Lisa Kane Low, personal communication, 1998). Many CNMs earn in excess of $60,000 per year; their salaries range between $25,000 and $85,000, with a mean of $55,000 (Bauer 1998:4). (The mean salary for obstetricians is $212,000.) Some CNMs are able to work pre-set hours with a reasonable number of days off, and accrue vacation and leave time and retirement benefits.

Box 2

THE INTERNATIONAL DEFINITION OF A MIDWIFE

A midwife is a person who, having been regularly admitted to a midwifery educational program duly recognized in the country in which it is located, has successfully completed the prescribed course of studies in midwifery and has acquired the requisite qualifications to be registered and/or legally licensed to practice midwifery.

She must be able to give the necessary supervision, care and advice to women during pregnancy, labour and the postpartum period, to conduct deliveries on her own responsibility, and to care for the newborn and the infant. This care includes preventative measures, the detection of abnormal conditions in mother and child, the procurement of medical assistance, and the execution of emergency measures in the absence of medical help.

She has an important task in health counseling and education, not only for the women, but also within the family and the community. The work should involve antenatal education and preparation for parenthood and extends to certain areas of gynecology, family planning and child care. She may practice in hospitals, clinics, health units, domiciliary conditions or in any other service.

(World Health Organization 1996)

Nurse-midwives primarily care for women around their reproductive functions, dealing mainly with pregnancy and birth, family planning, health screening, and management of common gynecological conditions. Although officially CNM practice is centered around the care of low-risk women, in fact many CNMs give high-quality, nurturing, and collaborative care under extremely difficult conditions in inner city hospitals to high-risk indigent women who otherwise would receive the dregs of our inadequate medical system. Their new core competencies (1997) expand their scope of practice into more general women's primary healthcare, should they wish to offer it.

Because most CNMs attend births in hospitals, they become part of hospital culture, learning it from the inside. Thus they are often able to generate significant cultural change. In hospitals across the country, CNMs have introduced alternative policies and techniques such as allowing women to eat or drink during labor, to get up and walk, to labor in water, and to room in with their babies after birth. CNMs have designed and opened in-hospital alternative birth centers, successfully lobbied for LDRPs (a single room for labor, delivery, recovery and the postpartum period) and offered breastfeeding education and support. Obstetricians and nurses who observe the benefits of CNM care are often inspired to change both their attitudes toward birth and the way they treat birthing women. Most CNMs find their work intrinsically rewarding: they thrive on the intimate connections they develop with their clients, often on the spot during labor or birth; on a client's positive response to their nurturing, empowering care; and on their ability to sometimes hold a holistic space in which a woman can freely birth the way she chooses, in spite of the medicalizing constraints of the hospital environment. CNMs have also been instrumental in developing out-of-hospital freestanding birth centers where they can regularly offer holistic midwifery care; a few of them (probably less than three percent[6]) attend births in homes.

Some states give CNMs clear legal prescriptive authority; in others, they are usually able to prescribe under a more limited arrangement such as standing physician orders. Within the parameters of nurse-midwifery, CNMs have plentiful opportunities to learn new skills: for two examples, in order to give their clients more continuity of care, many CNMs are learning and performing diagnostic ultrasound, and some are training to first-assist when their clients undergo cesarean sections. Some CNMs also incorporate alternative and complementary methods such as herbal, nutritional or homeopathic therapies. CNMs can advance professionally into directorships of programs, education or research positions, or can move into the growing field of public health. And their numbers are growing at a rapid rate, as is the percentage of births they attend. When I first started my midwifery research in 1994, there were 4,993 members of the ACNM; as of June 1998, there are 7,717 members (including students).

Paralleling the above gains are a particular set of losses. Although high salaries and team practices facilitate raising a family, they do not guarantee job security—virtually all CNMs are vulnerable to managed care cutbacks and physicians' resistance to competition. Participation in managed care often subjects CNMs to pressure to care for more women in less time with fewer resources. Because a standard for all CNMs is that they must practice in collaboration with physicians,[7] they can be prevented from practicing if the physician withdraws from that collaboration, or the hospital decides to deny them privileges. For example, a number of CNMs have invested heavily to open birth centers, only to be forced to close them when they lose their collaborating physician and cannot find another. Their opportunities to attend homebirths are similarly limited (see below). There is also the reality of the debt load associated with a university-based degree, which can go as high as $70,000 (some CNMs have government-funded scholarship assistance).

And although many nurse-midwifery educators make concerted efforts to train their students in a midwifery, not a medical, model of care, nurse-midwifery training is inevitably medicalized to some extent because it is primarily hospital-based. In effect CNMs are taught a duality of models and must learn to creatively balance them both (Cecilia Wachdorf, personal communication). Yet they must strive to create this balance inside a system that is heavily weighted toward the medical, not the midwifery, side. Once in practice, nurse-midwives must maintain good working and social relationships with physicians and nurses, usually must follow the policies of the hospitals in which they attend births, whether or not they agree with them, and must struggle to be included in HMOs and other managed care programs.

Many CNMs have told me how easily this inevitable medicalization slipslides into over-medicalization. I recently spent a day with a group of about seventy nurse-midwives in upstate New York. I asked how many of them feel that they are offering truly woman-centered, holistic midwifery care in the hospitals where they practice. Only about five hands went up, engendering a lively discussion about how these five manage to do it when the others want to but cannot for fear of losing their jobs.

Over-medicalization is the shadow side of nurse-midwifery education and practice, but it is very hard to generalize about. Some CNMs practice holistically, but humanistic caring and compassion are more constant features of nurse-midwifery care than the non-medicalized holistic approach.[8] Some CNMs, most especially those involved with high-risk patients, become extremely dependent on medical technologies and diagnostic techniques; some become as interventive as any obstetrician. Others who try to resist the overuse of these technologies that characterizes the medical approach to birth may end up succumbing to hospital pressure and end up not practicing the kind of midwifery they would like to practice. Frustration and burnout can often result. Many CNMs I have interviewed point out with sadness that the women they attend often insist on ultrasounds and epidurals. As I learned in my earlier research (Davis-Floyd 1992), it is a fact that the majority of American women feel safer when birth is medically controlled. Most women want a combination of high technology with humanistic care in which their opinions are considered and their decisions are respected. Nurse-midwives are able to offer this combination; several studies have shown that most women are satisfied with their nurse-midwifery care.

But not all. The promise of a woman-centered advocate is a compelling one for many nurse-midwifery clients who wish to avoid unnecessary intervention; if that promise is eclipsed by medicalization, it can be an unhappy surprise. Recently a number of letters and personal accounts from new mothers protesting their CNM care have come to my attention. These women counted on their CNMs to protect them from unnecessary intervention, but instead ended up with labor induction and/or augmentation, frequent or continuous use of the electronic fetal monitor, withholding of food and drink, too-hasty episiotomies, etc. When CNMs perform such interventions unnecessarily, which of course physicians are notorious for doing, consumers point to the over-medicalization of CNM practice and training. On a panel discussion at the 1997 MANA conference in Seattle, ACNM President Joyce Roberts seemed to accept this criticism as a necessary price to pay for higher gain:

> You ask, what is the risk of this formalized education? You say it is over-medicalized. I would say it need not be, but I would also add that the risk of not having it is not being able to practice in all the domains that the WHO definition says midwives practice in. [See box 2, page 75.] One has to weigh the risks of protecting themselves from over-medicalization and the realities of our healthcare system today, or take the consequences of limiting your practice to a very narrow domain.[9]

Such limitation has indeed been the choice of many MANA midwives. Although they are increasingly moving into the mainstream in a number of states, in general most have in the past consciously chosen to stay outside the dominant medical culture. This has resulted in a greater degree of marginalization, which many consider a worthy price to pay for maintaining autonomy, avoiding over-medicalization, and holding open the homebirth option. Nurse-midwives, who must practice with physician collaboration and under insurance restrictions, usually cannot provide homebirth services. Very few CNMs attend homebirths (see endnote 6), whereas MANA's 1,400 members primarily attend homebirths. The following section will discuss the upside and the downside of direct-entry midwifery as practiced by the members of MANA.

THE UPS AND DOWNS OF DIRECT-ENTRY MIDWIFERY [10]

In the United States, homebirths account for less than one percent of all births—a figure that has not changed nationally in over a decade (Rooks 1997). That percentage is higher in Oregon (around six percent) and rising in Florida, Washington and other states where midwifery is legal, but on a national level it is still minuscule. While many decry this low figure, Ina May Gaskin, the current president of MANA, points out that this low percentage of homebirths

> can be seen as an accomplishment, given the highly financed, highly organized efforts that American physicians over the course of this century have made toward stamping out homebirth altogether. We have not only maintained that steady rate, we have begun to experience what happens when a struggle such as this takes place over a generation. Given the opposition the medical profession has directed against midwifery, we in MANA believe that it has been an accomplishment for us to have survived at all! As more studies are carried out on the safety and efficacy of DEM practice, we believe that the percentage of homebirths will rise, not fall, during the years to come. We see the six-fold increase in homebirths in Oregon, where midwifery has long been

legal, as significant. We are still in the stage of being a "best-kept secret" when it comes to mainstream culture (Personal communication, 1998).

Direct-entry midwives are legal, regulated and licensed, registered, or certified in fourteen states (Alaska, Arkansas, Arizona, California, Colorado, Florida, Louisiana, Montana, New Hampshire, New Mexico, Oregon, South Carolina, Texas, Washington); legal through judicial interpretation or statutory inference, or a-legal (not legally defined but not specifically prohibited from practice) in nineteen states; effectively prohibited in eight states where licensure is required but unavailable; and illegal in nine states and the District of Columbia.[11] They can obtain insurance reimbursement from private companies in most states where they are licensed, and Medicaid (and sometimes managed care) reimbursement in Arkansas, Arizona, Oregon, Florida, Washington, New Mexico, South Carolina and Vermont. (In many other states licensed midwives are fighting for Medicaid and managed care reimbursement, with varied results. In most states, homebirth attended by direct-entry midwives is still an out-of-pocket expense.) They often work alone or in practices with one or two primary midwives,[12] and are almost always on call. For some, burnout is the result of this constant availability; others find this a viable way of life.

They are rewarded for their dedication by the excellent outcomes and untrammeled beauty of the out-of-hospital births they attend, by the empowerment their clients experience through having given birth on their own, and by the strengthening of the family that often results when birth takes place at home. Other rewards include the awareness that their work is helping to preserve homebirth as a viable option for American women[13] and that they are keeping holistic, independent midwifery alive and are furthering the preservation and development of its unique body of knowledge—a knowledge based on the wide variations in truly normal birth, which can only take place outside the artificial constraints of the hospital environment (see below). Many direct-entry midwives appreciate the flexibility they enjoy as independent practitioners: should they desire more time off, they can cut down on the number of clients they take on. In areas where interest in homebirth is steady or growing, they can choose to accept more clients until they build their practice to the level they desire. Thus their incomes vary widely: those who attend only a few births a year may make only a few thousand dollars, while some direct-entry midwives make upwards of $60,000 per year.

In short, direct-entry midwives (DEMs) face the challenges and reap the benefits of being self-employed entrepreneurs. Like some MDs, they run independent practices; their earning ability is not constrained by salaries but rather depends on their level of energy and their ability to attract clients (which itself is constrained by cultural attitudes toward homebirth). In states where they are licensed and regulated, they often serve as the sole proprietors of thriving businesses (at a time when many MDs are being forced to trade in their economically advantageous positions as independent practitioners for the rigid payment schedules of HMOs). Many DEMs make a good living, many do not, but all of them love their work. Most DEMs would not trade the challenges, tribulations, and rewards of their entrepreneurial practices for the constraints of working in a hospital setting.[14] Wanting to be where the majority of women are, some DEMs do desire to become qualified for hospital practice and go on to become CNMs; they usually retain their ideological commitment to MANA and to out-of-hospital birth (Ventre, Spindel and Bowland 1995).

In states where they are licensed, direct-entry midwives are gaining increasing respect from the physicians in their areas. In part this seems due both to their proactive creation of educational standards and protocols, their participation on licensing boards and agencies (for a midwife, the professional is always political), and to the documentation of their good outcomes that played a part in their obtaining licensure. In such places, DEMs are usually welcome to remain in the hospital with the clients they transport. But in other states where they are shut out of the system and are little understood, they may be actively persecuted by the legal and medical establishments. The possibility of prosecution may limit their ability to carry appropriate technologies. And even when they transport in a timely and appropriate manner, they may be banned at the hospital door and blamed by hospital personnel for "botched homebirths." Many medical practitioners, and some nurse-midwives, have serious concerns about the safety of direct-entry practice; they point to the fact that there *are* some DEMs in practice with truly inadequate training.[15] Thus when a DEM makes a mistake, no matter what her individual knowledge and skills, most people in the medical community are only too ready to assume that she is "ignorant" and "incompetent," and go on to assume that incompetence and lack of education characterize all midwives of her ilk—an irrational application of a damaging stereotype that has no basis in fact. Most direct-entry homebirth midwives have excellent midwifery educations, are highly skilled clinically, and are increasingly choosing to demonstrate their education and their competence through meeting the standards for CPM certification.

> For a midwife, the professional is always political.

THE PROFESSIONALIZATION OF LAY MIDWIFERY

The Midwives' Alliance of North America (MANA) was formed at a meeting held during an ACNM convention in 1982, called by Sister Angela Murdaugh, then president of the ACNM. She was acting in response to what she thought was a desire on the part of ACNM members to dialogue with "lay" midwives (see box 3). Her intention was to facilitate that dialogue, but others within ACNM hoped instead to convince the lay midwives to enter the ACNM fold. Nevertheless, the meeting that was called to generate dialogue evolved into the formation of MANA—an organization with an international scope (North America includes Canada and Mexico) that gave these midwives a sense of group identity and common cause. Why did they choose to form a new organization instead of becoming nurse-midwives and joining with ACNM? My observation is that it is because they believe deeply in the value of preserving their independent midwifery model of education and care in order to effectively serve the women who choose out-of-hospital birth, and they did not and do not believe this task can safely be left to the ACNM. MANA vice-president Anne Frye further explains:

Thirty years ago, non-nurse midwifery rejuvenated itself via a network of women with no prior experience who began to attend births as a direct result of community demand. At that time, nurse-midwifery was a little known profession with very few CNMs in practice compared to today—many of these early truly lay midwives did not even know there was an option, and many that did know rejected the idea that nursing had anything to offer midwifery. However, as the movement grew and these original "lay" midwives became more sophisticated in their understanding of the details of medical training and practice, they saw quite clearly that what they were seeing at homebirths often did not reflect what they were reading about and seeing in hospital birth. Understanding that they were developing a different knowledge system, over time they sought to develop educational methods and programs that would perpetuate that system, and to avoid incorporation into the more medicalized nurse-midwifery approach. (Personal communication 1998)

Emerging from the grassroots to serve an out-of-hospital clientele, for nearly four decades these women who started out in the late 1960s and early 1970s as "lay midwives" have educated themselves, attended births, trained apprentices, codified their unique body of knowledge in books and articles (see for examples Bruner 1998, Frye 1996, Davis 1997, Gaskin 1990), joined together to write appropriate standards for their out-of-hospital practices, lobbied for workable legislation, developed educational programs and state certification processes, and thrived in spite of the ill wishes and often active persecution of the medical establishment. They have organized themselves into a movement powerful beyond its small numbers because of the widespread public support it

---

Box 3

MY USAGE OF THE TERM "LAY"

Out of their self-made level of expertise, during the 1980s members of MANA began to reject the term "lay" midwife in favor of terms that better characterized their status; these included "empirical," independent," "traditional," and later the more professional term "direct-entry" (see Box 1).

But the general public and many in the healthcare professions have not caught up with these changes, and still refer to all DEMs as lay midwives. In this article I use the term "lay" only in the following cases: (1) when I am talking about nurse-midwives who still call direct-entry midwives "lay"; (2) when I am talking about licensed direct-entry midwives who call unlicensed direct-entry midwives "lay" (as in Washington state and elsewhere); (3) when I am talking about nurse-midwives who used to be, and used to call themselves "lay midwives"; and (4) when I am talking about a historical period in which MANA members referred to themselves as "lay." It should be noted that, in spite of the pejorative use of this term by some groups, having been a lay midwife at the beginnings of the midwifery renaissance is a strong source of pride for many midwives, even though they no longer use the term.

enjoys from the dedicated and numerous members of the alternative childbirth movement.

THE CREATION OF THE CERTIFIED PROFESSIONAL MIDWIFE (CPM)

When I was asked to speak at my first MANA conference in El Paso in 1991, there was an ongoing debate over the word "professional," which many of the midwives present were refusing to use because of its exclusionary connotations. Nevertheless, it was clear that they were evolving themselves as professional midwives with codified and cohesive body of knowledge and skills. During the Carnegie-sponsored Interorganizational Work Group (IWG) meetings between ACNM and MANA that took place in the early 1990s, delegations from both organizations worked to pinpoint their similarities, and looked (ultimately unsuccessfully) for ways of resolving their differences (see Rooks, this chapter). The ACNM delegates pointed out that non-nurse midwives lacked standards and methods for measuring competence. Anyone could hang out a shingle, call herself a midwife and join MANA.

Responding not only to such critiques from the outside, but also to problems within the homebirth community occasionally generated by midwives who did not practice appropriately, many MANA members felt a strong need for both means of standardizing midwifery education to ensure that homebirth midwives would share a common and established base of knowledge and skills and for clear mechanisms for peer review and professional discipline[16] (Pam Weaver, personal communication 1998). At the same time, MANA members were increasingly recognizing a need for a mechanism for proving the professional competency they had been developing that would help them interface with the medical system. These midwives, whom the ACNM still characterized as "lay," were feeling, acting and running businesses like professionals, and they perceived the potential value of a credential that would validate their knowledge of midwifery. (Those who had been the victims of medical persecution report being "forced" to this conclusion.)

The strong desire for such a credential on the part of many members of MANA was paralleled by great concern that the uniqueness of direct-entry midwifery as they had been developing it would become co-opted in the process of trying to achieve standardization and enter the mainstream. It was the powerful vision of one of the MANA representatives to the IWG, Sharon Wells, that it would be possible and indeed was the ideal time to create a certification process that preserved MANA's "Midwifery Model of Care," and that the preservation of this midwifery model—as developed by the midwives who founded MANA and as expressed in writing for the first time by sociologist Barbara Katz Rothman in 1982—would ultimately depend on the existence of this certification.

The concern felt by many MANA members about the possible dangers of co-option led to the gradual step-by-step development of certification, with great care being taken at each step to address these concerns. During the 1980s midwives in Oregon, California, Massachusetts, Colorado, New Mexico and New Hampshire had created and implemented their own certification processes in their respective states. The creation of national certification had been a topic of much discussion at the

1985 MANA business and open forum meetings (Elizabeth Davis, personal communication, 1998). In the late 1980s, these discussions crystallized into MANA's formation of an Interim Registry Board (which later evolved into the North American Registry of Midwives (NARM), whose charter was to develop an examination to test knowledge. The original intention was to develop a national registry of those who had passed this written examination. Over 400 midwives were eventually listed on this voluntary registry.

Once it existed, the NARM written exam was quickly picked up by midwifery associations and state agencies which had been needing such an exam but did not wish to develop it themselves. Perceiving the potential benefits, many in MANA intensified their call for a professional credential through which they could demonstrate not only their knowledge but also their experience, abilities and skills. This demand, in combination with the professionalizing impetus of the many state certifications, and the critiques stemming from the IWG meetings, the medical community, and even the homebirth midwifery community about the lack of standards for independent direct-entry midwifery, spurred the members of MANA and NARM to expand NARM into a full-fledged testing and certifying agency, designing, developing, and implementing the credential, the certified professional midwife (CPM). (For a detailed description of this process, see Houghton and Windom 1996b and Rooks 1997: 248-252.)

In 1991, the Midwifery Education and Accreditation Council (MEAC) was founded by the National Coalition of Midwifery Educators, a group of MANA midwives who had created or participated in direct-entry midwifery programs in the United States over the previous ten years. MEAC is responsible for the evaluation and accreditation of direct-entry educational programs; it has accredited or pre-accredited ten such programs to date. MEAC's stated mission is to improve the quality of direct-entry midwifery education, as well as support innovative and diverse midwifery education programs, including apprenticeship. (Structurally speaking, MEAC is the equivalent of ACNM's Division of Accreditation (DOA), and NARM is the equivalent of the ACNM Certification Council (ACC)). See Figure 1.

Figure 1.

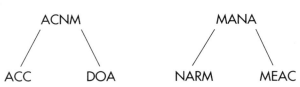

It is important to note that the ACNM is a professional organization: you must hold ACC (or ACNM[17]) certification as a CNM or a CM to be a full voting member,[18] and you must graduate from a DOA-accredited program and pass the ACC exam to receive that certification. In contrast, MANA is not a professional organization in the same sense, but rather an inclusive umbrella group that welcomes all midwives as members, certified or not. You do not have to be a member of MANA to receive CPM certification, nor do you have to graduate from a MEAC-accredited program. Anyone who declares herself to be a midwife can be a full voting member of MANA. Generally speaking, ACNM, whose membership is *exclusive*, has represented the profession of nurse-midwifery, whereas MANA, whose membership is *inclusive*, has represented the independent midwifery movement (a social phenomenon, not a profession) (Betty Anne Daviss, personal communication). Nevertheless, MANA is professionalizing, and it remains to be seen whether, as more and more members of MANA choose to become CPMs, MANA itself may (or may not!) evolve into a professional organization that requires CPM certification for voting membership.

In line with the concerns of many MANA members, the board members of NARM and MEAC and their many volunteer supporters were determined that the new CPM credential and all MEAC-accredited educational programs would not co-opt direct-entry midwifery by medicalizing its standards, but rather would fully reflect the "Midwifery Model of Care" (see box 4) to which MANA and its affiliates lay claim— independent, woman-centered, holistic, out-of-hospital midwifery. To ensure success in this endeavor, NARM designed and carried out a full-scale survey of practicing home-birth midwives to determine what these practicing midwives considered to be appropriate entry-level requirements. The survey, known as the *1995 NARM Job Analysis*, was sent to 3,000 midwives, 800 of whom sent in properly completed surveys (one-third of them were CNMs). This high return rate is remarkable, especially given the fact that these detailed surveys took up to twelve hours to fill out. The responses showed a high degree of consensus among all respondents, indicating strong agreement within the home-birth midwifery community about the knowledge and skills that should be required for safe entry-level out-of-hospital practice. On the basis of these responses, NARM designed its written and skills examinations, ensuring that CPM requirements are based on actual homebirth midwifery practice. In celebration of this accomplishment, and speaking for all those who participated in the development of CPM certification, during a 1997 panel discussion direct-entry midwives Pam Weaver and Elizabeth Davis exclaimed, "We did it! We actually managed to develop a certification

---

Box 4

THE MIDWIFERY MODEL OF CARE

The Midwifery Model of Care is based on the fact that pregnancy and birth are normal life events. The Midwifery Model of Care includes: monitoring the physical, psychological and social well-being of the mother throughout the childbearing cycle; providing the mother with individualized education, counseling and prenatal care, continuous hands-on assistance during labor and delivery, and postpartum support; minimizing technological interventions; and identifying and referring women who require obstetrical attention. The application of this woman-centered model has been proven to reduce the incidence of birth injury, trauma and cesarean section.

that encompasses everything we hold dear!" The first CPM, Abby Kinne of Ohio, received her certificate on November 10, 1994.

CPM certification is competency-based; *where* you gained your knowledge, skills, and experience is not the issue—*that you have them* is what counts. In keeping with MANA's values NARM has been as inclusive as possible, honoring multiple routes of entry into midwifery, including self-study, apprenticeship, private midwifery schools and university-affiliated programs, including those accredited by the ACNM. [19]

Thus the major criticism that ACNM educators level at NARM certification is that it is not tied to a required formal educational process that utilizes only standardized, accredited programs. Here we find the crux of the philosophical differences around educational issues that divide these two organizations. MANA members do not accept the argument that formal, standardized education is necessary to provide safe and competent practitioners. Citing recent trends in adult education in other fields, they stand behind their value on competency-based education. CPM certification has built into it what is known in adult education as a portfolio process (a portfolio is the formal documentation of a person's education through life experience). This documentation must be extensive and must demonstrate that the candidate meets NARM midwifery experience requirements (performance of seventy-five prenatal exams, attendance at twenty births as an active participant and twenty more as primary caregiver, etc.) as listed in the NARM publication *How to Become a CPM*. Knowledge is tested through the NARM Written Exam. Skills are verified in two ways: the candidate's educational supervisor or mentor must attest that she has achieved proficiency on each area listed on the *Skills, Knowledge, and Abilities Essential for Competent Practice Verification Form* provided in the CPM application packet, and the candidate must take a hands-on skills exam.

Because most midwives who took the early forms of the NARM written exam passed, the exam was criticized by CNMs and others as being too easy, a mere mechanism for "grandmothering in" all practicing midwives without any real testing of their abilities. It was not widely understood that the pilot project in which these early forms of the exam were tested was for experienced midwives only, who would be expected to pass. The fact that few did fail the early, less sophisticated versions of the NARM exam seemed to some leaders in the ACNM to justify their pre-existing view that they should not leave direct-entry certification up to MANA and NARM. (In this context, it is worth noting that, by report of an elderly nurse-midwife who took it, the earliest nurse-midwifery exam was given orally and was only half an hour long.) But over the ensuing three years, NARM hired an outside testing agency and created sophisticated, psychometrically valid, rigorous written and hands-on skills exams, which have proven to be effective screening mechanisms.

In 1997, the consumer group Citizens for Midwifery contracted with two specialists in competency-based education and testing at Ohio State University, Deborah Bingham Catri and Robert A. Mahlman, to carry out independent evaluations of the NARM process, including its exams. They each presented expert testimony to the Direct Entry

Midwifery Study Council (established by Ohio statute), copies of which are available through Citizens for Midwifery. Catri testified about competency-based education, and concluded from her analysis that the CPM process is in fact competency-based. Mahlman, a testing expert, reviewed the testing aspects of the certification process to determine if the examination and its development meet industry standards for high quality certification tests; he found that the quality was as good or better than comparable programs and that the procedures followed were based on established standards for this kind of testing. (Their testimonies are unpublished, but copies of the full texts as well as summaries are available from Citizens for Midwifery (1-888-CfM-4880) or may be downloaded from the Internet at <www.mana.org> or <www.cfmidwifery.org>.)

As of June 1998, there are approximately 400 CPMs, with about 150 applications in the works and more coming in every day (Sharon Wells, personal communication). The NARM exam has been accepted as the state direct-entry licensing exam in thirteen states and two Canadian provinces (Alberta and British Columbia), and the entire CPM certification process has been accepted as a route to licensure in two states (Oregon and Texas) and one Canadian province (Manitoba) and is under consideration in fifteen other states. It is important to remember that this process is very new. Contemporary comparisons between the ACNM and MANA fail to take into account the differences in the ages of these organizations. Founded in 1955, ACNM has had forty-three years to work out the kinks. MANA has had just sixteen years, and NARM and MEAC have been in their present form only since the early 1990s. There was a time when nurse-midwives were illegal in most states, a time when their certification exam was rudimentary, a time when they struggled to define their knowledge base and set practice standards, a time when they had to fight for legalization and licensure state by state as MANA and NARM are doing today. I recently paid a visit to Toronto, where I spoke with some of the midwives who had been instrumental in the legalization of direct-entry midwifery in Ontario. They told me they had been heavily criticized in the early stages of their process for deficiencies they needed only time and the benefits of their learning curve to correct. One of them said, "To criticize us for not getting it perfect from Day One is like criticizing a child for having growing pains." I felt the point was well-taken, in both countries.

ACNM educators also criticize the NARM process because it is not tied to specific standards of practice. Some clarification is in order. Both NARM and the ACC are certifying agencies and as such they certify that a given midwife has demonstrated mastery of a specified body of knowledge and skills. Neither NARM nor the ACC has any legal authority to enforce compliance regarding practice standards. Licenses for both CNMs and DEMs are granted by individual states based on regulatory statutes, and the rules under which each must practice (including standards of practice) are set and legally enforced by the regulatory board of the state in which they reside and are licensed. Both MANA and the ACNM have created documents regarding practice standards, values and ethics, which many midwives follow. Although the state sets the rules, the professional standards set by the ACNM and MANA do have the power to influence legislation and policy by serving as models; the exams created by the ACC and NARM are examples of resources these agencies can provide to states.

Whether or not CNMs, CMs, CPMs or licensed midwives (LMs) agree with or agree to abide by any specific standards of practice other than those determined by state law reflects their individual values and ethics. It should be noted that the practice setting (hospital, birth center, home) generally affects both the amount of scrutiny an individual midwife is subject to as well as the degree of freedom she has to provide highly individualized care. Practicing with a greater degree of freedom may be confused with a lack of practice standards when that is not the case. But greater freedom and less scrutiny do increase the importance of regular review and discussion with peers regarding practice techniques and standards (Susan Hodges, personal communication, 1998). For homebirth midwives, peer review, instead of operating only as a judgmental or disciplinary process, needs to and often does serve as an effective means for ongoing evaluation of their own practices from the perspectives of their midwifery community.

THE CREATION OF THE CERTIFIED MIDWIFE (CM)

One of the roots of ACNM's move into direct-entry certification can be traced to the development, twenty years ago, of the three-year masters' level program at Yale University that allows a fast track through one year of nursing into two years of midwifery training. Other roots lie in the vision and determination of key figures like Dorothea Lang, a former president of ACNM and a highly respected leader in nurse-midwifery, who became a nurse-midwife in order to move the profession of midwifery away from nursing. In recent years, this vision came to be more commonly shared among ACNM members for a set of specific reasons:

- Increasing numbers of currently practicing CNMs take the role of midwife as their primary professional identity ("I am not a nurse, I am a midwife!" is a statement I have heard countless times during my interviews, see also Scoggin 1996), including many who went to nursing school only to become qualified to enter a nurse-midwifery educational program—a requirement they resented at the time, and continue to regard as unnecessary. In addition, they resent being identified as nurses, licensed to practice under nurse practice acts, and regulated by state nursing boards. They wanted to provide a way for people who want to be midwives but don't want to be nurses to become educated in line with ACNM/DOA standards, and to be certified by the ACC.

- Physician assistants (PAs) and some nurse-practitioners with little obstetrical training have begun to attend births in many states (Burst 1995). CNMs see this as both an infringement on their territory and as potentially dangerous for birthing women, and they recognize that someone who is already a PA should not be required to become a nurse in order to receive midwifery training.

- Increasing numbers of young women want to become midwives through ACNM-accredited routes, but regard the subordinate status of nursing as a hindrance to their desire to be independent practitioners and the years of nursing training as an unnecessarily time-consuming impediment to their midwifery careers.

- Increasing numbers of CNMs were realizing that only specific aspects of nursing knowledge are relevant to providing quality midwifery care, and that this knowledge can be obtained outside of nursing training (Rooks 1998; Lisa Kane Low, personal communication).

- Many CNMs had no confidence in MANA's and/or NARM's ability in their early stages of development to impose high educational and competency standards on direct-entry midwives. They believed that the midwives certified by NARM would be "substandard," and would endanger the midwifery profession with their substandard practice. Thus they concluded that direct-entry certification should not be left to NARM, but should be taken on by the ACC.

In 1994, ACNM members voted overwhelmingly for the ACC to create a direct-entry certification process; in 1995, they chose CM (certified midwife) as the name of this new type of practitioner; and in May 1997, they passed a resolution making this new CM a full-fledged voting member of the College.[20] Only two DOA-accredited educational routes of entry to the CM credential are available: university-based programs and university-affiliated distance learning programs. These routes will not include apprenticeship programs or non-university-affiliated midwifery schools. CM entry-level requirements are based on entry-level CNM requirements; the exams taken by CMs and CNMs are essentially the same.[21] All DOA-accredited direct-entry programs must either lead to a baccalaureate degree or require one for acceptance into the program. After January 1999, all nurse-midwifery programs will have the same requirement. As noted previously, to date there are no pre-baccalaureate DOA-accredited direct-entry programs, although some nurse-midwifery certificate programs are investigating ways to offer the baccalaureate. Should ACNM educators choose to develop a bachelor's in midwifery, as has been done in Canada, this degree requirement could quickly become more supportive of many students' search for the most direct route into ACNM-certified midwifery.

At present, the only DOA-accredited direct-entry program currently operating is a two-year program located at the State University of New York (SUNY) Health Science Center on the Brooklyn campus in New York City (colloquially known as SUNY downstate). (Others are under development in Pennsylvania, Texas and elsewhere.) Entry requirements for SUNY downstate include obtaining a baccalaureate in any field if the student doesn't already have one[22] and taking courses to satisfy the basic science requirements. Through the establishment, eventually, of many such programs, ACNM direct-entry advocates seek to further the ACNM's stated goal of 10,000 ACC-certified midwives by 2001. Within a few years there will likely be distance learning programs like CNEP (a very successful at-distance nurse-midwifery program based at the Frontier Nursing Service in Hyden, Kentucky that allows students to remain in their communities, studying on computer and working with a local CNM preceptor) around the country for direct-entry students, so that they won't have to leave home.

Given that they are going to great lengths to make their version of direct-entry midwifery education more accessible, many ACNM members feel they have now "opened up" their profession, allowing easy ingress to all those who want to be midwives but don't want to be nurses. Thus some in ACNM feel more than justified in believing that ACNM should be the one and only national midwifery organization. Some of the key players I have interviewed insist that having two national organizations only divides and weakens midwifery, and would like MANA midwives to rally around their new direct-entry standard.

In contrast, many MANA members do not see ACNM's move into direct-entry as an opening up but rather as a closing down, an exclusionary move to redefine direct-entry on ACNM's terms and shut out MANA-style direct-entry midwifery. They insist that having two national professionally-oriented organizations, two certifying bodies (the ACC and NARM) and two accrediting bodies[23] (the DOA and MEAC) strengthens midwifery, keeping important options alive for midwifery education and practice that would vanish if MANA were to disappear. As soon as ACNM's plans for creating the CM became known, those in MANA who equate "direct-entry midwifery" with out-of-hospital training and birth reacted with outrage to what they perceived as incursion into an area they had spent years developing and a co-option of their chosen label (see box 1). They believed they were doing a very good job of defining "direct-entry midwifery" and of setting national standards for direct-entry education and practice. Anne Frye further explains:

> It seemed to us that nurse-midwives with no homebirth background teaching direct-entry students would be like direct-entry midwives suddenly deciding to open nurse-midwifery programs within hospitals.[24] This would not only be ludicrous, but also a reinvention of the wheel. And the fact that the ACNM thought they could do this without so much as consulting any "real" direct-entry midwives was, in the minds of many MANA members, only proof positive that they did not have any understanding of the uniqueness of direct-entry midwifery as practiced by the members of MANA, NARM and MEAC. To us it was clear that there are two distinct approaches to midwifery that both have value and which are similar in many ways but certainly not the same— a fact that calls for two different groups to oversee their ongoing development. (Personal communication, 1998)

In Frye's words we can again see the effects of the semantic confusion generated by both organizations' use of the same term (direct-entry) to refer to these two very different models. Frye indicates the desire felt by many MANA members to maintain separation between the realms of nurse-midwifery and direct-entry midwifery, with the ACNM and its affiliates in charge of standard-setting and credentialing for the nurse-midwifery realm, and MANA and its affiliates in charge of standard-setting and credentialing for the direct-entry realm. The conceptual neatness of this distinction was blurred when ACNM established its own "direct-entry" certification process (see endnote 10). Of course, ACNM never intended to create the same kind of direct-entry midwifery practiced by MANA members, but rather, as I noted above, is modeling its direct-entry educational programs on its existing nurse-midwifery programs to produce midwives who, while ideally qualified to practice in a range of settings, are *de facto* primarily qualified to practice in hospitals.

In contrast to the feelings of many of MANA's direct-entry members, others, most especially MANA's CNM members, welcomed ACNM's move into direct-entry education and certification, realizing that to some extent it *does* mean an opening of the College to new ways of thinking about and becoming a midwife. The existence of this entirely new kind of "direct-entry" midwife, the CM, represents fierce determination on the part of many committed CNMs to move their profession into a more autonomous position within the American healthcare system. The ACNM prime movers who created the CM faced down massive resistance from the nursing-oriented "old guard" members of the ACNM (and, in New York, from the nursing and medical professions) to bring her into existence. (There was tremendous controversy within the ACNM over this issue, as some CNMs believe deeply in the value of nursing training and feel that it would be suicidal for the ACNM to give it up. Indeed, a group of CNMs threatened to secede if the college changed its name to the American College of Midwives.) And they will have to face down opposition from state agencies and legislatures all over the country as they fight to obtain legal status for the CM in all fifty states. It seemed to me as an anthropologist that such an enterprise could be self-defeating in an already marginal group, so I interviewed many of those most involved in creating the CM about their motives for pushing the boundaries of their vulnerable profession (just as I had interviewed many of the prime movers in NARM and MANA about their motives for creating the CPM).

During my interviews with these prime movers within ACNM, their level of commitment to this new kind of midwife became clear. They envisioned her as a way of rapidly expanding their numbers, since she would graduate from one of the numerous new programs educators would eventually design and offer around the country. The existence of this credential would be a way of incorporating PAs into the midwifery fold, and also of incorporating the many foreign-trained midwives living in the United States who did not have nursing training. They envisioned that the CM would be an open door to the "lay" midwives who had been vociferously protesting CNM nursing requirements. Or she might simply be someone with a baccalaureate degree who wanted to become a midwife but did not want to become a nurse. She would graduate with the same skills as CNMs, but without having her life derailed by a lengthy passage through nursing training,[25] much of which is viewed as irrelevant to midwifery. She would be likely to have more independence of thought and spirit than those who had been socialized into a nursing model,[26] she would be more likely to work in freestanding birth centers and/or to attend homebirths,[27] and she would be a pioneer who would help reconstitute midwifery as an autonomous profession and the midwife as a skilled, highly educated primary care professional. Because her existence would help solidify midwifery as an autonomous profession unattached to nursing, she would help nurse-midwives "get out from under the thumb" of nursing boards, hopefully to be regulated by their own midwifery boards in every state.[28]

ACNM has risked much and will risk more in the future to achieve this transcendent vision of an expanded and more autonomous midwifery profession. Although at this date of writing (May 1998) there are only seven CMs, all of whom are licensed only in New York, the mere potential that they represent has caused

Helen Varney Burst to change the name of her classic textbook from *Varney's Nurse-Midwifery* to *Varney's Midwifery*, and has generated a serious movement within the College to change its name from the American College of Nurse-Midwives to the American College of Midwifery (see endnote 20).

CONFLICT IN NEW YORK

New York was the first state to legalize and legitimate the CM. Up until 1992, nurse-midwives in New York practiced under an obscure clause in the Sanitation Code, were granted permits, not licenses, to practice and had no prescriptive privileges. In the early 1980s a committed group of CNMs began to lobby for a midwifery bill that would establish them as an independent profession regulated by New York's Department of Education, give them real licenses to practice, grant them prescriptive privileges, *and* expand their profession by allowing direct-entry midwives with training deemed equivalent to that of nurses by the state to be licensed as well. It took them ten years of intense effort to get such a bill passed. Had this group of women concentrated only on nurse-midwives, they could have had their bill five years earlier. But they were deeply dedicated to their vision of direct-entry midwifery (that is, to creating a category of practitioners trained in midwifery, not in nursing, who would enter the profession through university-affiliated DOA-accredited direct-entry programs) as a means of expanding and growing and broadening their profession, and so they hung on for an extra five years, fighting not only the New York Medical Association but also the New York Nursing Association for the right to legitimize both their profession and this new kind of direct-entry midwife. They were thrilled when, after a last minute flurry of intense lobbying, they succeeded in pushing their bill through, and in establishing, for the first time in New York history, a state midwifery board through which they could regulate themselves.

This bill—the New York Professional Midwifery Practice Act, which most CNMs lauded as ground-breaking, the wave of the future—turned the practice of unlicensed midwifery from a misdemeanor to a felony and made it impossible for almost all the practicing direct-entry midwives in New York, all of whom were attending homebirths, to obtain licensure.[29] Seeking inclusion in the law, the Midwives Alliance of New York (MANY) had hired a lobbying firm, established a relationship with a senate sponsor, and organized consumer grassroots lobbying efforts (Sharon Wells, personal communication 1998). Believing that they had succeeded, MANY members mobilized to support the Practice Act. But eleventh-hour changes to the bill left them completely shut out (Wells 1992; personal communication 1998),[30] leading to much bitterness and disenchantment in the New York direct-entry midwifery community and, for a time, to the issuing of cease and desist orders to around ten of its members, to the arrest/and or prosecution of three, and to the harassment and investigation of some homebirth clients.[31]

Watching ACNM and its affiliates the ACC and the DOA establish a new direct-entry certification, set standards for accrediting direct-entry programs, and grant pre-accreditation to one such program—SUNY downstate in New York City—all using a hospital-based model of midwifery and without consulting any practicing direct-entry midwives, these experienced New York midwives saw themselves and their independent model of direct-entry midwifery ignored and discounted in the ACNM process. They note the emphasis ACNM has placed on making its direct-entry midwifery education exactly equivalent to the training CNMs receive, and are suspicious that in spite of the desire of their creators that CMs be trained in out-of-hospital settings (see endnote 27), the CM will be just another overly medicalized practitioner. From the point of view of the nurse-midwifery educators who designed the new direct-entry program, there was no need to consult any of New York's practicing direct-entry midwives, whom they thought of as "lay," as they never intended to model the SUNY downstate program on "lay midwifery" practice or education.

The fundamental disagreements between these groups in New York have led not only to bitterness and enmity, but also to much loss of livelihood and great reduction in the availability of midwife-attended homebirth in New York state, as many DEMs have either stopped practicing or left New York to practice in friendlier climes. (Out of the over 600 CNMs in New York, only a handful attend homebirths.)

In this type of polarized situation, Midwifery Today often works to play a unifying role, generating dialogue between nurse- and direct-entry midwives at Midwifery Today conferences, and offering opportunities across the country for each group to learn more about the other. For one example, many of the direct-entry and nurse-midwifery students currently enrolled at SUNY downstate attended the Midwifery Today conference in Salem, Massachusetts in March 1998 and seem to be developing a philosophy supportive of both sides of this new direct-entry equation.

HOMEBIRTH: PRESERVING THE FULL RANGE OF THE SPECTRUM OF CARE

A prevalent perception among nurse-midwifery educators is that midwifery is midwifery. Said one: "We teach midwifery, not homebirth or hospital birth, but midwifery. The setting is irrelevant to how midwifery should be taught." But this perception is contradicted by my interviews with thirty nurse-midwifery students, most of whom had just completed their education. They feel, and I have observed, that the setting of birth has a great deal to do with what they learn and how they practice. Consider this student's description (paraphrased from an interview) of a hospital birth she recently attended:

> By the time I got to this woman, her labor was kind of stalled and she was just wild, writhing around, pulling out her IV. I didn't know what to do with her, I simply didn't know what to do. So I called in the OB, who pitted her and got her contractions stabilized, got her under control and her labor back on track. Once she was back on track and pushing, I felt like I could handle the birth.
>
> Q. You say you didn't know what to do with her. What would you have done if you had been at home with no OB to call?
>
> Oh, I would have done everything differently! I would have put my arms around her and asked her what she was feeling. I would have gotten her up, given her something to drink, helped her take a shower or walk around. We

would have gotten to the bottom of her emotional issues before we tried any-thing else.

Q. So it sounds like you *did* know what to do with her! Why didn't you do that, instead of calling the OB?

Because the circumstances didn't allow it. There was no space for me to con-nect with her at that level.

This student nurse-midwife is reporting on her exposure to the dual models of medicine and midwifery. In this case, as she does, we can attribute her decision to turn over control to a physician and to follow the medical approach to the fact that she is still a student and has not yet matured into a sense of autonomy. Trained and capable of operating in both models, she prefers the midwifery approach as she would be free to apply it at home. But, constrained by her environment, she is practicing (and thus internalizing) the medical way. Calling in the doctor or "pitting" a stalled labor can get her out of a difficult situation once, twice, three times without affect-ing her too much. But by the time she has taken this approach forty or fifty times, will she even remember that she once knew another way?

A poignant commentary on this student nurse-midwife's (SNM) experience is provided by CNM Fran Ventre. She writes:

After practicing as a "lay midwife" for several years, I had the same experience in nurse-midwifery school at DC General Hospital as the student quoted above. The difference was a nurturing caring faculty person who, when I was at sea, asked me the same question, "What would you do at a homebirth?" After easily rattling off the same things the student said, my teacher replied, "Well, why don't you just do that now?" (Personal communication 1998).

The contrast between Fran's experience and the experience of my student-inter-viewee provides an excellent example of the individual variations in nurse-midwifery training and thus of the difficulty in trying to explain it in generalized ways. While some programs and some preceptors stress this more holistic approach, in other pro-grams students may find that approach difficult or impossible to apply.

The perceptions of my nurse-midwifery student interviewees of the overall qual-ity of their educational programs were overwhelmingly positive; most gave their program a 7 or an 8 on a 1 to 10 scale. The two to three points off were, in almost every case, protests against the lack of opportunity to experience homebirth; this lack was one of the two major criticisms that all these students voiced about their nurse-midwifery training. (The other was a sense of being inadequately prepared to do primary healthcare.) While ACNM officially sanctions homebirth, the reality is that few CNMS (see endnote 6) attend homebirths: most cannot get physician collaboration or insurance for homebirth, and few receive adequate training for homebirth practice.[32] As noted above, nurse-midwifery educators feel that CNM and CM training will be adequate in any setting. But MANA midwives disagree, insisting that hospital-based training makes midwives too afraid of birth and too dependent on technology and support personnel to be qualified for independent homebirth practice.

Samantha's experience illustrates a very important point: the members of the ACNM and MANA need each other.

One CNM who agrees with them is Samantha McCormick. Samantha told me that her three years as an obstetrical nurse in a high-risk hospital in New York left her terrified of birth, and that her year in Columbia University's nurse-midwifery program did not allay those fears. In an effort to develop confidence in herself and in the birth process, she interned at a nurse-midwifery program in Cooperstown, New York renowned for its holistic approach. After two months there, she still did not feel confident, so she decided to apprentice with Shari Daniels, a direct-entry midwife who used to run a midwifery program in El Paso, Texas and who at that time was taking groups of midwives to do births at Victoria Jubilee Hospital in Kingston, Jamaica. Her apprenticeship with Shari finally gave Samantha the trust in birth and the courage to handle emergencies in the self-reliant way characterized by homebirth midwifery for which she had been searching.

Samantha's experience illustrates a very important point: the members of the ACNM and MANA need each other. While CNMs are giving midwifery care to thousands of women in the high-tech world of hospitals, the members of MANA are holding open a spectrum for that care that the ACNM alone cannot preserve. (Fewer than 200 CNMs attend homebirths—a task that the other 7,717 members of the college are not undertaking.) Although many ACNM educators would like their students to have the full range of out-of-hospital experience, offering it as part of clinical training is often made impossible by their collaborating physicians, by hospital and insurance policies—the costs of liability coverage would usually be prohibitive—and by the limited number of homebirths attended by CNMs. Consider the following email request received by Abby Kinne CPM, a direct-entry midwife in Ohio:

Hi Abby! I had a very disappointing meeting with the director of my nurse-midwifery program. After inquiring about spending time with a lay midwife for clinical experience she informed me that the ACNM has policies and guidelines that prohibit me from being involved (participating or observing) with lay midwives while I am a student at a nurse-midwifery program. I am so frustrated—how do I provide the option of homebirth to my future clients without any experience? She did say that if I could find a CNM that does homebirth I could spend time with her—that would be OK! The only one I know of is in Cincinnati (and I cannot do clinicals there; the University of Cincinnati has that site). Do you know of any CNMs around Ohio or out-of-state that do homebirths??? I REALLY want to get some homebirth experience before I graduate!!

As of this writing, her search for an Ohio CNM who does homebirths has been unsuccessful. In her email message, she added:

Otherwise, I was told that once I am a CNM ut practicing on my own, I can do whatever I want, and that I will have to wait until then to get my experience!!!

In response to this latter remark, another midwife wrote back:

This is hardly true. A CNM must be lucky enough to find an OB/GYN (in Ohio anyway) who supports her and her philosophy of care 150 percent and will be willing to go to bat for her whenever administrators/ bureaucrats begin to question what she is doing; and they WILL question what she is doing unless she practices according to strict standards.

These sorts of exchanges take place on the Internet almost daily. For MANA members, they confirm what they already deeply believe: that their independent, holistic, home-based style of midwifery is unique and special, that it will not be taught in ACNM programs, direct-entry or not, and that it is up to them to preserve what they have to offer, which will be lost if they allow themselves to be subsumed by the ACNM. When I queried direct-entry students about why they chose not to become CNMs, they unanimously responded that they did not want to participate in the medicalization of women and birth, but rather to be agents of their emancipation from that medicalization. When I asked them how they felt about not serving the vast majority of women who give birth in hospitals, they responded that they believe that each midwife who learns homebirth will be a magnet attracting more women away from the hospital, and helping to create home and birth center birth as increasingly viable alternatives. Beyond learning the technicalities of midwifery care, they see their mission as (1) internalizing an attitude of profound respect for the sacredness of birth and women's bodies and fostering this attitude in others; (2) preserving the practice of holistic midwifery, and preserving and furthering its body of knowledge; and (3) preserving and expanding women's options for out-of-hospital birth. They believe passionately in the worth of this mission.

They are confirmed in this belief by the members of the newly birthed Bridge Club. Originally conceived by Fran Ventre (a CNM who is also one of the founding members of MANA), the Bridge Club was spontaneously formed at the 1997 MANA conference in Seattle by a group of CNMs who are also members or supporters of MANA.[33] (Many of them had practiced as lay midwives before they became CNMs.) If ACNM-style midwifery were truly superior in all ways, this Bridge Club might have formed to work within MANA to convince more MANA members of the inadequacy of their training and to encourage them to apply for entry into ACNM-accredited programs. But instead, the members of the Bridge Club are trying to convince the ACNM Board that there is something ineffable and precious about MANA-style midwifery, something that must be preserved and would be lost if all independent midwives decided to become CNMs or CMs, something that is preserved by NARM certification and that ACNM should at best support or at least do nothing to undermine. Many of these women have learned both models with their bodies, hearts, and minds; they seem most qualified to speak to the relative merits of each model. Supporting the CM, they also support the CPM, and advocate for the complementary co-existence of both. With one voice they insist on the value of preserving independent out-of-hospital midwifery and apprenticeship training, as the CPM credential seeks to do.

Didactic and Experiential Learning: New Combinations in Midwifery Training

What is so important about apprenticeship, you may ask? To understand that, it is important to understand the difference between *experiential* and *didactic* learning. Didactic instruction is linear, logical, sequential, and often abstract, involving graphs, charts, diagrams and rote memorization. Experiential learning is learning with the whole being, not just with the mind.[34] This is the oldest and most effective method of human learning. It is how children learn to function in their cultures—they simply participate, absorbing the rhythms, patterns, conceptual categories and techniques of daily life, along with their underlying system of values and beliefs. Whereas it is obvious when didactic training is taking place—someone is clearly being taught by someone else or is studying alone—experiential learning is often invisible: you can't see it happening so you don't know it's there.

In all types of contemporary midwifery training in the U.S., both experiential and didactic learning are brought into play.

Apprenticeship in traditional societies takes place through just this sort of experiential, whole-being learning (Jordan 1993; Singleton 1989). For example, the master potter might say to the apprentice, "bring me a lump of clay." The apprentice complies, and is told the clay is too hard. S/he tries again, and is told it is too soft. Getting it right the third time, the apprentice has just learned the right texture of clay for this type of pot at this moment in its making, but all the master potter has done is to save herself a trip! When Western anthropologists and filmmakers have tried to film apprenticeship training and record how it takes place, they have often found themselves stymied. Applying didactic models, they look for physical and especially verbal interactions between apprentice and teacher, waiting for the teacher to "teach." But such moments of didactic instruction are relatively rare in traditional apprenticeships—most learning takes place as the apprentice simply participates in the task at hand, absorbing through doing (Coy 1989, Lave and Wenger 1991). Thus how or what the apprentice learns is often not visible to the didactically trained eye, nor easily put into logically sequenced words.

An example of the difference between didactic and experiential training in midwifery is provided by Charis Smith, a student nurse-midwife enrolled in a distance learning CNM program who is simultaneously apprenticing with a pair of direct-entry midwives in her community. (I have used a pseudonym instead of her real name because, like the Ohio SNM, she was explicitly forbidden by the head of her program to work with "lay" midwives.) Thus Charis is experiencing the difference between didactic and experiential styles of education first-hand. She comments,

> I had been reading for school about fetal positioning and where what parts should be and how to feel them and types of pelvises. I thought that having that information stored in my head would help my hands figure out what they

were doing. The next morning I went to [my direct-entry mentors'] clinic to do prenatal exams. They told me to put my hands on the mother's tummy and assess the baby's position. I was trying to think my way through feeling the baby. I felt totally lost. [The midwife] told me to erase everything from my head. To get rid of any ideas that I might have about where the baby should be and close my eyes and feel the baby through my fingers and hands. Let the baby tell me where she is. The same idea with fetal heart tones. She told me not to think about what they should be while I am listening with the fetoscope. Rather, close my eyes and feel the beat in my ears and in my body. At first all I was hearing were the trucks going by in the street below, Mom's belly gurgling, and the kids playing on the floor next to me. As I shut that off and tried to feel what was coming through, the babe's heartbeat jumped right out at me, clear as can be. And like feeling the baby, I could feel the presence of this child right through my ears and into my being.

In all types of contemporary midwifery training in the United States, both experiential and didactic learning are brought into play. Linear didactic instruction, for example, is often creatively combined with non-linear methods such as the case study approach, which combines experiential learning with synthesis of new information and critical thinking and analysis. While didactic teaching is most strongly emphasized in university-based nurse-midwifery programs, it also plays an important role in private midwifery schools and even, nowadays, in apprenticeship (see below). Experiential learning is most strongly emphasized in apprenticeship, but it also constitutes a major part of nurse-midwifery training, under a different name and in a different form—preceptorship.

The number of preceptors involved in the education of a given SNM can vary widely. Many SNMs work with more than one preceptor, which some nurse-midwifery educators see as an advantage. Others work closely with only one preceptor and gain very little experience with other practice styles. Nurse-midwifery educators generally value one-on-one learning, but feel that it must take place within the structured didactic framework of a formal, university-affiliated program. Aspects of such programs that they consider to be important include specific criteria for entrance into the program, structured learning objectives that work to ensure that every student masters the necessary body of knowledge, formalized didactic instruction, clinical experience with more than one clinical instructor and involvement of several faculty members in judgment about the student's ability to provide safe, effective beginning level midwifery care, which the director of the program must attest to in order for the graduate to be eligible for the ACC exam (Judith Rooks, personal communication), since the ACC does not test skills (Peter Johnson, personal communication 1998). Most ACNM accredited programs are based on a modular format that places responsibility for learning in the hands of the student (Johnson and Fullerton 1998). The use of modules is predicated on the concept of adult learning, which takes an individualized approach to mastery of the needed knowledge or information (Lisa Kane Low, personal communication 1998).

The small but growing number of private direct-entry midwifery schools around the country essentially include all of these above components as well; like nurse-midwifery programs, they combine didactic with experiential training, often in a modular format. MEAC-accredited schools and programs have specific entrance criteria, incorporate learning objectives and formal instruction, and offer varied clinical experiences; their faculty members regularly evaluate student competency. Here we can see the transformations in midwifery being wrought in the 1990s: the differing approaches of nurse-midwives and direct-entry midwives to midwifery education these days form not a dichotomy but a seamless continuum. One end of this continuum is defined by formal university programs; the other by pure apprenticeship and self-study. The middle range moves from at-distance university-affiliated programs (like CNEP and SUNY Stonybrook) to college-based direct-entry programs (like the program at Miami-Dade Community College in Florida) to private midwifery schools with entrance requirements, faculty, and formal curricula (like Seattle Midwifery School, the Florida School of Traditional Midwifery, the Utah School of Midwifery and Birthingway Midwifery School in Oregon). (See my overview of types of midwifery training, next article.)

And these days, even apprenticeship training is moving toward that middle range. In many cities, senior midwives take turns teaching weekly classes for all of their apprentices, adding the didactic element to traditional apprenticeship. The Utah School of Midwifery and the Midwifery Institute of California have both developed distance-learning/apprenticeship programs in modules that can be adapted for use by mentors and apprentices anywhere in the country. The modular form ensures that learning objectives can be formally set, and that what the apprentice learns can be tracked and evaluated, so these two have become the first apprenticeship programs to receive MEAC accreditation.[35] And increasingly, midwives serving as mentors are using the NARM Test Specifications in the *Candidate Information Bulletin* as a guideline for the apprenticeship training process, in order to ensure that their apprentices will be fully prepared to achieve CPM certification. NARM certification also requires that there be more than one midwife who evaluates the abilities of the student: all CPM candidates must pass not only a written examination but a hands-on skills exam administered by an experienced midwife trained to serve as a NARM Qualified Evaluator.

Given the increasing convergence of didactic and experiential models in direct-entry midwifery training, it is important to ask why MANA, NARM and MEAC have gone to such lengths to preserve stand-alone apprenticeship as a valid route. My observation is that they honor it for the connective and embodied experiential learning it provides, but most especially for the deep trust in women and in birth that it builds. The apprenticeship training that produces many of today's direct-entry midwives takes many creative and original forms, but fundamentally involves attending births with one or more practicing midwives, assisting them in myriad ways, observing the way they interact with and care for pregnant, laboring and postpartal women, watching and helping them deal with emergencies, and talking endlessly with them about every detail of their care. During countless hours jointly spent in prenatal exams, home labors and births, postpartum visits, the routine maintenance of equipment and office space, and the mundane necessities of running a business, doing everything together from cervical checks to cooking, labor support to laundry, pelvic exams to paying bills, the mentor and apprentice develop a connective and intimate relationship that facilitates rapid and integrated learning within a context of trust in one's teacher and one's self.

Birth is a fundamentally successful natural process that turns out well with very little intervention most of the time; thus, apprentice-trained midwives are mostly exposed to women working hard and successfully giving birth. Although they have opportunities to experience pathology and emergency management over the course of their apprenticeship training, these incidences form the periodic punctuation, not the defining ethos, of their clinical experience. Thus apprentice-trained midwives generally develop a strong faith not only in themselves, but also in the inherent trustworthiness of the birth process and in women's ability to give birth. They can and very often do include as part of their training a stint in a high-volume program either overseas or in the United States (such as the MEAC-accredited program offered at Maternidad La Luz in El Paso), where they will encounter many complications, but this exposure takes place against an already-established background of trust in the power of women and in the normal process of birth.

> Birth is a fundamentally successful natural process that turns out well with very little intervention most of the time.

The relationships between student nurse-midwives and their preceptor(s), while often rich, rewarding, and mutually supportive, seldom take on the particular depth and intensity of the apprentice-mentor relationship, which some nurse-midwifery educators criticize as too all-encompassing. Another difference is that SNMs' exposure to complications in childbirth can vary widely. Some who train in settings where patients with complications are quickly transferred out may graduate without ever having seen shoulder dystocia, a postpartum hemorrhage or true fetal distress. Others who train in high-volume, high-risk settings may be exposed in rapid succession to multiple complications. Many CNM educators make concerted efforts to minimize exposure to pathology until later in student training, but in some settings that can be difficult to achieve. (Many CNM educational programs offer clinical experience in the care of indigent women, who have a higher incidence of complications.) In addition, as we have seen, the standard of care in the hospital environment in which SNMs receive most of their clinical experience is based on a medicalized, technological approach to birth which itself often creates pathology—too much monitoring leads to too many cesarean sections, too much haste leads to too many episiotomies, etc. Tension prevails, rather than trust. Thus the hospital norm is to intervene to prevent possible complications, rather than to wait patiently for the natural process of birth to unfold.

CNMs are educated to deal with a wide variety of "normal variations" in childbirth, and in certain settings must deal with many complications themselves. But, as we have seen, the majority of CNMs work in large hospitals where help is generally readily available should an emergency arise that is outside their competence or comfort level. At home, if a complication arises, the mother must either be transported to the hospital or the midwife and her partner must handle the problem on site. If the complication develops when birth is imminent or so rapidly that transport is out of the question, homebirth midwives must have the skills to deal with it themselves. Thus they tend to develop an independence of thought, a strong self-reliance, a sense of trust in birth and a self-confidence in the face of crisis that nurse-midwives trained only in hospitals may lack.[36] The most common criticism leveled at nurse-midwifery training by the direct-entry midwives I have interviewed is that it produces midwives who are afraid of birth. Knowing that fear itself can generate birth complications, these direct-entry midwives fiercely defend apprenticeship, which they honor for its production of midwives who truly trust birth and the women who give birth—to which many CNMs would respond that lack of formalized training will not bring recognition in the technocracy, and will result in the narrow scope of practice and cultural marginalization Joyce Roberts described above.

Again the waters are muddy here: this is true in many places, but not all—in California, for example, full scope well-woman care is in the new direct-entry licensure law as a valid part of direct-entry practice, all of the 100 or so California licensed midwives, including those who were apprenticeship trained, passed a rigorous challenge examination based on the Seattle Midwifery School's formal educational program, and a few licensed midwives in California and Florida who are apprenticeship-trained and practice primarily at home now have hospital privileges as well. This California situation, though a bare beginning, indicates some of the long-term possibilities for increasing convergence between these two midwifery systems.

MY DREAM

I see in this present dispute over the proper nature of direct-entry midwifery two completely different world views that stem from disparate histories, disparate values, disparate perceptions of the nature of midwifery and the meaning of midwifery care—in short, disparate midwifery cultures. It seems almost impossible for these two cultural systems to agree (a situation that is particularly hard on those who are members of both). Everything the ACNM does makes perfect sense if one accepts the belief and value system of the ACNM. Everything MANA does makes perfect sense if one accepts MANA's belief and value system. These belief systems are not just intellectually understood but are felt, lived, experienced, expressed in myriad aspects of life, from the kinds of clothes midwives wear to the kinds of conventions they put on.

MANA has long been an irritating thorn in the ACNM's side. Faced with bigger issues, from recalcitrant physicians to managed care, since MANA's inception many ACNM members have wished it would just go away. Indeed, by her own report Sister Angela was almost subjected to impeachment proceedings for having called the initial meeting. Sixteen years later, although MANA's supporters within ACNM have grown in number, some CNMs are still wishing MANA would disappear. At the very least, many of those in the ACNM wish that all non-ACNM midwives would just accept ACNM as the one and only standard-setting organization for midwifery, and study for ACC certification. As noted above, these CNMs strongly believe that it harms midwifery to have two major national organizations, and that it would help midwifery to speak with one unified voice—i.e., theirs.

In the fall of 1997, I facilitated a panel at the MANA conference in Seattle entitled "ACNM and MANA: A Direct-Entry Dialogue." In the most dramatic moment of that panel, I asked ACNM President Joyce Roberts if she could support CPMs and CMs to be legal and licensed side by side in all fifty states. I was grateful that she courageously and honestly answered with a straightforward "No," as it helped to clarify to the MANA midwives that President Roberts' intention, and that of many in power in the ACNM, is to advance their direct-entry certification and to establish the ACNM as the only recognized standard-setting midwifery organization. (This was hard for some MANA midwives, whose own philosophy is so much more inclusive, to believe.) It is important to understand that President Roberts and many of her colleagues *quite sincerely* believe that would be the best for midwifery; they honestly see their standard as superior. Everything in their training and experience (not to mention the values of the wider culture) tells them that university degrees and university education produce midwives who will be both more qualified and more empowered to function effectively in the technocracy and to make needed changes in the healthcare system.[37] Of course, the members of MANA and its affiliates believe equally deeply in the superiority of their CPM certification as the standard for out-of-hospital birth, in the value of diversity in educational routes and practice styles and in the importance of holding open more options for out-of-hospital birth.

Thus it seems clear that for the present, MANA and its affiliates may have to fight not only against the medical profession but also against some state ACNM chapters to establish MEAC accreditation and NARM certification as legitimate in a given state.[38] This is a tragic situation, a major waste of energy that could be much better spent, and I hope it will not last for very long. It is a point of extreme sorrow to me that many midwives in MANA, NARM, and MEAC feel that in some states they are engaged in a war in which the ACNM is on the wrong side. We must remember that MANA is not threatening the survival of the ACNM, so there is no need to defend the ACNM from being subsumed by MANA, whereas MANA midwives fear that as the ACNM works to legalize the CM in all fifty states, the members involved in this legislative effort will be branding the CPM as an inferior credential and, openly or subtly, will encourage state legislators to make the CM the *only* legal and licensed direct-entry credential.

As I discussed with members of MANA and NARM the possibilities for peaceful co-existence of the two credentials (their desired goal), I have been told various times, with deep feeling, "This is not a tea party, it is a war. We are in a war for our survival." These MANA midwives have realized that they cannot defend all of direct-entry midwifery in state legislatures; they can only defend their CPM credential. Thus they are increasingly coming to interpret their survival as independent practitioners, and the survival of their out-of-hospital Midwifery Model of Care, as dependent on the legitimation of that credential. Although some prominent members of ACNM have stressed to me that they are not fighting MANA, that is not the experience of MANA members who watch other CNMs subtly or overtly denigrate the CPM in state legislatures and elsewhere, insisting that ACNM should be the only organization to "set the standard" for direct-entry midwifery.

> Let us not
> make the
> mistake of believing
> that the existence of
> one weakens the other
> and is bad for
> midwifery, but rather
> let us understand that
> each strengthens
> the other.

I prefer to dream a different dream. In my dream, all parties choose to reject the kind of rigid and hierarchical thinking that assumes there can be only one standard, so that if there are two, that has to mean that one is better and the other is worse. There is more than one good way to do something good! A number of states have already been successfully modeling a dual system of midwifery for more than ten years, including Oregon, Washington, New Mexico, Arizona and Texas. As an anthropologist I say, for the immediate future let there be two kinds of certified direct-entry midwives: two educational standards, two national certifications, two certifying bodies, two accrediting bodies (see endnote 23). Let us not make the mistake of believing that the existence of one weakens the other and is bad for midwifery, but rather let us understand that each strengthens the other. The existence of ACC-certified midwives (CNMs and CMs) opens the techno-medical realm of the hospital to midwifery care where it is most urgently needed. And the existence of the strong independent midwifery movement that MANA represents lengthens the spectrum of midwifery care, keeping a wide range of out-of-hospital options open for midwifery practice that would shrink considerably if the field should narrow down to CNMs and CMs. (Again, only about 200 CNMs attend homebirths; most of them are members of MANA and draw much of their inspiration and support from that wellspring.)

The fact that MANA midwives are working hard to preserve apprenticeship, to develop innovative new educational models, and to codify and strengthen their holistic, out-of-hospital midwifery model of care means that all that is precious about who they are and how they practice will grow as a strong and viable part of American midwifery. These models and these midwives will be available now and in the future as a resource that any CNM will be able to tap should she wish to learn how to attend homebirths, or simply to strengthen her sense of independence and self-confidence.[39] Like the thousands of women in hospitals who will benefit from the care offered by CNMs and CMs, thousands of mothers who want out-of-hospital birth will benefit from CPM care. As their value becomes recognized, CPMs will eventually be able to obtain licensure and regulation in every state, as well as insurance reimbursement. Clearly, today's MANA midwives strongly desire to move beyond marginalization—the theme of the 1998 MANA conference in Traverse City, Michigan will be "Midwifery in the Mainstream." They aren't there yet, but through development of their own direct-entry certification and accreditation processes have taken several major steps in that direction. With a little luck, I envision that five or ten years from now CPMs will be recognized and respected practitioners, legal and licensed in all fifty states, whose specialty is out-of-hospital birth, most especially homebirth. The prospective CPM statistical data collection project that is currently being worked out will be successfully completed; these data will demonstrate the safety and efficacy of CPM practice, and effectively refute the stereotypes of ignorance and incompetence that homebirth midwives have long suffered under.[40]

Meanwhile, in my dream CNMs and CMs will continue to increase their numbers and their presence at in-hospital, birth center and homebirths. As envisioned by many of the prime movers in the creation of the CM, the new CMs will indeed be more independent-minded. Never having been through nursing training, they will not internalize a sense of structural subordination to physicians, and thus will help to recreate ACNM-style midwifery as an increasingly autonomous profession. They will expand the scope and scale of midwifery practice. Their independence of thought will attract many CMs to out-of-hospital birth; many of them will work in birth centers and attend homebirths, often working in tandem with CPMs. It will be in the trust and intimacy of these individual relationships between direct-entry midwives that the two opposed meanings of the term "direct-entry" will finally converge.

Under siege from the advancing army of holistic practitioners and from the unified legislative front the midwives will present, MDs will lose legislative clout as their petty "because I said so" tactics to maintain their hegemony in each state are exposed, and midwives will increasingly be able to control their own destinies. Since a strong desire of many nurse-midwives at present is to get out from under regulation by nursing boards (see endnote 28), we can predict the emergence of midwifery boards in some, if not all, states. By the time this starts to happen, in my vision nurse-midwives will have gotten over their doubts about the NARM process and will understand the benefits that can accrue to each group from working together and presenting a united legislative front. Perhaps one obstetrician, one pediatrician, and one consumer will sit on these boards in advisory capacities, but they will mostly consist of midwives: one CNM, one CM and two CPMs, so that balance between ACNM's and MANA's philosophies and styles will be created and maintained.

Rather than opposing the legalization and regulation of CPMs, in my vision ACNM will support them in every state, working to educate legislators about the importance of providing trained professionals for the women who choose homebirth, affirming the value of the NARM process, and demonstrating the benefits that accrue to mothers and babies when (1) CNMs and CMs collaborate with CPMs, receiving their clients at the hospital door and assuring continuity of care by welcoming the CPM to continue to serve her client in the hospital as caregiver or doula; and (2) CPMs train interested CMs and CNMs in out-of-hospital birth. Physicians will be able to observe for themselves the benefits to mothers when midwives work together in such mutually supportive ways.

I have found in interviews that MDs' perceptions of direct-entry midwives are greatly influenced by what the CNMs they work with tell them. When the CNMs speak favorably of the homebirth midwives, the doctors tend to welcome their transports and treat both the midwives and the homebirth mothers with more respect. CNMs who denigrate the direct-entry midwives in their communities may well be harming mothers who will need their care. During my three years of research into the development of direct-entry midwifery in the United States, I have found that the CNMs who have little or no exposure to independent direct-entry midwives are the ones most likely to perceive them as uneducated and unsafe. In contrast, CNMs who have worked or interacted socially with DEMs tend to have great respect for their knowledge, training and practice styles. The more regular the interaction, the better they tend to understand each other and get along. So in my dream, monthly potluck dinners, joint regional conferences, Internet chat groups and mutual friendships will keep communication lines open between nurse- and direct-entry midwives, even when they don't practice together. But increasingly, they will establish joint practices owned by the midwives themselves (sometimes even hiring physicians, as Elizabeth Gillmore CPM has done in Taos, New Mexico), and make common cause.[41]

UNITY IN DIVERSITY

At the individual level, there are countless interlinkages between these two national organizations which seem on the surface of things to be so diametrically opposed. Consider the following:

- Most CNMs and DEMs share basic values and beliefs about the normalcy of birth and the importance of woman-centered, non-interventive care for facilitating women's ability to give birth.

- The midwives of MANA *and* of the ACNM are vulnerable and culturally marginal groups jointly attending only a small fraction of American births. Because most of them try to offer connective, nurturing care that honors the normalcy of women's individual rhythms, they—nurse- and direct-entry midwives alike—are subject to harassment and persecution for failing to adhere to conventional medical norms.

- From the 1970s on, CNMs have played an important role in the development of direct-entry midwifery; some CNMs have trained direct-entry apprentices and taught in direct-entry programs and schools.

- Likewise, DEMs have introduced some nurse-midwives to the magic of home-birth, and the holistic philosophy and writings of DEMs like Ina May Gaskin, Elizabeth Davis, Jan Tritten and many others have inspired countless students to enter midwifery, including many SNMs.

- MANA was created at an ACNM convention, and one-third of MANA's members are and have always been CNMs.

- Approximately one-fifteenth of ACNM's members belong to MANA, and a significant number of nurse-midwives were direct-entry midwives before they became CNMs.

- CNMs always attend MANA conferences for a "dip in the holistic spring," as several of them have expressed it, and MANA always has a presence at ACNM conventions, in the interests of exchanging information, working together and improving relationships between the two groups.

- The presidents of MANA and the ACNM make a point of attending each other's annual convention; indeed, for several years in the recent past the president of MANA was also a CNM.

- In part, CPM certification was created in response to criticism from ACNM regarding the lack of standards for direct-entry midwifery education. In part, CM certification was created in response to direct-entry midwives' criticism of the CNM educational nursing requirement (Scoggin 1996:41).

- Across the country, there are hundreds of occurrences of interdependence between CNMs and DEMs. For example, I have heard numerous stories of hospitals that suddenly become willing to hire CNMs after direct-entry midwives open a birthing center nearby. Sometimes, direct-entry midwives and nurse-midwives work together in private practices; often, they create informal collaborative arrangements that benefit them both.

My point about the intense interlinkages between MANA and the ACNM on the individual level is reinforced by the fact that the first person in the world to receive CM certification was already a CPM. Her name is Linda Schutt—she was trained in England and practiced midwifery both in Africa and in New York, illegally, as an independent homebirth midwife for years before she challenged the new CM process under the new New York law. Linda has been a member of MANA since 1983 and of ACNM since 1995. Julia Lange Kessler provides another example of these interlinkages: as a CPM in the second CM class at SUNY downstate, she sees herself not as exclusively aligned with one camp or the other, but as a bridge builder between them. So do many of the former direct-entry midwives who became CNMs, retaining their independent midwifery knowledge and spirit and their memberships in MANA. They include the 112 members of ACNM's new Bridge Club, which is urging the ACNM to rethink both its attitudes and its policies toward the CPM, and to find the path toward peaceful and mutually supportive co-existence—a petition I am happy to support.

I personally would like to see much more of this sort of bridge building. I would like some CPMs to go on for ACC certification when it can serve their needs, and I would like some CNMs and CMs to go on for NARM certification when it can serve them and their clients. It benefits both midwifery and women for midwives from both groups to expand their scopes of practice and knowledge bases. I want CM programs accredited by the ACNM to also seek MEAC accreditation, and look forward to the day when the ACNM will recognize the excellence of MEAC-accredited programs and offer them ways to obtain ACNM accreditation as

> I want CM programs accredited by the ACNM to also seek MEAC accreditation, and look forward to the day when the ACNM will recognize the excellence of MEAC-accredited programs and offer them ways to obtain ACNM accreditation as well.

CHOOSING YOUR PATH:
SOME ADVICE FROM AN ANTHROPOLOGICAL ACTIVIST
WHO SUPPORTS ALL SIDES OF THIS MIDWIFERY STORY

If you, my reader, would like to become a midwife and are confused, as you well may be, about what path to take, I advise you to research all available options and pick the one that will best set you up to be the kind of midwife you most want to be, serving the clientele that you most want to serve (see "Types of Midwifery Training," next article). I also advise you to remember that the choice does not have to be an exclusive one. Many students, as I noted above, are creatively combining didactic training with apprenticeship; a few are even enrolled in at-distance nurse-midwifery programs and are at the same time participating in apprenticeships with homebirth direct-entry midwives. Such enterprises are risky; not only can they result in expulsion from the nurse-midwifery program, but also, getting training simultaneously from opposite ends of the spectrum can be intellectually disjunctive and emotionally trying. Those who do attempt this mixture, like Charis Smith, are aware of the dangers but seem to find it a valuable combination that gives them the best of both worlds (see endnote 26).

> It is damaging to midwifery for some midwives to destructively criticize other midwives and their training.

Whichever path(s) you pick, I ask you most earnestly to honor all paths to midwifery education and practice. Don't pick one and then tout it as the best or the only acceptable route. I would be so happy never again to hear direct-entry midwives criticize nurse-midwives as "medwives" and "physician extenders," or listen to nurse-midwives level charges of incompetence or ignorance at direct-entry midwives who choose not to walk through ACNM's "open door." *It is damaging to midwifery for some midwives to destructively criticize other midwives and their training.*

Once in practice, if you find yourself interacting, perhaps working, with a midwife whose training and orientation are different from yours (e.g., you are a DEM and she is a CNM, or vice-versa) and seem to you to be problematic (I have heard that story from *both* sides), I ask you not to badmouth her but if at all possible to work with her and the other midwifery colleagues in your community through peer review to understand where she is coming from and to either expand her skills or your understanding, as appropriate. Sometimes (not always) what at first glance appears to be bad practice may, in fact, reflect a totally different way of doing things that you have not been exposed to before. It may only seem "wrong" because you are unfamiliar with it. Therefore, beware of rumor and gossip about how another midwife practices. If you have questions about a midwife's practice, try to address your questions directly to her and encourage others to do the same. Offer her your own expertise and be open to what she has to teach you. Help her or let her help you connect with others who may be able to act as teachers. Unless *the peer review consensus* is that she truly presents a danger to her clients, don't turn her in or lobby for legislation that works against her; you may find out one day that what she knows is lifesaving to one of your own clients (see endnote 13). In the words of a song I often hear midwives sing:

> *Humble yourself in the sight of your sister*
> *You need to bow down low and*
> *Humble yourself in the sight of your sister*
> *You need to know what she knows and*
> *We shall lift each other up, higher and higher*
> *We shall lift each other up!*

As we debate the relative merits of the various models of direct-entry education and practice, let us keep our eyes on the prize, which is not a better future for midwifery but rather better healthcare for mothers and babies. While I understand that many in ACNM believe that this better care can only be offered by midwives trained in DOA-accredited programs, I don't agree that this kind of limitation is best. Midwives are the only caregivers who can keep open the full spectrum of choice for birthing women in hospitals, in freestanding birth centers and at home. Midwives must go where the mothers are, and that includes the mothers who give birth in hospitals where most CPMs cannot go, as well as the mothers who choose homebirth whom most CNMs cannot serve. Let us honor all kinds of mothers, and create midwives who can offer them all kinds of choices.

ACKNOWLEDGMENTS

The research on which this article is based was funded by the Wenner-Gren Foundation for Anthropological Research, Grant # 6015, and I would like to extend my appreciation to Wenner-Gren for its support. The following midwives have offered me invaluable editorial assistance: Alice Bailes CNM, Mary Ann Baul CPM, Kate Bowland CNM, Pat Burkhardt CNM, Katherine Camacho Carr CNM, Elizabeth Davis CPM, Diane Holzer CPM, Anne Frye CPM, Ina May Gaskin CPM, Deborah Kaley CPM, Peter Johnson CNM, Lisa Kane Low CNM, Elaine Mielcarski CNM, Joyce Roberts CNM, Judith Rooks CNM, Linda Schutt CM, Holly Scholles CPM, Cecilia Wachdorf CNM, Fran Ventre CNM, Ruth Walsh CPM, Pam Weaver CPM and Sharon Wells CPM. I also extend my thanks to Susan Hodges, Pam Maurath and Jo Anne Myers-Ciecko for their helpful suggestions and to *Midwifery Today* editor Joel Southern for his patience, trust and heartwarming encouragement.

NOTES

1. As of this date of writing (June 1998), there are presently 7,717 members of the ACNM. MANA has 1,400 active members, so the total membership for both groups

is 9,117. But one-third of MANA members are CNMs, and most of them are also members of the ACNM. (About one-fifteenth of ACNM's members belong to MANA.) So it is very difficult to tell how many active members of each group there are without counting some of them twice. This figure of 8,700 is my best guess! Also, it is important to remember that there are many practicing homebirth midwives who are not members of MANA. We do not have exact figures on these midwives, many of whom are members of religious groups, but there are probably at least as many of them as there are members of MANA, and possibly as many as 4,000 or more.

2. Nurses usually classify nurse-midwifery as an advanced form of nursing, but many nurse-midwives do not consider it to be so. Rather they say that they are cross-trained in two professions, nursing and midwifery—a subtle but important difference (Judith Rooks, personal communication). Furthermore, the ACNM official definition of a nurse-midwife is someone who is "educated in the two disciplines of nursing and midwifery"—wording that provides firmer grounds for ACNM to distance itself from nursing than coding nurse-midwifery as advanced nursing (Lisa Kane Low, personal communication 1998).

3. A *technocracy* is a society organized around an ideology of technological progress. The general evolutionary thrust in a technocracy is upward, toward ever less dependence on nature and ever "higher" levels of educational and technological development.

4. This decision was controversial and was opposed by a number of prominent members of the ACNM (Lichtman 1996; Rooks and Carr 1995) who believed that requiring degrees would limit the accessibility of midwifery education. These researchers pointed out that there was no evidence that CNMs with degrees were safer or more effective midwives than those prepared through certificate programs. In fact, two studies showed that certificate graduates scored higher on the ACC exam than did CNMs who graduated with master's degrees (Fullerton and Severino 1995) and spent more time in clinical practicums and course work directly related to midwifery practice than did master's candidates (Sulz et al. 1983).

5. Requiring the baccalaureate could restrict the number of nurses eligible to become CNMs; 65 percent of nurses do not have a baccalaureate degree (Roberts 1995:152; Bureau of Health Professions, Division of Nursing, 1997). Thus it will be important for nurse-midwifery certificate programs, which lead only to associate degrees, to create viable ways for their students to obtain the bachelor's degree. (Currently a bachelor's in midwifery does not exist in the United States, but I believe that it should, as should the master's and the Ph.D.)

6. ACNM conducted a membership survey in 1994 which showed that 137 out of 2,789 respondents attended homebirth, or 4.9 percent. This is not a definitive figure, of course, but exact numbers are not available. According to Alice Bailes, Chair of the Home Birth Section of the ACNM, at present fewer than 200 CNMs attend home-births. Out of the current total membership of 7,717, that is less than three percent. Primary factors keeping nurse-midwives away from homebirth include the unavailability of both malpractice insurance and physician collaboration for homebirth.

7. State regulations defining the nature of this collaboration vary widely. In some

states, such as New York, CNMs must have written practice agreements signed by a specific physician; in other states, such as New Mexico, they are not tied to any individual MD. For more information, see Rooks 1997: 205-210.

8. In *From Doctor to Healer: The Transformative Journey* (1998), Robbie Davis-Floyd and Gloria St. John delineate the three major paradigms that define the contemporary medical spectrum in the United States: the technocratic, humanistic and holistic models of medicine. The technocratic model defines the body as a machine, stresses mind-body and patient-practitioner separation, and insists on a short-term aggressive, interventive approach. The humanistic model softens these hard edges, stressing the connection of mind and body, a mutually considerate and respectful partnership between patient and practitioner, the importance of individualized, compassionate care and prevention of illness instead of aggressive intervention for a short-term cure. The humanistic model can be applied in an intensely techno-medical context; care can be humanistic at the same time as it is technological. The more radical holistic paradigm defines the body as an energy field, stressing the oneness of the body, mind, and spirit and of client and practitioner, and suggesting an all-encompassing long-term approach to healing that involves self-responsibility and consideration of the emotional and spiritual aspects of illness as well as their physiological dimensions. (For more information, see Davis-Floyd and St. John 1998.)

9. MANA midwives believe that a "narrow domain" would be created should training options be limited to university-affiliated programs. Current MANA President Ina May Gaskin notes that

> university-affiliated programs are not considered essential in most European countries. To make them so ignores the possibility that if the ACNM stood in solidarity with MANA on this issue, we might really open a door wide enough to rapidly and significantly increase the number of working midwives in this country. The ACNM often points to how many new CNMs there are, but they often neglect to note how many CNMs are not actually practicing as midwives.

An ACNM membership survey in 1994 revealed that out of the 4,399 respondents, 71.3 percent were in active clinical practice.

10. Common usage in midwifery parlance has for some years now contrasted "nurse-midwives" with "direct-entry" midwives when the topic is the difference between ACC-certified midwives and others. I follow this usage here. But this distinction between nurse- and direct-entry midwives will not hold for long. Right now there are only seven ACC-certified direct-entry midwives (CMs). But as their numbers increase, the term "direct-entry" will come to apply to both ACNM-certified and non-ACNM-certified midwives, and will cease to be useful as a means of distinguishing between the two groups. At that point, will "direct-entry" come to include only non-nurse midwives with a professional credential (CM, CPM, LM)? Or will it also continue to apply to non-nurse, non-licensed, non-certified midwives?

11. Here is the complete breakdown, as of June 1998:

[Editor's note: See also the Direct-entry Program Chart in the Resource section.]

Regulated states: AK, AR, AZ, CA, CO, FL, LA, MT, NH, NM, OR, SC, TX,

WA. (Fourteen states)

Unregulated but practice legally (by judicial interpretation or statutory inference, or simply not prohibited): nineteen states: CT, ID, IL (though current legal cases may change IL to illegal), KS, MA, ME, MI, MS, NE, NV, ND, OK, SD, TN, UT, VT, WI, WV, WY. (PA used to be on this list but a recent legal opinion discovered a change in the medical law several years ago definitively makes DEMs illegal in PA.)

License required but unavailable: eight states: AL, *DE, GA, HI, MN, NJ, *NY, *RI.

> *Note: In DE and RI a single midwife in each state has been "grandmothered" in, but no new DEMs will be licensed according to the law. In New York, as in Washington state, licensure is available only to direct-entry midwives who can demonstrate that their education meets the education requirements of the law. But in New York, these requirements are too stringent for most practicing direct-entry midwives to meet. Ironically, in Washington state, requirements for direct-entry licensure would be too stringent for the New York CMs to meet—they include three years of midwifery education and attendance as primary midwife under supervision (see note 12) at fifty births. The SUNY downstate direct-entry program is only two years long, and requires attendance as primary at only twenty births. (Its students are expected to practice with supervision for a period of time after certification, whereas Seattle Midwifery School's students are expected to be fully qualified to practice on their own upon graduation.)

Prohibited by statute or judicial interpretation, ten states (including DC): DC, IN, IA, KY, MD, MO, NC, OH, PA, VA.

It is interesting to note the geographic distribution—ALL illegal states and states where a license is required but unavailable are in the eastern half of the country (except for HI). Also, DEMs practice legally in many more states than they are illegal—thirty-three legal states vs. eighteen "illegal" (fifty-one because Washington DC has been included as an "illegal" state").

(My thanks to Susan Hodges, President of Citizens for Midwifery (CfM), for most of the above information.)

12. According to the NARM publication *How To Become a CPM* (1998:4), "The primary midwife has full responsibility for provision of all aspects of midwifery care (prenatal, intrapartal and postpartal) without the need for supervisory personnel."

13. Most midwives I have interviewed, CNMs and DEMs alike, insist that unless a midwife has attended homebirths, she cannot understand the vast qualitative difference between births at home, where the woman's own rhythms hold sway, and birth in the hospital, where institutional rhythms are constantly superimposed. It is impossible to understand the ebbs and flows of normal birth in hospitals where labor is highly regimented and regulated. For example, in the hospital, "normal" labors are supposed to take less than twenty-four hours. If labor does not steadily progress within the allotted time period, Pitocin is administered and ultimately a cesarean may be performed. Homebirth experience expands a midwife's understanding of what "normal" means. At home, where personal, not institutional, rhythms prevail, "normal" labors may stop and start, and can take one hour or three days. Mothers will eat and drink as much as they like to keep up their strength; in the hospital, these options are usually denied.

14. In states where they have licensure, some DEMs do apply for hospital privileges, of which a very few have been granted. (I personally know of one in Louisiana, two in Florida and two in California.) Certainly most DEMs would like to be able to accompany their clients into the hospital should they require transport, and to continue to serve them there. Were hospital privileges more readily available to licensed midwives, as they are in Canada, no one really knows what percentage of DEMs would choose to practice in hospitals.

15. While this statement is true, any attention given to the mistakes made by some DEMs must be counterbalanced by the acknowledgment that hospital practitioners also often make mistakes, and "botched hospital births" are an all too common occurrence. It is also important to note that CNMs and even MDs who attend homebirths are often subjected to the same stereotyping process when they transport their clients to the hospital.

16. Midwifery works best when midwives act as team players. A few midwives who work outside the peer review consensus in their communities do sometimes present real problems for midwifery in that community and real dangers to parents. In such cases, when peer review is not effective, action is generally taken by the state. The dangers presented by such practitioners, who are sometimes referred to as "renegade midwives," constitute one of the major reasons why many MANA members have come to believe in the importance of some degree of standardization of education to meet established criteria for professional certification.

17. The ACC is relatively new; all CNMs certified before 1992 were certified by the ACNM. The ACC was created as a separate organization in order to comply with antitrust laws that require separation between a professional organization and its certification process (Lisa Kane Low, personal communication).

18. Technically speaking, you do not have to be a member of the ACNM to take the ACNM examination and be certified by the ACC as a CNM; but this is rare. Over 90 percent of CNMs belong to the ACNM.

19. Until recently, CNMs who wished to obtain NARM certification did not need to take the NARM written or skills exam, but, in addition to meeting other criteria, did have to document attendance as primary caregiver at ten out-of-hospital births, and three courses of continuity of care (which means they have to be the primary midwife for at least three women whom they follow throughout pregnancy, birth and the postpartum period). Continuity of care is sometimes difficult to achieve during nurse-midwifery training, and sometimes even during direct-entry training in high-volume clinics like the ones in El Paso, where women often appear in labor with no prior prenatal visits. Nevertheless, documenting continuity of care with at least three clients is a NARM requirement because members of MANA, NARM and MEAC consider it to be an essential ingredient of out-of-hospital midwifery practice. (There is a qualitative difference in the relationship a midwife has with a client whom she sees all the way through the childbearing experience.)

DOA-accredited programs must demonstrate that they encompass the ACNM Core Competencies (see the Resource Section), which require that CNMs and CMs provide care "on a continuous and comprehensive basis"; no specific numbers are required.

The CPM credential, which qualifies midwives to attend out-of-hospital birth, reflects a different body of knowledge than the knowledge CNMs and CMs attain. Recently, the NARM board decided to add the CM to their application form as a route of entry, but to require from this point on that all CMs and CNMs applying for NARM certification take the NARM written exam, in addition to attending 10 out-of-hospital births and documenting the care of three women throughout their pregnancies (continuity of care), to ensure that all CPMs will share a common body of knowledge and expertise in the MANA Midwifery Model of Care (see box 4).

20. A major issue that accompanied the acceptance of the CM as a voting member of the college was the issue of a possible name change, from the American College of Nurse-Midwives to (1) the American College of Nurse-Midwives and Midwives (ACNM) or (2) the American College of Midwives (ACM). Very few people liked option 1, as it is so unwieldy; a majority of the membership voted in a survey that they prefer option 2. The motion for a name change was defeated by a narrow margin at the 1997 Boston convention, and subsequent motions asked for alternative name options and for the implications of a name change to be considered and explained at the 1998 convention in San Francisco. During the San Francisco convention, yet another option was added: the American College of Midwifery. This is the preferred option of the ACNM board, because it would name the profession, not the practitioner, and thus would easily encompass both nurse- and direct-entry midwives without invalidating or giving primacy to either one. (Additionally, it has a historical precedent: in 1968, the American Association of Nurse-Midwives (formed in Kentucky in 1929) merged with the American College of Nurse-Midwifery (which had been formed in 1955) to become the American College of Nurse-Midwives (Roberts 1995:145).) A motion to put the name-change issue to a mail vote by the fall of 1998 passed by a large majority.

21. The ACC exam is based on Task Analyses, the latest two of which were carried out in 1985 and 1993–1994. This latest Task Analysis is based on multiple sources, examples of which include "state statutes and regulations which define the practice of nurse-midwifery and midwifery in those jurisdictions, the ACNM Core Competencies, the MANA Task List, and relevant contemporary literature describing nurse-midwifery and midwifery practice" (Judith Fullerton, personal communication, 1998). These task analyses are revised every five to seven years; a new Task Analysis Research Project is currently underway.

22. In New York, ACNM members have worked to make the baccalaureate requirement as easy as possible to meet: Empire State College will give a great deal of credit to individual students for life experience, which helps to minimize the number of courses that need to be taken for the baccalaureate degree. Twenty-two hours of credit are currently available at Empire State College for having a CPM (Julia Lange Kessler, personal communication).

23. Some professions, including medicine, have two national accrediting bodies. The following examples are taken from *Nationally Recognized Accrediting Agencies and Associations*, published by the U.S. Department of Education, 1996. Two agencies accredit Allied Health Programs: the Accrediting Bureau of Health Education

Schools and the Commission on Accreditation of Allied Health Education Programs. Emergency Medical Services are accredited by the Joint Review Committee on Education Programs for the EMT-Paramedic, and the Commission on Accreditation of Allied Health Education Programs. Occupational education has the Accrediting Commission of Career Schools and Colleges of Technology and the Council on Occupational Education, as well as the American Occupational Therapy Association. Christian colleges are accredited by the Accrediting Association of Bible Colleges, the Transnational Association of Christian Colleges and Schools, the Association for Clinical Pastoral Education, Inc. and the Association of Theological Schools in the United States and Canada. Medical Laboratory Technician Education is accredited by the Accrediting Bureau of Health Education Schools and the National Accrediting Agency for Clinical Laboratory Sciences. Programs leading to the M.D. degree are accredited by the Liaison Committee on Medical Education of the Council on Medical Education of the (1) American Medical Association and (2) Association of American Medical Colleges. (Mary Ann Baul, personal communication, 1998)

24. This generalization has important exceptions. Some nurse-midwives have long been involved in direct-entry education. For example, Katherine Camacho Carr, CNM, taught the first class at Seattle Midwifery School and has kept on teaching there for years. She says, "We are all midwives and must teach each other!" (Personal communication 1998)

25. The length of the passage through nursing varies considerably, depending on the kind of nursing training undertaken and the requirements of the program. Students I have interviewed who entered nursing training specifically to become midwives usually spend about a year and a half learning to be nurses. Those who enter master's level nursing programs can take much longer. Many pre-midwifery nursing students are repeatedly told by nurses that one should not become a midwife without several years of practice as a labor and delivery nurse. (A strong characteristic of the culture of nursing is to regard those who have practiced for less than two years as not having really practiced at all.) Those who take this advice seriously can find themselves "stuck" in a nursing job for years before they can get back on the midwifery track. The fastest passage through nursing is found in three-year post-baccalaureate nurse-midwifery programs such as the one directed by Helen Varney Burst at Yale: only one year is spent in nursing training.

26. I do not mean to denigrate nurses here. Many nurses show great independence of thought, develop innovative programs and styles of care and treat patients holistically. But all the midwifery students I have interviewed noted a strong difference between their socialization as nurses and their socialization as midwives. They report that as nurses they were expected to defer to doctors, to mute their opinions or express them subtly, and to know and keep to their place in the medical hierarchy. As nurse-midwives they find themselves above nurses in the hospital hierarchy and are encouraged by their educators to develop more autonomous, collaborative, nonsubordinate relationships with physicians. (Nursing students are often taught the same thing, but physicians are not—they continue to be taught to treat nurses as

subordinate, which makes it difficult for nurses to establish themselves as collaborative equals.)

27. ACNM/DOA standards for the accreditation of direct-entry midwifery education programs say that the program must have "a patient population large and diverse enough in both in-hospital and out-of-hospital settings that students can acquire the elements contained within the 'Skills, Knowledge, Competencies and Health Sciences Prerequisite to Midwifery Practice' document." "Out-of-hospital" could be technically interpreted to mean, for example, Planned Parenthood clinics where prenatal and well-woman care is provided, but the intent of most of my CNM interviewees is that the CM will have the skills and experience to attend out-of-hospital birth. Apparently, the intent of the DOA requirements is somewhat different. DOA head Helen Varney Burst (1995:291-292) stressed that ACNM was not creating certification for MANA-style direct-entry midwives, but rather for "healthcare professionals," and that hospital experience would be a requirement for ACNM's new CMs. According to Laura Slattery at ACNM headquarters (personal communication), DOA-accredited direct-entry programs do not have to require out-of-hospital experience. The issue as Slattery explained it was that because nurse-midwifery programs require a credential, the RN, it was assumed that applicants already had experience in hospital birth because of their familiarity with the hospital. But it could not be assumed that CM applicants had ever worked in a hospital, so the exposure to hospital birth during their training, which they must have, may be the only exposure they get. (The criteria for nurse- and direct-entry programs are presently under evaluation and are being merged, so that as of July 1998 there will be only one set of criteria for both.)

28. Most nurse-midwives are regulated by state boards of nursing, yet surveys conducted in 1991 and 1995 showed that in only eight states did CNMs have designated places on those boards (DeClerq et al. 1998). New York and Utah were the only states in which CNMs constituted a majority of the board members; in most states there was not even a formal route for them to provide input. Interviews in both surveys suggested conflicts between the content of CNM education and certification and the nursing boards' definitions of CNM scope of practice. "This lack of control of their own regulatory boards is in sharp contrast to the traditional physician dominance on the boards that regulate medical practice" (Declerq et al. 1998:193).

29. The law states that to be eligible for licensure, direct-entry midwives must have an education "equivalent to that of nursing" and must pass through a state-accredited midwifery program or demonstrate an equivalent education, and must pass the state licensing exam (which through special contractual agreement with the ACC is essentially the same exam as that given to CNMs; those who pass the exam are awarded the CM along with their New York midwifery license). Many of the practicing DEMs in New York were eager to take the exam, but were not eligible do so because they could not meet the education requirements.

30. New York CNMs insist that the Professional Midwifery Practice Act would never have passed had the DEMs been included. But the DEMs vehemently disagree, insisting that they had legislative backing for a version of the bill in the New York

Senate that did everything both the DEMs and the CNMs wanted. When it was about to be brought before the House, under circumstances too complex to go into here, the bill was suddenly and drastically changed. The direct-entry midwives who had invested five years lobbying for the Professional Midwifery Practice Act felt betrayed by the CNMs. The CNMs in turn insist that the changes were necessary compromises to get the bill past the opposition posed by the nursing and medical associations. More detailed discussion of this difficult and painful chapter in midwifery history is beyond the scope of this chapter. I will soon begin work on a lengthy article on this subject, entitled "Birth of a Dream, Death of a Dream: The Development of Direct-Entry Midwifery in New York."

31. Pat Burkhart, CNM, a member of the New York Midwifery Board, notes that:

We nurse-midwives in New York state who were working desperately to obtain passage of the bill were focused on fighting off the state medical and nursing societies and did not stop to consider the ultimate consequences of legalizing ACNM-certified direct-entry midwives. Once the law passed and was being implemented, most of us were shocked to realize that the practice of unlicensed midwifery had been transformed into a felony. When the members of the new Board of Midwifery became aware that the state attorney's office had begun prosecuting unlicensed midwives, we were appalled and we did not understand why they were doing so. We were told that complaints from consumers were what led to the prosecutions, but our further investigations did not completely verify that statement. We talked with the state attorney's office, asking them to back off and insisting that unless there was clear indication of a need to investigate a particular midwife, there was no reason to enforce a law just to enforce a law. The situation has calmed down considerably since then, but those were very trying times. (Personal communication, 1998)

32. It is important to note that homebirth experience *is* available to nurse-midwifery students, albeit on a very limited basis. Alice Bailes, Chair of the ACNM Home Birth Section, notes that the ten students in Georgetown University's midwifery program have the opportunity to experience out-of-hospital birth at four birthing centers and in one CNM-run homebirth practice in the Washington metropolitan area. Students in the University of Pennsylvania's midwifery program have an opportunity to do their integration in CNM Rondi Anderson's homebirth practice among the Amish. Most of the 180 or so CNMs who attend homebirth try to offer clinical opportunities for students whenever possible. Students who want homebirth experience would do well to explore these options before picking their training program. Bailes is presently engaged in compiling a database of available opportunities for SNMs and SMs to gain clinical experience in homebirth, which she plans to make available by spring 1999. For more information, contact Alice Bailes at Birth Care and Women's Health (703-549-5070) or at home (703-243-0189). (Alice Bailes, personal communication, 1998)

33. Earlier meetings of the Bridge Club had taken place, but had not led to any type of ongoing organization or plan of action.

34. In Chapter 7 of *Birth in Four Cultures* (1993), Brigitte Jordan provides an outstanding and useful discussion of the differences between experiential and didactic learning.

35. To date, MEAC has given full accreditation to Seattle Midwifery School, the Utah School of Midwifery and Maternidad La Luz in El Paso, Texas, and pre-accreditation to the Midwifery Institute of California, the Oregon School of Midwifery, Birthingway Midwifery School in Oregon and the Sage Femme Midwifery School in Oregon and California. Pre-accredited programs have met all standards and requirements for full accreditation but have not yet graduated enough students to demonstrate success consistent with their missions.

The members of MEAC, all of whom are deeply involved in direct-entry midwifery education, have designed their evaluation process in full accordance with the specifications of the U.S. Department of Education (US DOE) (which recognizes both categories of accreditation and pre-accreditation), and they plan to apply for DOE recognition for MEAC in the latter part of 1998. (The ACNM's DOA, which has had DOE recognition for nurse-midwifery programs since 1982 (Roberts 1991), has already applied once for US DOE recognition to accredit direct-entry programs; their application was refused on the basis that they have no experience with direct-entry programs. After they graduate the necessary number of students, they will apply again, and are on track for receiving DOE recognition.) Much is riding on the success of MEAC's application: if they succeed, all MEAC-accredited programs will be qualified to apply for approval to give out government-funded grants and loans to students. This will help increase accessibility to midwifery education and further MEAC's goal, which is to improve the quality of that education while preserving its diversity. US DOE recognition will also put MEAC on the same level as the DOA in the eyes of federal state agencies. The US DOE officially welcomes the existence of dual routes to accreditation within a given profession as long as all criteria and standards are met. (Mary Ann Baul, personal communication 1998)

An additional benefit of MEAC's gaining US DOE recognition may be that all graduates of MEAC-accredited programs, including apprenticeship programs, will meet the international definition of a midwife (see above), whether or not they are recognized in the states in which they are located. At present, all direct-entry midwives currently licensed by their jurisdictions who graduated from educational programs recognized by that jurisdiction are understood to meet the international definition and are thereby qualified to hold membership in the International Confederation of Midwives, which many of them do. The narrow interpretation of the international definition published by the WHO in *Care in Normal Birth* reads as follows: ". . . the international definition of a midwife, according to WHO, ICM and FIGO (the International Federation of Obstetricians and Gynaecologists), is quite simple: if the education programme is recognized by the government that licenses the midwife to practice, that person is a midwife." But the exact wording of the definition is less specific: "A midwife is a person who, having been regularly admitted to a midwifery educational program duly recognized in the country in which it is located, has successfully completed the prescribed course of studies in midwifery and has acquired the requisite qualifications to be registered and/or legally licensed to practice midwifery." This definition does not specify that the midwife is licensed, only that she has graduated from a program "duly recognized in the country where it is located." Thus, a case could clearly be made that if MEAC gains US DOE recognition (which would mean that MEAC-accredited programs will be "duly recognized in the country in which [they] are located"), graduates of MEAC-accredited programs will conform to the international definition, even if they practice in states in which they are illegal. This would add additional strength to the refutation of the claim that only ACNM-certified midwives meet that definition, and would work to legitimize the apprenticeship route to midwifery (for those apprenticeship programs that achieve MEAC accreditation) and to preserve the diversity of private midwifery education programs.

36. Most direct-entry midwives I have interviewed seem to understand the fine line between confidence and over-confidence, between self-reliance and knowing your limitations, between trusting birth while remaining aware of its risks. Most complications occur to low risk women, because most women are low risk. Good training and a good balance between trust in women and birth, and level-headed, informed awareness are essential components of any brand of midwifery. (In addition, it is important to note that CNMs trained to work in homes, birth centers, Level I community hospitals, or high-risk tertiary care hospitals where they practice with a great deal of autonomy tend to develop the same skills and sense of self-reliance as independent homebirth midwives.)

37. Everything, that is, except their own data. In *Midwifery and Childbirth in America*, Judith Rooks also points out that:

> there is no evidence that nurse-midwives with masters' degrees provide safer, more effective or more satisfying care to women. Nor are CNMs with master's degrees more likely than certificate program graduates to pass the national nurse-midwifery certification examination. A 1995 study of factors associated with higher scores on the national certification examination found that graduates of certificate nurse-midwifery education programs had a higher average score on the test than graduates of master's degree programs (Fullerton and Severino). In addition, a 1985 study of factors affecting the level of success experienced by individual CNMs found no association between type of nurse-midwifery education and the level of professional success. (Haas and Rooks 1997:172)

38. Their fight will be an inclusive one—plans are underway for including the CM as yet another route to NARM certification (see note 13). In other words, in states where the CM has no legality but the CPM does, a CM could become a CPM and be licensed as such.

39. It is important to remember that most of the 200 or so CNMs who attend homebirth are MANA members. These homebirth CNMs, who constitute less than three percent of their national organization, draw inspiration, support, courage, and companionship from MANA; they find that their independent and holistic model of birth is given louder voice and more definitive shape in MANA than in ACNM.

40. The MANA database being compiled by a Canadian epidemiologist already

has data on 10,000 births turned in by MANA midwives on the extremely detailed MANA data form. These data, which are as yet unpublished, show excellent outcomes, but because they are voluntary, they are not as statistically valid as would be a prospective study of every outcome of every birth attended by a CPM in a given year. Plans are underway to carry out such a study in the year 2000.

41. Late-breaking news: The common cause I envision may come soon. At work on the final draft of this chapter, I have just received word that during the Board meeting held in May 1998, the ACNM Board of Directors, following a convention vote by ACNM members, voted to establish another joint ACNM-MANA work group, to be composed of four representatives from each organization. The purpose of this group as the ACNM BOD conceives it will be three-fold: (1) to create appropriate language for a model state practice act that would encompass both new direct-entry certifications; (2) to explore the possible mutual articulation of ACNM and MANA-style models of education (in other words, how could the gaps between these models be bridged without a student having to repeat large portions of her education? That is, if you are a CPM, what might be a streamlined way to become a CNM or a CM, and vice-versa. If you are a graduate of a MEAC-accredited program, how might a DOA-accredited program give you credit for that, and vice-versa?; and (3) to develop new and better ways for ACNM and MANA to communicate and continue to work together. This ACNM initiative is the result of a motion put on the convention floor by the members of the new Bridge Club, which passed by a large majority. It reflects the good will many ACNM members feel toward MANA, and now awaits MANA's response.

REFERENCES

Arms, Suzanne. 1996. *Immaculate Deception: Myth, Magic, and Birth*. Berkeley, CA: Celestial Arts.

Bailes, Alice. 1998. Personal communication. Alice Bailes CNM is cofounder, co-owner, and co-director of Birth Care and Women's Health, a practice that specializes in home and birth center births in the DC metropolitan area. She has been attending homebirths for over 25 years, and currently serves as the Chair of the ACNM Home Birth Section.

Baul, Mary Ann. 1998. Personal communication. Mary Ann Baul CPM is a direct-entry midwife and educator in Flagstaff, Arizona who currently serves as the Executive Secretary of MEAC.

Bauer, J.C. 1998. *Not What the Doctor Ordered*. 2nd edition. New York: McGraw Hill.

Bruner, Joseph P., Susan B. Drummond, Anna L. Meenan, and Ina May Gaskin. 1998. "All-Fours Maneuver for Reducing Shoulder Dystocia During Labor," *Journal of Reproductive Medicine* 43:439-443.

Burkhart, Patricia. 1998. Personal communication. Patricia Burkhart is Director of the Nurse-Midwifery Education Program at New York University and currently serves as Vice-Chair of the New York State Midwifery Board.

Burst, Helen Varney. 1995. "An Update on the Credentialing of Midwives by the ACNM." *Journal of Nurse-Midwifery* 40(3):290-296.

Carr, Katherine Camacho. 1998. Personal communication. Katherine Camacho Carr CNM is a nurse-midwifery educator living in Seattle, Washington who currently serves as vice-president of the ACNM. She has joined the faculty of the SUNY downstate program to work on developing a direct-entry distance curriculum.

Chester, Penfield. 1997. *Sisters on a Journey: Portraits of American Midwives.* New Brunswick NJ: Rutgers University Press.

Coy, Michael W., ed. 1989. *Apprenticeship: From Theory to Method and Back Again.* New York: SUNY Series in the Anthropology of Work.

Davis, Elizabeth. 1997. *Heart and Hands: A Midwife's Guide to Pregnancy and Birth,* 3rd edition. Berkeley, Calif: Celestial Arts.

—Personal communication 1998. Elizabeth Davis CPM, a direct-entry midwife in Windsor, California, is a renowned midwifery educator, international lecturer and author of numerous articles and books.

Davis-Floyd, Robbie E. 1992. *Birth as an American Rite of Passage.* Berkeley: University of California Press.

Davis-Floyd, Robbie E., and Gloria St. John. 1998. *From Doctor to Healer: The Transformative Journey.* New Brunswick, NJ: Rutgers University Press.

Donegan, Jane B. 1978. *Women and Men Midwives: Medicine, Morality and Misogyny in Early America.* Westport, Conn: Greenwood Press.

Donnison, Jean. 1977. *Midwives and Medical Men: A History of Inter-Professional Rivalries and Women's Rights.* New York: Schocken Books.

Frye, Anne. 1995. *Holistic Midwifery: A Comprehensive Textbook for Midwives in Home Birth Practice.* Volume I, *Care During Pregnancy,* by Anne Frye. Portland, OR: Labyrs Press.

—1998. Personal communication. Anne Frye, CPM, a direct-entry midwife in Portland, Oregon, is author of several midwifery texts and currently serves as vice-president of MANA.

Fullerton, Judith T, and R. Severino. 1995. "Factors That Predict Performance on the National Certification Examination." *Journal of Nurse-Midwifery* 40:19-25.

Fullerton, Judith. 1998. Personal communication. Judith Fullerton, CNM, is professor of nursing in the Department of Family Health Care, School of Nursing, University of Texas Health Sciences Center in San Antonio. A former test consultant to the ACNM Division of Competency Assessment and the ACNM Certification Council (ACC), she is the immediate past chair of the ACC Research Committee. She currently serves as a member of that committee.

Gaskin, Ina May. 1990. *Spiritual Midwifery.* 3rd edition. Summertown TN: The Book Publishing Company.

—1998. Personal communication. Ina May Gaskin, CPM, is a direct-entry midwife on the Farm in Summertown, Tennessee, editor and publisher of the *Birth Gazette,* and author of two books and numerous articles. She is often referred to as "the most famous midwife in North America."

Goer, Henci. 1995. *Obstetric Myths versus Research Realities.* Westport CT: Bergin and Garvey.

Haas, J. E., and Judith P. Rooks. 1986. "National Survey of Factors Contributing to and Hindering the Successful Practice of Nurse-Midwifery: Summary of the American College of Nurse-Midwives Foundation Study. *Journal of Nurse-Midwifery* 32(5):212-215.

Hodges, Susan. 1998. Personal communication. Susan Hodges is president of Citizens for Midwifery, a consumer organization.

Houghton, Pansy, and Kate Windom. 1996a. *1995 Job Analysis of the Role of Direct-Entry Midwives.* North American Registry of Midwives.

—1996b. *Executive Summary of the 1995 Job Analysis of the Role of Direct-Entry Midwives.* Copies can be obtained from the NARM Education and Advocacy Department (1-888-842-4784).

Jackson, Marcia E., and Alice Bailes. 1997. ACNM *Handbook on Home Birth Practice.* Washington, DC: ACNM.

Jordan, Brigitte. 1993. *Birth in Four Cultures.* 4th edition, revised and expanded by Robbie Davis-Floyd. Prospect Heights, Ohio: Waveland Press.

Leavitt, Judith. 1986. *Brought to Bed: Childbearing in America 1750-1950.* New York: Oxford University Press.

Lichtman, Ronnie. 1996. "Entry-Level Degrees for Midwifery Practice." *Journal of Nurse-Midwifery* 21(1):47-49.

Litoff, Judy Barrett. 1978. *American Midwives: 1860 to the Present.* Westport, Conn.: Greenwood Press.

—1986. *The American Midwife Debate: A Sourcebook on Its Modern Origins.* New York: Greenwood Press.

Lisa Kane Low, CNM, is on faculty in the Nurse-Midwifery Program of the University of Michigan and is a Ph.D. candidate in Women's Health and Women's Studies. She is also currently in clinical practice at the University of Michigan Hospital.

MacDorman, M. and G. Singh. 1998. "Midwifery Care, Social and Medical Risk Factors, and Birth Outcomes in the U.S.A." *Journal of Epidemiology and Community Health* 52:310-317.

Roberts, Joyce E. 1991. "An Overview of Nurse-Midwifery Education and Accreditation." *Journal of Nurse-Midwifery* 36(6): 373-376.

—1995. "The Role of Graduate Education in Midwifery in the USA." In *Issues in Midwifery,* ed. Tricia Murphy Black. Edinburgh: Churchill Livingstone.

Rooks, Judith P. 1997. *Midwifery and Childbirth in America.* Philadelphia: Temple University Press.

1998. "Unity in Midwifery? Realities and Alternatives. *Journal of Nurse-Midwifery*, in press.

—1998. Personal communication. Judith Pence Rooks CNM is an epidemiologist and public health expert living in Portland, Oregon. She has authored more than fifty scientific and professional papers, and is past-president of the ACNM.

Rooks, Judith P. and Katherine Camacho Carr. 1995. "Criteria for Accreditation of Direct-Entry Midwifery Education." *Journal of Nurse-Midwifery* 40(3):297-303.

Rooks, Judith P., Katherine Camacho Carr, and Irene Sandvold. 1991. "The Importance of Non-Master's Degree Options in Nurse-Midwifery Education." *Journal of Nurse Midwifery* 36:124-130.

Rothman, Barbara Katz. 1982. *In Labor: Women and Power in the Birthplace*. New York: W.W. Norton.

Scoggin, Janet. 1996. "How Nurse-Midwives Define Themselves in Relation to Nursing, Medicine, and Midwifery." *Journal of Nurse-Midwifery* 41(1):36-42.

Singleton, John. 1989. "Deconstructing Apprenticeship Models in Folkcraft Pottery: Traditional Arts and Alternative Careers in Mashiko Workshops." In *Redefining the Artisan: Traditional Technicians in Changing Societies*, Paul H. Greenough, ed. Papers from the First Conference on Artists, Artisans, and Traditional Technologists in Development, April 14-16, 1989. Center for International and Comparative Studies, University of Iowa.

Slattery, Laura. 1998. Personal communication. Laura Slattery CNM is education manager for the ACNM.

Sulz, H.A., O. M. Henry, L. J. Kinyon, G.M. Buck, B. Bullough. 1983. "Nurse-Practitioners: A Decade of Change, Part II." *Nursing Outlook* 31:216-9.

U.S. Department of Education. 1996. *Nationally Recognized Accrediting Agencies and Associations*. Washington D.C.: US DOE.

Varney, Helen. 1997. *Varney's Midwifery*. 3rd ed., Sudbury, Mass. : Jones and Bartlett Publishers.

Ventre, Fran. 1998. Personal communication. Fran Ventre CNM was a licensed lay midwife in Maryland and is one of the founding mothers of both MANA and the ACNM Bridge Club. She has worked in the full range of birth settings, and is presently planning a birth center in Brooklyn, New York.

Ventre, Fran, Peggy Garland Spindel, and Kate Bowland. 1995. "The Transition from Lay Midwife to Certified Nurse-Midwife in the United States." *Journal of Nurse-Midwifery* 40:428-438.

Wachdorf, Cecilia M. 1998. Personal communication. Cecilia Wachdorf CNM is engaged in clinical practice in the Tampa Bay area of Florida while working on her PhD in Public Health–Maternal-Child Health at the University of South Florida.

Weaver, Pam. 1998. Personal communication. Pam Weaver CPM is a practicing direct-entry midwife in Alaska. She is co-author of the *Practical Skills Guide for*

Midwifery, and currently serves as the NARM Board liaison to state legislatures and agencies.

Wells, Sharon. 1992. "The New York Legislative Sellout." *Birth Gazette* 8(4):32-33.

Wells, Sharon. 1998. Personal communication. Sharon Wells CPM has been a practicing midwife for seventeen years. She served as founder and administrator of The North Florida School of Midwifery, was a founding mother and the first president of the Midwives Alliance of New York (MANY), and currently serves as certification coordinator for the North American Registry of Midwives.

Wertz, Richard W., and Dorothy C. Wertz. 1989 (orig. pub. 1977). *Lying-In: A History of Childbirth in America*, 2nd edition. New Haven: Yale University Press.

World Health Organization. 1996. *Care in Normal Birth*, Report of the Technical Working Group of the Maternal and Newborn Health/Safe Motherhood Unit, Family and Reproductive Health. WHO, Geneva.

Robbie Davis-Floyd, PhD, is a research fellow in the Department of Anthropology at the University of Texas, Austin. She is author of Birth as an American Rite of Passage *(1992), co-author of* From Doctor to Healer: The Transformative Journey *(1998), and coeditor of* Childbirth and Authoritative Knowledge: Cross-Cultural Perspectives *(1997),* Intuition: The Inside Story *(1997) and* Cyborg Babies: From Techno-Sex to Techno-Tots *(1998). She lectures nationally and internationally on these and related topics. Her current research investigates contemporary transformations in midwifery in the United States and Mexico. Books in progress include* Midwives in the Mainstream: The Politics of Change; *a coedited collection on* Midwives in Mexico: Continuity, Controversy, and Change; *and* The Power of Ritual.

TYPES OF MIDWIFERY TRAINING:
AN ANTHROPOLOGICAL OVERVIEW

by Robbie Davis-Floyd, PhD

Potential midwives reading this book will want help in picking their educational path. Hoping to be of assistance, I offer the following brief overview. (More thorough and detailed overviews can be found in Frye 1995: 22-26 and Rooks 1997:164-178, 258-268.) As I worked on this overview, I found it extremely difficult to make any kind of generalization that I could be sure was true. The differences between types of midwifery training are no longer easy to define: what I witnessed as I talked to midwives about this article was what anthropologists might call an elision between models of midwifery training (to elide in linguistics means "to slur over in pronunciation"). As you will see below, these models are increasingly blurring into each other.

The only hard and fast distinction I can make is the one between programs accredited by the ACNM's Division of Accreditation (DOA) and programs accredited by MANA's affiliate, the Midwifery Education and Accreditation Council (MEAC). In terms of experience and longevity, these two are not appropriately comparable: the DOA (under various names) has been in operation since 1957. During that time, it has accredited well over fifty nurse-midwifery programs and has pre-accredited two direct-entry programs.[1] MEAC has been in existence only since the early 1990s; it has accredited or pre-accredited seven programs. If comparisons are to be made, it would be fairer to compare MEAC to the DOA as it was during its first decade. But this overview is not intended as an evaluation of either the DOA or MEAC, and I need a way of organizing the programs I will compare. Accordingly, I have organized this overview into two sections based on the distinction between DOA- and MEAC-accredited programs. Where I have enough information, I present the upside and the downside of each educational route.

Some of the information I present comes from the sixty interviews I have conducted over the past four years with both direct-entry and nurse-midwifery students or recent graduates. I make an effort to talk with them wherever I find them—I do not pretend that my sample here is representative. I include this kind of anecdotal information to help prospective students know in advance what to watch out for, so they can work to obtain the best education possible through their chosen route.

The background knowledge necessary for a full understanding of this overview can be found in the preceding article on "The Ups and Downs of Nurse- and Direct-Entry Midwifery: An Anthropological Perspective." In what follows, the reader's familiarity with the information presented in that article is assumed. It is important to remember that first and foremost, the aspiring midwife should look clearly at her personal and career goals, her family and financial situation and her learning style. Having taken stock, she should then explore all the options that offer what she needs.

ACNM DOA–ACCREDITED PROGRAMS

Fifty programs accredited by the ACNM's Division of Accreditation were in operation at the end of 1997. All of them are university-affiliated or university-based, and all qualify their students to practice at a safe, beginning level, caring for women during pregnancy, birth, and the postpartum period (and now across the life cycle), and equipping them to participate in healthcare institutions (hospitals, birth centers and managed care organizations) and sometimes to manage private practices. The majority of faculty in these programs must be CNMs; faculty positions can also be held by experts in a given area, including MDs, PhDs, nurse-practitioners, etc. Clinical supervision is always the responsibility of CNMs or CMs. In-hospital training is the norm. The availability and depth of both didactic teaching about and clinical experience in out-of-hospital birth can vary considerably from program to program. Out-of-hospital clinical experience is not required for certification or for program accreditation.

Every program includes specific criteria for entrance, structured learning objectives that work to ensure that every student masters the required body of knowledge, formalized didactic instruction, clinical experience with more than one clinical instructor, and involvement of several faculty members in judgment about the student's ability to provide safe, effective beginning level midwifery care. (An update on the status and number of DOA-accredited programs is published every year in the *Journal of Nurse-Midwifery*, and is available on the Internet at <www.acnm.org>. For up-to-the-minute information, contact the ACNM national office at (202) 728-9860 and ask to speak to staff members from the DOA.) Nurse-midwifery educators have long been leaders in educational innovation, and they continue to develop and refine creative and interactive learning and teaching methodologies. [2]

While most DOA-accredited programs are well-established and solidly funded, like all academic programs some are subject to sudden budget cuts, departmental reorganizations and streamlining procedures. It is important to research the refund policies, educational and disciplinary policies, reputation, and success rate of a school thoroughly before enrolling. Talk to enrolled students and graduates. Are they receiving or did they get what they expected? Are they happy with their education? Were all policies, fees and expectations disclosed to them?

UNIVERSITY-BASED PROGRAMS

Upside: This kind of training is in alignment with the values, beliefs and status consciousness of mainstream society; it is culturally thought of as the bottom line for white-collar professions. As a socially valued educational pathway, it carries concomitant benefits, including social recognition and prestige, easy access to government loans, and straightforward routes to advanced degrees, which bring prestige and salary raises and empower their recipients to teach, to start new programs, to effect changes in legislation and to carry out research on client needs and various aspects of midwifery care. (In general, the higher the level of university training of a group of professionals, the higher the social prestige of the entire profession.) Being present on a university campus enables students to learn about and participate in a wide variety of learning experiences and gives them access to excellent libraries and other resources. University students have the opportunity to gain a liberal arts base in disciplines designed to expose the student to different points of view and ways of understanding the world, including the humanities, psychology, sociology and the basic sciences, with the ultimate goal of making the student a "well-rounded" person.

While didactic learning is usually primary in universities, midwifery training, like training in other healthcare professions, always includes some form of preceptorship, in which students are exposed to one-on-one experiential learning with more than one preceptor. Because the clinical parts of university-based midwifery training are mostly carried out in hospitals (some university programs make an effort to provide their students with some—albeit limited—out-of-hospital experience), students also are exposed to and develop expertise in dealing with individuals of diverse socio-cultural and economic backgrounds, a wide range of birth complications and unusual health conditions, and the latest and newest in medical technologies. Educators generally work with students to help them develop a critical sense of which technologies have efficacy, under which circumstances, and which ones do not. (The only currently operating DOA-accredited direct-entry program is university-based, at the SUNY-Brooklyn Health Science Center in New York City, aka SUNY downstate.)

I have interviewed students from university-based programs across the country, including New York University and Columbia University in New York, the University of Pennsylvania in Philadephia, Case Western University in Ohio and the University of California in San Francisco; for the most part, they rate their programs very highly, usually giving them an 8 on a 10-point scale.

Downside: The vast majority of university-based programs require that the student leave home for an extended period to attend, and almost all still require nursing training, including the fast-track programs at Yale, Columbia and UCSF. The thirty students I have interviewed about their nurse-midwifery educational experiences were unanimous in agreeing about the downside of nursing training: it socializes them into an attitude of subordination in the medical hierarchy that they must work to overcome once they begin clinical study as midwives. It can also derail their lives and career goals: there is a strong ethic in nursing that (1) you are not really a nurse unless you have practiced for at least three or four years, so students are expected by their nursing instructors to "put in their time"; and that (2) you shouldn't become a nurse-midwife without practicing as a labor and delivery nurse for several years first. The required nursing education can be completed in most programs within a year and a half, but some of the students I interviewed reported being heavily pressured to practice as nurses for an extended period before entering midwifery training. Some succumbed, some resisted, but all resented the pressure and the nursing belief that you are not well-qualified to be a midwife if you haven't practiced as a nurse. Much less of this sort of pressure is experienced by students who enter the fast-track programs mentioned above, which are designed to make their students nurses solely so that they can become midwives; in such programs a briefer (one year) passage through nursing is the norm.

Tuitions in university-based programs range widely. Some university programs have tuitions of under $20,000. Three students I interviewed graduated with debts in student loans of over $100,000. More common were debts of around $70,000. If money is a major issue, the prospective student would do well to shop around. Some students manage to go through their entire nurse-midwifery education without incurring debt. They may participate in work-study programs or work part-time, often as nurses, and apply for scholarships and grants. (Cecilia Wachdorf, personal communication)

A criticism often leveled at university training is that its standardization stifles individual creativity. I have not found this criticism to apply to the nurse-midwifery students I have interviewed. In our conversations, it was clear that they are accustomed to thinking "out of the box." They reported that this kind of unbounded thinking is strongly encouraged by most of their teachers. Nevertheless, a very real downside to university-based nurse-midwifery education is that training offered in large cultural institutions such as universities will inevitably reflect hegemonic philosophies and practices. In the cultural realm of birth, the patriarchal medical model is hegemonic; midwifery training carried out in such institutions will inevitably incorporate many elements of a highly medicalized, patriarchal and technocratic approach to birth. Thus, midwives will often be required to intervene in birth in ways contrary to the midwifery model in order to successfully graduate.

For example, some SNMs (student nurse-midwives) have discussed with me in interviews their distress over the unnecessary interventions they are often asked to perform. They report that they are usually able to resist cutting unnecessary episiotomies (four of my most recent interviewees had only cut one during their entire training), but that there is no way to get out of applying the other interventions that are standard in most hospitals, such as routine monitoring, labor induction and augmentation, IV administration, analgesia, etc. The early exposure to birth complications that many student midwives experience often makes them afraid of birth—a fear that can translate into overdependence on medical technologies and a lack of the confidence needed to become guardians and guides of the natural process of birth. It is important to know that the level of medicalization of nurse-midwifery education varies from program to program. Some university-based programs are highly humanistic and woman-centered in their approach; others are far more oriented toward technomedicine.

The graduates of university-based programs with whom I have spoken generally appreciate their training and value their technical skills. Some also express a fear of all the things that can go wrong at birth, note their dependence on support from other hospital personnel, and wonder how that fear and that dependence will affect their development as midwives.

Some students complained that they were ill-prepared for the private practices they tried to open because they were not taught business skills or how to deal with insurance forms and companies. Several recent grads have told me that they had tried to attend homebirths, but soon realized that they were totally unprepared for out-of-hospital practice. Indeed, lack of homebirth training opportunities was a major complaint voiced by all my student interviewees.

The second most serious complaint, also voiced by all my interviewees, was that during their training, their potential role as primary healthcare providers was heavily stressed, but upon graduation, none of them felt qualified to provide primary healthcare. (Some of their instructors have told me that they shouldn't worry: having obtained the theory and the knowledge in school, they will gain the necessary experience after graduation.) Two complained that they did not get enough practice in neonatal resuscitation and infant examinations, because those were taken care of by neonatal nurses in the hospitals where they were trained. And four complained about an abusive instructor or preceptor. (Since faculty in such programs are continuously evaluated, it is unlikely that such situations are allowed to continue.)

Another major source of stress was reported by SNMs who enter programs in which clinical and didactic components are separated in time. About half of my interviewees were in programs in which they studied didactically for a year before gaining any clinical experience. They found this both frustrating—a further delay in their desire to practice midwifery—and "disconnecting." They struggled to learn the didactics in isolation, often finding that the information made no sense in the absence of hands-on experience. Then later when they gained the hands-on experience, they had to link it back to a piece of information they had intellectually acquired over a year earlier. In group discussions between my interviewees, there was unanimous agreement that those who had been in programs in which clinical and didactic work happen in tandem from Day One had received a much more viable and rewarding training experience.

University-Affiliated Distance Learning Programs [3]

Upside: These programs creatively combine formalized, modular education with community-based and at-home learning. They allow the midwife to learn in evaluable components, interacting via computer (and occasionally in person) with other students and with various faculty members, and to be preceptored one-on-one by a nurse-midwife in her community. Unlike the situation in university-based training programs where each student has a variety of preceptors, the student-preceptor relationship in distance programs may be a much closer one, more like the intimate, trusting relationships developed in apprenticeship training. Such a relationship can be an extremely productive context within which to develop both midwifery skills and self-confidence. And it is often supplemented by exposure to other preceptors when the student is trained in multiple sites. Distance programs also combine some of the advantages of university-based education (social prestige and status, access to advanced degrees), with the advantages, especially for women with children or other family demands, of becoming a nurse-midwife without having to leave home for more than brief periods every year. And they are more likely to include training for out-of-hospital birth than most university-based programs.

The largest DOA-accredited distance learning program is the Community-based Nurse-midwifery Educational Program, better known as CNEP. It was specifically designed "in response to the need to prepare more nurse-midwives, to prepare nurse-midwives for practice in birth centers, and to make it easier for women living in small towns and rural areas to become CNMs" (Rooks 1997: 167). This program has been extremely successful. From its inception it tapped into a large pool of obstetrical nurses who wanted to become nurse-midwives but were not free to leave home for the necessary two years of study. For the same reasons, it has also attracted many direct-entry midwives who wanted to become CNMs. By reputation, the CNMs produced by the CNEP program acquire the same level of technical expertise as other CNMs, yet are also among the most holistically oriented and least medicalized of nurse-midwives, and tend to be very community-oriented. (For a detailed description of the CNEP program, see Rooks 1997:167-170 and the article on CNEP in Chapter 4 of this book.) I have interviewed five recent CNEP graduates; all were in general very happy with their learning experience (the downside exceptions are described below).

A number of other DOA-accredited programs also offer distance tracks for nurse-midwifery students; check with ACNM for up-to-date information. I have not studied these programs, and thus cannot speak to their individual pros and cons. Should DOA-accredited distance programs for direct-entry students be developed, I'm sure they will be very successful; there are many women who want to be midwives but cannot leave home to study and do not want to become nurses. (SUNY downstate has recently hired a new faculty member to develop a distance direct-entry program.)

Downside: A student's ability to enter a distance program will depend on whether she can find a CNM who practices within driving distance willing to serve as her preceptor. Should this one-on-one relationship not prove to be a compatible one, the student may have difficulties completing her training. I have been told of two incidences in which this preceptor-student relationship was extremely trying for the student; such problems seem rare, however.

Perhaps the major problem with distance programs is the sense of isolation students often experience—the feeling that "I am all alone with my computer." Distance students often try to organize study groups with other students within driving distance, which sometimes works and sometimes doesn't. "Nobody walks you through it," said one student. "Nobody spoon-feeds you the information. You've got to be highly motivated to do the work on your own." (This is also true in modular university-based programs in which the students must creatively problem-solve. "Spoon-feeding" is most common in programs based around the didactic lecture format.) For those who are highly motivated, such programs can be ideal. One of my CNEP interviewees, who had no family and "really got into it," reported that she "whizzed through" the program. But the other four reported major difficulties in staying on track. They noted that those who are not so self-disciplined, or who try to work full- or part-time as nurses, have a family life, and still complete the CNEP program, often have bouts of succumbing to panic and despair. A common reaction is to avoid the computer for days or weeks at a time. Failing to log in regularly, my interviewees reported that they fell more and more behind, then were afraid to log in and find out how far everyone else had progressed. Each one of the four thought that she was the only one who had let this happen; all were surprised to find how much company they had had without knowing it! In the end, they all "got their act together" and got through; their advice to others is to "stay in touch with total regularity" and to report and ask for help with any problems. The help is there, they said, but you have to ask for it. [4]

All five CNEP graduates reported that, as in some university-based programs discussed above, their didactic and clinical work was completely separate. The first year of study is spent on computer; none of them were allowed to begin clinical work with their preceptors until the second year. Those who were working as labor and delivery nurses didn't mind this disjuncture so much, but those with little nursing experience, or who had not worked as nurses for some time, did find the same problems with this disjuncture that I describe above. On the other hand, there is value in working full time with a preceptor, which enables the student to offer and to learn about the importance of continuity of care, as opposed to participating in more structured university-based programs, where students' busy schedules often do not allow them to stay the course with a given client.

Another downside of distance programs as of this writing is that all current DOA-accredited distance programs still require nursing training as a prerequisite (this will soon change). I do not have information about other potential downsides to distance programs; I have only interviewed a few CNEP graduates, who were all very happy with their education. I suggest that any students seeking to enter a particular distance program talk to a number of its graduates.

MEAC-ACCREDITED PROGRAMS

All MEAC-accredited programs qualify their students to practice at a safe, beginning level, caring for women during pregnancy, birth and the postpartum period, and equipping them to run independent midwifery practices. Most faculty in these programs are direct-entry midwives; some are CNMs. These programs prepare direct-entry midwives primarily for out-of-hospital practice. Hospital training is available in only a few such programs; such training is generally not required for certification or for program accreditation. All comply with MEAC standards relating to midwifery philosophy, curriculum, faculty, students, facilities and resources, credit hours, student services and resources, admissions and enrollment policies, financial management and student success in relation to mission (Mary Ann Baul, personal communication). These programs have undergone comprehensive study and peer examination, which have ascertained that the program directors have set structured learning objectives, provided services that enable students to meet those objectives, and can, in fact, show that graduates have benefited from the learning experiences provided.

Every MEAC-accredited program offers a combination of formalized didactic instruction and one-on-one clinical experience, usually with more than one clinical instructor, and involvement of several faculty members in judgment about the student's ability to provide safe, effective midwifery care from the prenatal through the postpartum period in out-of-hospital settings. MEAC accreditation indicates that the school adheres to established criteria, policies and standards, thereby providing an assurance of quality for employers, educators, government officials and the public (Mary Ann Baul, personal communication). (For more detailed and up-to-date information about MEAC-accredited programs, contact MEAC, 220 W. Birch,

Flagstaff, AZ 86001, or electronically at amabaul@aol.com and/or see listings published annually in the MANA News.) MEAC educators are developing flexible,
creative and innovative models for on-site and distance learning that creatively
combine didactic instruction and self-paced learning with apprenticeship.

One of the factors prospective students should evaluate is the financial stability
and resources of the program. All accredited programs must have refund policies, and
policies to finish training their enrolled students even if the school must close. It is
important to research the policies, reputation and success rate of a program thoroughly before enrolling. Talk to enrolled students and graduates. Are they receiving
or did they get what they expected? Were all policies, fees, and expectations disclosed
to them? Are they happy with their education?

College- or University-based Direct-entry Programs:

Confounding my attempts to use "university-based" to distinguish DOA- from
MEAC-accredited programs is the Miami-Dade Community College in Miami,
Florida, which offers a three-year program (opened in 1996) leading to an associate in
science degree in midwifery. In addition to didactic training in the basic sciences and
humanities, the program includes a strong apprenticeship component. Additionally,
students have access to high-tech equipment and a variety of clinical experiences in
hospitals, public health facilities, birth centers and homebirth practices in Florida and
at a high-volume hospital in Jamaica. Since ACNM will soon require the baccalaureate, this community college model, which combines the advantages of a college education with a deeply held commitment to independent midwifery, seems especially
appropriate for replication elsewhere.

Further blurring the boundaries between DOA-accredited and other programs,
Bastyr University in Seattle, Washington offers midwifery training for naturopathic
physicians in a program that blends these two complementary professions. I mention it
only for its uniqueness; it does not properly belong in this discussion as it has not sought
MEAC accreditation, but rather is accredited by the naturopathic accrediting body.

Private Midwifery Schools,
Some of which are Degree-granting:

Upside: Private schools can create and teach any model of midwifery they please,
free of the hegemonic influence of technomedicine that is pervasive in university-
based training. They can offer highly tailored, focused and formalized combinations
of apprenticeship and didactic training that can meet established standards and be
easily and continually evaluated, while at the same time keeping their philosophy
and practice holistic and woman-centered. They usually offer courses not only in
clinical training but also in midwifery philosophy and the practical side of how to run
a midwifery business. And, unlike one-on-one apprenticeships, students in these
schools have exposure to several primary faculty members who are in teaching positions because of their demonstrated expertise, and can interact with and learn from
each other. Some schools offer extensive additional training in herbs, homeopathy

and/or other forms of alternative medicine. Most educators in these schools seek to imbue their students not only with technical knowledge but also with a philosophy that stresses the importance of honoring and respecting the sacredness of women's bodies and the ever-present spiritual dimensions of pregnancy and birth.

Two of the private schools that are MEAC-accredited or in the process of becoming so offer advanced degrees recognized by the states in which they operate: the Utah School of Midwifery in Springville, Utah, which offers the bachelor's and master's degrees; and the National College of Midwifery in Taos, New Mexico, which offers degrees all the way up to the PhD. Both of these programs have strong apprenticeship components and are extremely affordable.

Downside: Some private midwifery schools are expensive and thus out of the reach of many potential students, while others are quite affordable: the tuitions of the MEAC-accredited private schools range from $8,000 to $22,000 (for the whole program). The expense of these private programs can be quite a lot higher than the expense incurred in an apprenticeship. Universities may be equally or more expensive, but federal loans and grants are often available to help with university tuition; such aid is generally not available to students in private programs. (It will become available if MEAC is successful in gaining Department of Education recognition—see the preceding article, endnote 35.)

Like university programs, private schools require moving from one's home to the location of the school (unless they have a distance education element). They are often organized around the strong personalities of one or a few experienced midwives and will inevitably reflect their individual values and styles. Many private midwifery schools have an "overseas" component, which is an added expense. Like some nurse-midwifery programs, midwifery schools are continually challenged to find enough births, especially out-of-hospital births, to meet the experiential needs of students. Students may be "placed" with a midwife for an apprenticeship for a period of time. Usually this works well, because mentors are allowed to choose the students they wish to work with. I have heard of three instances of problems between the mentor and the student involving personality conflicts or the imposition of unusual and extreme duties. Such occurrences are rare: in accredited schools all mentors and faculty are evaluated and students have opportunity for feedback and grievance procedures, so that abusive or extremely demanding relationships are not allowed to continue.

Another problem faced by private schools is the fact that taking the middle ground of combining formalized education with MANA's holistic midwifery model can subject them to criticism from both sides: (1) many in ACNM denigrate them as "trade schools" that do not guarantee the broad education that university training does; and (2) some proponents of apprenticeship training occasionally criticize them for offering a didactic approach that over-emphasizes what can go wrong and, like university-based CNM programs, can sometimes produce midwives who fear birth.

While the caveats are many, the rewards can also be great: the seven graduates of private midwifery schools whom I have interviewed generally seem thrilled with the individualized education they have received and the holistic, woman-centered philosophy that permeates their education.

DISTANCE LEARNING PROGRAMS (SEE ENDNOTE 3), WHICH NOW INCLUDE APPRENTICESHIP:

Distance direct-entry programs like the National College of Midwifery in Taos (which has applied for MEAC accreditation) and the two MEAC-accredited distance programs offered by the Utah School of Midwifery and the Midwifery Institute of California will no doubt form a major part of the wave of the future in direct-entry education. Whether under the aegis of MANA or the ACNM, the benefits of programs that allow student midwives to remain in their own communities are clear.

APPRENTICESHIP

Upside: Midwifery educator Sharon Wells provides the following apt description of apprenticeship:

> This student is in an experientially based educational setting that is client-centered. This student's education is self-paced, self-motivated and community-oriented. The learning occurs within the setting of the midwifery practice and not at a separate clinical site. Most learning is experiential and/or problem solving in nature. The didactic occurs by self-study, guided study courses or workshops. The educational focus is upon normal pregnancy, labor, delivery, postpartum and the newborn. This midwifery student learns continuity of care, counseling skills and to trust her own intuition in addition to her midwifery skills. The length of this educational process depends upon the apprentice and the midwife, but usually lasts from two to four years. The mentor may suggest using core competencies and a skills check list if they are available. "Graduation" occurs when the senior midwife and the apprentice think the apprentice is ready to function as a midwife safely on her own. Most births occur at home.[5]

Apprenticeship learning involves the whole human being—body, emotions, mind, spirit—and therefore is the most powerful form of learning there is. We all learn to be full members of our cultures through this kind of experiential learning. Pure apprenticeship learning is connection-based, as opposed to didactic learning which can seem to take place in a vacuum, with no apparent connection to anything. If the apprentice attends a birth with her mentor, for example, during which the woman hemorrhages, the apprentice will spend the next day studying every book she can find on postpartum hemorrhage and quizzing her mentor about its management. She knows, in an immediate and visceral sense, why this knowledge matters.[6]

Because birth turns out well most of the time, apprentices attending home and birth center births usually are not exposed early on to pathology, and have the time to build up a profound trust in the process of birth and in women's ability to give birth. Their training gives them a much broader experience of the wide range "normal" birth can take when it is not technologically controlled. (See preceding article, endnote 13.) The establishment of this kind of trust can have a great deal to do with the relationship between the apprentice and her mentor. I have interviewed a number of apprentices and mentors around the country, and am always impressed by the special quality of their relationship. Most mentors care deeply about the apprentices they take on, get to know them intimately, become committed to making sure they obtain the best education possible, and work to bolster the student's trust both in birth and in herself as she learns.

To fear birth is to generate complications that result from the fear. Midwives who trust birth profoundly tend to help women give birth more effectively: to trust a woman to give birth is to help her trust herself—this is part of the magic and the great strength of apprenticeship training. Another part of that magic and strength is continuity of care. In high-volume programs, continuity of care can be very hard to achieve. But it constitutes part of the essence of apprenticeship training, where the student accompanies her mentor not only to the birth of a given client but also to every prenatal and postpartum visit. It is apprenticeship training that establishes the midwifery ideal for continuity of care, an ideal that other training programs do the best they can to emulate.

As Wells indicates above, pure apprenticeship training, which includes few didactic elements, is increasingly rare. Today's apprentices are developing experiential trust in birth and learning continuity of care in the context of semi-structured curricula that their mentors design to make sure the training meets the standards set by NARM. These curricula include a tremendous amount of reading and often involve weekly classes taught by midwives in their communities, which may be supplemented with college courses in the basic sciences and other relevant areas. Many apprentices complete their training by working in high-volume clinics in the United States or the Third World where they can be exposed to multiple complications of birth and can learn to deal with them effectively.

An additional benefit is that apprenticeship is both financially and geographically accessible. Women who do not have the money or the mobility to attend a private school or university-based program can still learn how to be competent practitioners and build an economically viable business to support their families while serving their communities.

Downside: Apprenticeship learning, because it is so fluid, can be hard to evaluate for efficacy. The success of the process can depend on the skills of the mentor; having just one person involved can offer opportunities for subjectivity that are reduced when several faculty members have had experience with a student. Pure apprenticeship is only as excellent as the teacher and the student make it. If the learner is not motivated, the greatest teachers cannot help her. If the teacher is not a good teacher, the learner will be challenged to obtain the needed education. There is the additional risk that the learner may not be able to judge whether she is getting a quality, thorough preparation. If the student has only one mentor, and if that mentor is deficient either in knowledge, clinical judgment, skills or the ability to interact with clients, the student can be at risk, and therefore the future clients she may serve. If the apprentice does not learn sufficient skills for entry-level practice, then moves to a different community, there may be no one to judge her competence. These are in fact some of the reasons why many direct-entry educators are working to combine apprenticeships with more didactic models.

Apprenticeships can span the spectrum from inspiring, loving mentorships to abusive, traumatic relationships. (Of course, so can clinical preceptorships within universities, much like what residents/interns go through in the last years of medical school.) Abusive student-mentor relationships should under no circumstances be allowed to continue. In a school or university setting the student will be helped to end such a relationship and will be encouraged to give feedback so that other students will not have to endure the same. Ending one-on-one apprenticeships without such institutional support can be more difficult for the student. (On the positive side, I have interviewed over twenty apprentices and many of their mentors across the country, and in general find this to be a very special and mutually nurturant relationship in which the mentor is almost always deeply committed to responsibly working with and caring for her student.) Most experienced direct-entry midwives take very seriously their obligation to mentor the students seeking to follow in their footsteps. But at present there are relatively few experienced direct-entry midwives available to serve as mentors. As their numbers increase, more student options will obviously become available. Students should know that many apprentices work with more than one mentor, sometimes traveling to live with their second mentor for extended periods, in order to ensure that they have exposure to more than one style of practice.[7]

Until recently, apprenticeship training in midwifery carried no certification and had no standards—in part, CPM certification was developed to address this lack. Apprenticeship training alone is in general not recognized in the technocracy as a valid educational route in most professions, although because of its unique combination of intimacy and efficacy, there is a growing trend in adult education toward re-valuing apprenticeship (aka mentorship) as a viable educational style for the 21st century.[8]

And as I hope all the above has made clear, there is also a growing convergence between experiential apprenticeship models and more formalized didactic midwifery education. Good luck, and don't forget to honor your sisters and their educational choices!

ENDNOTES

1. The two direct-entry programs I know of that have been pre-accredited by the DOA are at SUNY-Brooklyn and at Education Program Associates (EPA) in San Jose, California. Due to financial difficulties, the entire EPA program, including both its nursing and direct-entry tracks, has been closed.

2. Johnson, Peter G. and Judith T. Fullerton. "Midwifery Education Models: A Contemporary Review." *Journal of Nurse-Midwifery* 43 (4); Sept/Oct 1998, in press.

3. Mary Ann Baul, the Executive Secretary of MEAC, provided the following useful overview of distance learning:

Distance learning, in order to be effective, should offer a complete program, in as much depth and with the opportunity for student support as in an onsite program. It should be collaborative (that is, there should be interaction between faculty and students, and even better, interaction among different students in the program, whether real-time or time-delayed). It should have specific learning outcomes for each course, and a way to evaluate those outcomes based on standards. Its faculty should be well-qualified as both instructors and also have training in distance learning and education technologies. There should be a strong commitment by the program to provide support for both faculty and student services. The program should have very clear expectations and guidelines, with appropriate access to needed resources. It should be evaluated as to its efficacy regularly, by students, administrators and instructors. Of course, there is no way to learn midwifery solely by distance education. There must be a very strong, highly supported and guided preceptor or mentor in the student's community in order to teach her the clinical skills required to complement the didactic learning at a distance. There are five types of distance learning, with upsides and downsides to each type. They appeal to and are successful for different types of learners. I will list them and briefly go over benefits and disadvantages.

a. Correspondence courses. These are paper-based, so they don't require a lot of technology, but students taking them rarely talk to faculty or other students. Such courses may not have deadlines, so student must be very motivated with lots of self-discipline to finish the program.

b. Mentored or directed study. Can also be paper based, or partly on computer, but student has communication with a faculty member. Usually there are fewer deadlines or scheduled interactions than in on-site programs, so again, students must be very self-directed and motivated.

c. Online education. Here, students use a variety of interactive technologies, such as logging on to a chat room, to discuss ideas and work on projects with other students, as well as doing outside reading and assignments. There are regularly scheduled times for work together and with instructors, which are very good for interaction with other students and faculty. However, this can be very time-consuming, and the technology can be challenging and complex. The student will have great need for technological support to get the work done, unless she has excellent computer skills.

d. Internet-based education. This is where the instructor speaks to the student over the Internet (like television), but then is also able to interact with the student and expect assignments within limited time periods. (SUNY-Stonybrook's entire distance program is available via the Internet.) The instructor guides the student to research on the Internet. The technology can also be intimidating to the student here.

e. Video correspondence. An instructor is taped on site giving a class. The video is sent to the distance student, along with reading and work assignments. The upside is that the student gets to see hands-on demonstrations and note how other students are reacting to the instructor. The downside is that her particular questions may not be answered.

The two distance learning types most commonly used in direct-entry midwifery education are correspondence and directed study; online education is sure to follow. Nurse-midwifery programs like CNEP make extensive use of online education, Internet chat groups and bulletin boards, etc. Students should know that completion or success rates are higher for students who have scheduled class periods, clear assignments and deadlines, as well as interactions with other students and teachers for support during the learning process. If distance learning encompasses these components, the student has a better chance of succeeding. (Mary Ann Baul, personal communication 1998)

4. Researchers Carr, Fullerton, Severino and McHugh (1996) found that the degree of dedication to the program of study, the amount of time students set aside to study, and whether or not the students had a study partner were all significant predictors of whether individuals would drop out or would complete the distance program in which they were enrolled. (Katherine C. Carr, Judith Fullerton, R. Severino, and M. Kate McHugh. 1996. Barriers to Completion of a Nurse-Midwifery Distance Education Program." *Journal of Distance Education* 9:111-131.)

5. Sharon Wells, "Caught in the Middle of the Maternity Care Crisis and a Political-Educational Debate," *Birth Gazette*, Spring 1993 9 (2):16-19.

6. Nurse-midwifery educators point out that this kind of connected learning is not unique to apprenticeship, but is a common feature of nurse-midwifery education as well. I find that it is a question of emphasis—nurse-midwifery programs stress didactic learning according to a pre-set study schedule; aside from that, the student is also free, if she has time, to study whatever she likes on her own and to discuss whatever comes up with her preceptor. Apprenticeship programs stress experiential learning according to the rhythms of individual women and individual births; didactic learning takes place away from the client and thus tends to be less immediately connected to the situation at hand. But some university-based programs utilize a case study approach, which combines experiential learning with synthesis of new information and critical thinking and analysis.

7. An example of the eclectic form many contemporary apprenticeships take is provided by well-known childbirth educator and author Nancy Wainer Cohen, who underwent two years of apprenticeship training with a midwife in Boston where she lives, interspersed with periodic trips to Michigan for weeks at a time to apprentice with Valerie El Halta. Toward the end of this process, she spent eight weeks in El Paso at Casa de Nacimiento and two weeks with Shari Daniels in Jamaica; in both places, she attended many births in short order and learned to deal with a wide range of complications.

8. An example comes from the high-tech computer industry, in which many young people without college degrees are receiving on-the-job training from mentors within a given company in specialized computer skills not taught in universities. (Kate Bowland, personal communication)

This article was written especially for this book.

Robbie Davis-Floyd, PhD, is a research fellow in the Department of Anthropology at the University of Texas, Austin. She is author of Birth as an American Rite of Passage *(1992), co-author of* From Doctor to Healer: The Transformative Journey *(1998), and coeditor of* Childbirth and Authoritative Knowledge: Cross-Cultural Perspectives *(1997),* Intuition: The Inside Story *(1997) and* Cyborg Babies: From Techno-Sex to Techno-Tots *(1998). She lectures nationally and internationally on these and related topics. Her current research investigates contemporary transformations in midwifery in the United States and Mexico. Books in progress include* Midwives in the Mainstream: The Politics of Change; *a coedited collection on* Midwives in Mexico: Continuity, Controversy, and Change; *and* The Power of Ritual.

NARM

Compiled by Cher Mikkola from articles by Robert A. Mahlman & Deborah B. Catri, PhD

idwives from across the United States have come together to define and establish standards for national certification through the North American Registry of Midwives (NARM) program, founded in 1987. It is the first certifying body to offer both a national examination and a national validation process for professional direct-entry midwives who come to their practices through multiple educational routes of entry. NARM currently administers a written examination which tests entry-level midwifery knowledge. A certification process added entry-level qualifications, including experience requirements and an assessment of clinical skills, to the written examination for those wishing to become certified professional midwives (CPM). Certification validates mastery of entry-level skills and knowledge vital to responsible practice of midwifery and indicates the CPM has sufficient knowledge and experience to train and mentor new and future midwives. NARM certification recognizes the efficacy of competency-based education, and the testing and certification procedure has been rigorously established according to standard testing criteria under the guidance of an established qualifying body.

WHAT IS COMPETENCY-BASED EDUCATION?

Qualification for the Registry is based on competency based education (CBE), a mode which stresses performance in an actual work situation. A minimum level of competency based on specified criteria must be met. Competency implies performance at a stated level or criterion specific for an occupational area. It has also been generally described as achievement of the knowledge, skills and attitudes (KSA) required to perform a given task. All three learning domains—affective, cognitive and psychomotor—are involved.

Several standards identify a competency-based program: competencies are role-relevant and determined through job analysis; criteria used to assess competencies state explicit levels of mastery under specified conditions; competencies are specified to students prior to instruction; criterion-referenced measures are used to assess achievement; and a system exists for documenting the competencies.

The advantages of CBE are numerous. Learning tasks are clearly stated; criteria used to assess competencies are based on performance objectives specified in advance; students are often provided with immediate feedback on their progress; emphasis is placed on the student's ability to perform rather than on knowledge alone; assessment strives for objectivity; it is more cost effective, relevant, flexible and self-satisfying than traditional forms of education, and it is closely based on specific job requirements so that the education is relevant. Potential disadvantages do exist, however. For example, it is possible that adequate evaluation methodology and instrumentation is lacking; there may be difficulty in identifying and validating essential competencies; and there may be difficulty in identifying with instructional management.

NARM Certification Procedures: Establishing Criteria

In order to offer certification to direct-entry midwives, criteria and a method of establishing criteria had to be established. A job analysis forms the foundation for this process, and the description provided for the qualifying body in this case, Schroeder Measurement Technologies (SMT), was deemed to be especially comprehensive. The large sample of midwives who completed the task analysis included a broad representation of individuals.

Next, the task analysis survey was used to identify the tasks crucial to performance of the job of entry-level, direct-entry midwifery. These critical tasks defined the content specifications for both the written and performance components of the certification assessment procedures. These specifications are used to create test items to measure the knowledge, skills and abilities (KSAs) needed to demonstrate minimum proficiency. This is essential to test fairness and ultimately to the protection of public health and safety. The combined use of detailed job analysis and task analysis information as primary test specifications represents the "best practice" methodology in the development of certification assessments.

Criteria were thoroughly reviewed by the item writing team and the NARM board. The tests should measure the KSAs needed for minimum proficiency as defined by the NARM board. The minimum proficiency needed to protect the safety of the public is defined by a panel of experts within the occupation. Widely accepted procedures were used to determine pass-fail cut scores on both the written and performance components. SMT took significant precautions to minimize error inherent in these judgments. It still takes time, however, to collect empirical evidence that can describe the performance of the tests relevant to cut scores, so that data will become more available as time goes on.

The certification process incorporates information and procedures to ensure accuracy and fairness in testing. These include well-defined test specifications provided to the candidates; thorough standardization of test administration procedures; training for qualified evaluators to administer performance assessments; feedback to examinees regarding test performance; automatic rescoring of tests resulting near the cut scores; adequate procedures for test review and retesting for failing candidates; and procedures for appeal for those not meeting certification requirements. In addition, screening of applicants performed via rigorous prerequisites should ensure that only individuals with appropriate training and experience will be allowed to even attempt the certification assessments.

Job Relevance

The most vital test of the quality of any employment testing system is job relevance, which is established by showing a direct link between job analysis information and the employment testing system. Job relevance is also established via judgments by Subject Matter Experts (SMEs) regarding the relationship between the test or test items and the job. For a certification test to be fair, it must measure KSAs critical to the specific job in question, not those expected to be possessed by some "ideal" candidate that are over and above what are needed to perform the job. An entry-level certification test must measure entry-level skills rather than those expected of individuals with many years of experience.

The procedures followed by SMT were clearly based on established standards for educational and psychological testing as set forth by the American Educational Research Association, American Psychological Association and the National Council on Measurement in Education.

STRENGTHS AND WEAKNESSES OF NARM CERTIFICATION PROCEDURES

The identified strengths of the NARM certification procedure are numerous. First, it is a multi-hurdle process that ensures candidates hold the necessary KSAs to perform the role of entry-level midwifery. Certification applicants must meet stringent prerequisites before testing: In the realm of experience they should have attended a minimum of twenty births, a minimum of seventy-five prenatal examinations, twenty newborn examinations and forty postpartum examinations. They must have documentation of relevant education. As to their skills, they must provide evidence from a preceptor/supervisor/mentor that proficiency has been attained for each skill listed in a comprehensive skill list; they must hold a current CPR certificate; and they must provide detailed reference forms completed by two clients and a professional. Applicants must pass the written certification test and then pass a performance-based certification assessment.

Second of its strengths, as seen earlier, is that the certification procedure is based on very thorough and appropriate job analysis. Third, adequate training was given to item writers when the test was devised; that is, substantial attention was paid to test writing specifications and to the level of knowledge that the test is designed to measure. Other strengths are an appropriate content validation/item review; high quality cut score setting procedures; appropriate training for qualified evaluators for administering performance assessments; and high-quality test administration procedures.

To date there are also some perceived weaknesses in the NARM test, of a kind that is to be expected in a newly developed certification system. Strong evidence is not yet provided regarding whether or not the test is capable of discriminating among competent vs. incompetent candidates because empirical evidence has not yet been provided—the initial examinees completing the assessments are described as "extremely experienced compared to the minimum experience requirements established to take the examination." This type of data takes time and resources to collect. A more appropriate sample, especially for piloting, would have included individuals expected to be classified as non-competent. But given the stringent prerequisites to candidacy for certification, it is unlikely that many non-competent individuals will advance to the testing stages of certification. Moreover, a thorough piloting of the assessments before live administration would have been desirable.

According to Ohio State University's Vocational Instructional Material Laboratory Associate Director of Assessment Robert A. Mahlman, "the overall quality of the processes used by Schroeder Measurement Technologies, Inc. to develop certification tests and testing procedures is very high and represents best practice within industry standards. I would venture to say that the quality is at least as good as comparable certification programs and likely better than most."

MEETING THE CRITERIA

The certified professional midwife certification process has carefully met the competency-based education criteria in five general areas: First, it meets the CBE characteristic that competencies are to be demonstrated by the student as role relevant and determined through job analysis. The 1995 Job Analysis of the Role of Direct-Entry Midwives was developed through a strong, research-based job analysis process that serves to identify KSAs necessary to perform as a direct-entry midwife; and accreditation of direct-entry midwifery education programs' standards published by Midwifery Education Accreditation Council (MEAC) require that "curriculum is consistent with the current MANA Midwifery Core Competencies and NARM Certification."

The second CBE characteristic, that criteria employed in assessing competencies explicitly state levels of mastery under specified conditions, was met when core competencies were defined for a minimally proficient direct-entry midwife through panel discussions with subject matter experts during the job analysis process.

The third CBE characteristic, that competencies are specified to students prior to instruction, was met when clear documentation of competencies were provided from two sources: "Candidates Information Bulletin" published by NARM and "Practical Skills Guide for Midwifery" written by Pam Weaver and Sharon K. Evans and published by Morningstar Publishing Company.

The fourth CBE characteristic, that criterion-referenced measures are to be used to measure the achievement of competencies, was met when the CPM program incorporated cognitive and performance assessment and was clearly criterion-referenced back to the 1995 "Job Analysis of the Role of Direct-Entry Midwives."

The fifth CBE characteristic, that a system exists for documenting the competencies achieved by each student, was addressed when documentation of competency attainment was set up to begin with the preceptor/supervisor/mentor verification which requires sign off through a notarized form for each competency; a national certificate as a CPM is earned by passing the national CPM examination; and narrative reports are given to unsuccessful exam candidates which list areas of strengths to weaknesses.

NARM certification is answering the needs of a nation currently in a maternity care crisis. It has succeeded in defining the scope of midwifery practice and offered a certified group of practitioners from whom women can choose quality midwifery care. The public now has a growing body of practitioners whose skills and knowledge are verified according to a single set of standards, making it easier for those who are seeking an alternative to hospital-based midwifery care to understand and confirm the skills of the midwives they interview. As well, NARM has lent its support to the preservation and protection of midwifery for the future by helping significantly increase the number of midwives entering the field.

This article was compiled especially for this book.

Cher Mikkola has been an editor at Midwifery Today for twelve years and is also a freelance writer, editor and proofreader. She lives in Eugene, Oregon with her family.

Deborah B. Catri, PhD, is the Director of Assessment at the Vocational Instructional Materials Laboratory at Ohio State University.

Robert A. Mahlman is the Associate Director of Assessment at the Vocational Instructional Materials Laboratory at Ohio State University.

For more information from the North American Registry of Midwives (NARM): Call toll-free 1(888) 84-Birth (842-4784). A request form for the NARM Certification Application Packet and Candidate Information Bulletin can be found in the Resource section of this book, page 308.

HUMBLED IN THE POWER
OF WOMEN GIVING BIRTH

by Jan Tritten

There is a kind of strong uncompromising midwife who comes up through the community, perhaps by apprenticeship, often through self-study with other like minded aspiring midwives. Or as one mentor termed it, "midwives in waiting." This is the midwife who has a deep call to be a midwife but does not necessarily fit in the mold of today's Western society. We used to call ourselves lay midwives and many of us still wear that noble title as a banner that says, "I won't compromise the woman's choice for medical protocol." We knew a midwifery in the 1970s that was powerful and uncompromising. The greatest teachers were the women and babies.

Our own births and experiences breastfeeding our babies gave most of us the strength to follow the calling. Our calling to be with women was as strong as the need to eat. Every cell in our body said, "Be a midwife, help the women, help the babies." We had to be a midwife at any cost. Our whole body, heart and mind desired to help women have their babies. We were driven. We ate up all information like starved children. Deep in our souls we trusted birth. When you partner deeply with a woman around her birth there isn't a medical or cultural influence that can overpower that relationship. A doctor once said, "I wish I could just be there with the woman and her family, but instead I am there with the hospital administration, law suits, standards of practice and a whole medical culture."

When I am with a woman there is she and her baby, her family and our relationship including everything I have learned from other birthing moms and midwives. There is also our dear Creator, God, the ancient ones, and the deep knowledge that women can do this, indeed are designed perfectly to do this. We know that this is a holy event, a sacrament as Ina May Gaskin says. We know this is the most important event and transition in a woman's life. Nothing will ever be as important for this woman as this pregnancy and birth. We are acutely aware of our awesome responsibility and gift to be a midwife. We are there as her protector, her mom, one who loves her more at that moment than all but her family. We are her family in the ancient way that women birthed for a million years. We will do whatever is necessary to serve her and her baby toward completing the task of getting born and started well. For the duration of the pregnancy and birth we are partners of heart, soul and information. The ultimate decisions are hers. We just tell her all we know at this point. Tomorrow we will know a lot more because we will have learned from her. We will never know it all because we are always learning from the women, babies and families. We are humbled in the power of women giving birth. We are humbled that God called us.

The women are unfettered by the culture because we trust and they trust. When they don't trust they can borrow some of ours. When we don't trust we borrow some of theirs or each other's. We go with them to that ancient and primal place where we all know that "babies come out."

We aren't ignorant or blind in our trust. We sharpen our knowledge and skills constantly. We hunger to know every way there is to handle shoulder dystocia, hemorrhage or prolonged labor. We read voraciously, we ask each other, doctors and whoever knows something that might help our mom or her baby. We also know that most of the birth information in standard obstetrical books must be challenged because it was noted in a time, like now, of rampant drug use in birth. We still look for every helpful pearl in those books, but we are rewriting the textbooks with our knowledge of pregnant and birthing women. We work on knowing normal so well that we know when something is abnormal. More importantly we know our individual women so well that we know when something is wrong. Midwifery is about relationships. Without relationship there is no midwifery as we know it; it becomes something else. Midwife means "with woman" and you have to be truly with her on every level to be practicing authentic midwifery, as my friend Dr. John Stevenson terms it.

A midwife must have autonomy in her practice to be able to really serve women well. To the degree we lose that, we lose midwifery. As we get more absorbed by titles, any title besides midwife, we seem to lose our autonomy. We work to become accepted by the medical culture but we often lose the ability to stand outside and make decisions with the women. More demons such as standards of practice enter our birth room. You absolutely have to individualize birth. Every woman is different. Every birth is different. As we become stamped and approved, and as we become a profession, we often step away from the women.

If we allow the word "profession" to imply "I have knowledge, you don't," if we ever feel superior to, or separate from the woman, we hamper our ability to help that woman. I have watched professional midwifery conferences turn almost entirely to self-centeredness, not woman-centeredness. The talk is about the profession of midwives—the pay, benefits, stresses, losing or keeping jobs. When you aren't working for the woman, you are working for the wrong thing. These meetings are not about birth, women, babies or pregnancy, they are about how to keep the profession going. That attitude will kill the profession because it must be with and about birthing women. We must center on how to be a better midwife, not a gainfully employed one. Every compromise with the medical culture erodes a little of why we became midwives.

I know deep in my heart that as we become the ones accepted in the culture, there will be others who come up from the fringes to challenge our compromise. They will do that if we become co-opted. They will be the lay midwives of the next century. As editor and mother of *Midwifery Today* I am committed to hold that space open for them and always work to decriminalize midwifery. We cannot serve both birthing women and the medical culture.

Jan Tritten became a homebirth midwife in 1976, following the homebirth of her second child. Her first was born in the hospital, and the difference between the two births sent her into her midwifery career. She retired from active midwifery in 1989 in order to devote her time to her work as founder and editor of Midwifery Today and The Birthkit. Changing the way birth is done is her calling.

Direct-Entry Midwifery

" . . . the greatest portion of any midwifery education should be experiential in nature, with midwives teaching midwifery, not obstetrical technology. Aspiring midwives would ultimately apprentice to birth, respecting women as the true experts in giving birth, and babies in being born. Women and their babies would be regarded as the primary teachers of birthing."

—Carolyn Steiger

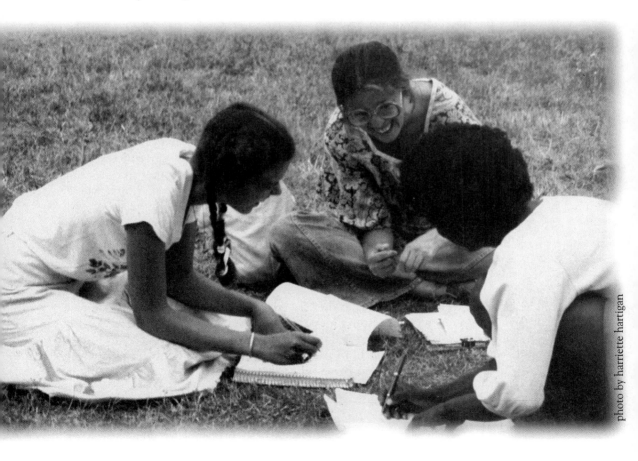

photo by harriette hartigan

A ROSE BY ANY OTHER NAME

by Jan Tritten

There is a battle going on for the very soul of midwifery.

Just because we call the work we do "midwifery" doesn't mean that's what it is. I can put a steel spike in a crystal vase and call it a rose; it doesn't mean that's its true identity. The foundation of the future of midwifery—or, the lack of a recognizable midwifery profession—is being laid right now. We personally choose on which side of the line we will fall: Are you going to be a midwife, protector of normal birth, or a practitioner who relies on medicine and technology (including the clock) to manage birthing women and their babies? Can you gaze into your own soul and conscience at the end of your day and say, "I served and helped empower women in their birthing process," or do you admit, "I served the medical establishment"? Do you practice in the midwifery way of encouragement, counseling, and imparting accurate information? Do you understand the full beauty but precariousness (a wrong word or damaging innuendo can do irreparable harm) of pregnancy and birth?

As time marches on and technology seduces us more and more, and while young women continue to be uninformed or misinformed, some midwives increasingly agree to surrender the midwifery model of with-woman care, which demands that we take time, give attention, and use love and compassion. Education and research give you a good foundation, but don't give up your intuition and your heart. Technology is there to assist when it is truly needed, and thank goodness for that, but it doesn't need to creep into our practices and supersede our womanly, human skills.

The medical model is insidious. We have adopted it not because it is ethical or accurate, but because we are still trying to please the men in power. We think that by making ourselves acceptable to them, we'll carve out a place for ourselves in the healthcare system. We'll be as good as they are so they'll hire us. We give up the truth that says we learn primarily from birthing women, babies and other midwives, for the lie of the medical model which changes constantly, where ego reigns, and where compassion takes a back seat. In the end, we are sacrificing women and babies; we are sacrificing midwifery.

What happens to the few who won't be co-opted? They are prosecuted as heretics for not bowing down to the god of medical technology! They are burned at the stake for their truth. In New York state, they are being wiped out. In Australia, my friend Maggie is being prosecuted. All over the United States they are threatened, prosecuted and persecuted. In the United Kingdom they are refused insurance or payment. In much of the rest of Europe, they don't stand a chance to even begin. The very best are forced to stop practicing. The Canadian government has forced Inuit women to be evacuated from their families and communities to fly several hours to the south to have their babies in Western-style hospitals. Only one Inuit community has fought successfully to regain their right to birth at home in their own culture, with attendants from their own community.

In the United States the dominant Western, white culture annihilated the custodians of this land, the Native Americans and the Mexicans. When there were only a few individuals remaining of those great Indian nations, the dominant white, Western culture finished the kill by stamping out their cultures and working to "rehabilitate" their few remaining ways.

Sound familiar? It reminds me of what is happening in midwifery and birth. The powerful, dominant, wealthy, male medical culture is working hard to wipe out what little is left of our women's ways of knowing and birthing. They use shiny instruments and shiny words to blind us to our own wisdom. They remove women from their families and community cultures and force them to birth within the medical paradigm. Many of those practitioners who bravely resist are arrested and prosecuted.

Midwives who practice real midwifery are the change agents; they are a threat to the livelihood of the medical model because they speak the truth of women and their babies, and try not to compromise for a license to practice or a piece of the pie. They convince women that they can birth, breastfeed and mother their children against all cultural odds. And their outcomes in birth and postpartum cannot be matched for family satisfaction and for safety.

So, where are you going with medicalized education and practice? Is your practice a steel spike you call a rose, or is it really a rose? To fit into the medical model is to be its handmaiden. Eldridge Cleaver once said, "You are either part of the problem or part of the solution." If you are already working within the medical birth system, good! Fight within it to bring it into line. Insist on finding ways to serve the women where you are. Go a step further and support your sisters who are on the firing line for all of us. If you do not work within the medical sphere, continue to do your good work and be wary of falling into the subtle, seductive trap of medical intervention. Hold your ground. And let's all remember what midwifery truly means: "with woman."

This article first appeared as an editorial in Midwifery Today Issue No. 40.

Jan Tritten became a homebirth midwife in 1976, following the homebirth of her second child. Her first was born in the hospital, and the difference between the two births sent her into her midwifery career. She retired from active midwifery in 1989 in order to devote her time to her work as founder and editor of Midwifery Today and The Birthkit. Changing the way birth is done is her calling.

THE HONOR, JOY, POWER AND CHALLENGE OF COMMUNITY, INDEPENDENT MIDWIFERY

by Judy Luce

Disclaimer: There are wonderful, dedicated, compassionate midwives working in every setting, often against almost insurmountable odds, who have arrived where they are by a variety of routes. However institutions do exist and are very powerful, and knowledge and ways of knowing have powerfully political dimensions. We need to be able to address institutional problems and aberrations but not attack those persons in those institutions, many of whom are working mightily hard for change. And we need to view knowledge—who controls it, how it is acquired and what is considered legitimate—as the political questions they are. I have often not measured up to the ideal I see possible in independent midwifery, which some now call a form of direct-entry midwifery. In fact, I feel that I am continually growing and changing and am self-critical of the degree to which I have been co-opted or have held on to practices that maintain my self importance. Birth and women continue to be my teacher. Nevertheless, I believe deeply in the ideas I am setting forth, and my vision of midwifery which I know is shared by many others.

I have been an independent midwife for nearly twenty-three years. I learned birth from birth, from the awesome physical and spiritual unfolding that birth is with its varied rhythms and expressions. I acquired skills through apprenticeship (I watched, listened, reflected with other women on my experience, read, questioned). Frequently I am asked if I were to live my life over would I choose this route and what are its pros and cons? I think of the question: route to what? Midwifery was a calling—a vocation—a calling rooted in my own experiences of giving birth and the passion born in me to want to make it possible for others to be able to birth at home as I had with my third child, Damara.

In talking about my personal journey, the advantages and disadvantages of this way of becoming and being a midwife will be addressed. I became a midwife because the experience of pain and violation, followed by an experience of empowerment, led me beyond myself. I became a midwife because women asked me to be present with them at their births; because the midwife who attended my birth asked if I would assist her; because a community of women existed in the 1960s and 1970s who were challenging the medicalization of birth, their bodies and their deepest life experiences. Many women experienced medicalized birth as violating, intrusive and physically and emotionally painful and the medicalized view of birth as distorting. They judged medicalized childbirth practices to be too often damaging and dangerous. My midwifery was born from that widespread, diverse group of women who desired to reclaim birth as their own, who knew with every fiber of their being that they could give birth, and that birth, for most women, was an expression of health and vitality and a powerful manifestation of their strength and creativity, of the awesome power of life renewing itself. I was born as a midwife on the tidal wave of that movement.

When I have been asked over the years what kind of midwife I was, I would say, "lay," "community" or "independent," depending on what seemed most appropriate. I certainly never referred to myself as a "professional" midwife or a "direct-entry" midwife. I am proud of being a "lay" midwife. George Bernard Shaw said once that all professionalization represents a conspiracy against the laity and, if anything, I see myself in collaboration, or better, communion with, the women I accompany on their journeys through pregnancy and birth into motherhood. I never doubted the value of what I brought to these women—in fact, I make different contributions to each woman and family depending on their unique situations—but I always recognize women as the experts about their bodies, their pregnancies, their births and their needs. I don't support perineums, as the silly bumper sticker reads, I support women. I affirm their health, the wisdom they often don't even know they have, their bodies, the normalcy of pregnancy, the rightness of the birth process, the uniqueness of their labors. And I use my knowledge and experience to help women achieve and maintain health and make corrections when deficiencies exist or balance is upset. Women's bodies, hearts and minds need to be nurtured and nourished during pregnancy. In situations where women need more care and attention I feel I am returning the woman's power and wisdom to herself.

I call myself a "community" midwife, not simply because I have lived and worked in particular communities, but because, as a midwife, I feel part of a community of women—childbearing women and midwives—who span the ages and those who are connected to each other today. I want to honor the wisdom and experience and power that comes from that collectivity—a wisdom that precedes our "scientific" understanding of birth. Ways of learning are tied to power. I learned birth from birth; I was empowered, educated and inspired by pregnant women and the stories of their births (I listened to any woman who would tell me her story and read every story I could find). They midwifed and continue to midwife me into existence as a midwife. Most of what I bring to the women I attend—I love the medieval image of a woman surrounded by her attendants—has been given to me by others. My own experience acts as a magnet to draw out the birth experiences of other women. I teach and inspire with birth stories and at each birth I am made new. Critical reading for any aspiring midwife is Brigitte Jordan's "Cosmopolitical Obstetrics: Some Insights from the Training of Traditional Midwives" (*Social Science and Medicine*. Vol. 28. No. 9, pp. 925-944), also included in the revised edition of *Birth in Four Cultures*. This is my bible of apprenticeship training and represents the best understanding of the colonization of birth and women's bodies by the Western bio-medical model. Make no mistake: this is not about traditional birth attendants somewhere else; this is about us.

I don't see myself as a "baby catcher" as much as a cultural worker. I help women carve out a space apart from the medical culture of birth and dominant cultural attitudes toward women and birth within which they, with their partners and loved ones, can welcome and receive their own babies. I do think the ability of anyone to function in this role is tied to an apprenticeship learning of midwifery. It takes time and discipline to learn this way and works best when you have already experienced pregnancy and birth, are a part of a community of women reflecting upon and learning from their experiences, and are steeped in a personal knowledge of childbearing, childrearing and mothering. So much of the knowledge essential for midwifery does come from within and colors everything else that is learned.

As an independent midwife who is not and has never been regulated by local authorities, I have the privilege of being as independent as possible of the medicalized culture that dominates birth with its disembodied, clinical language, its fragmented and fragmenting, supposedly "scientific" approaches that are so devoid of spirit and soul, and the institutions that rob us of our identities as healthy strong, powerful women by their narrow focus and distorted gaze. What this independence gives me is the freedom to be with women, to represent their interests, to listen to what they are telling me they "know" about their bodies and ability to birth, and to support their choices. I am able to honor their ways of "knowing" and my own, not as complementary or synergistic, but as central/core/essential. Being an independent, community midwife allows me the most autonomy, and makes it possible for my primary accountability and allegiance to rest with women and a community of midwives who share my beliefs and values and philosophy of birth, of life and of death. It allows me not to have to hold conflicting worlds within me—the risk based medical approach and the personal, holistic, individually responsive approach of the the best midwifery.

In seeking recognition in the mainstream and the respectability that comes with following traditional routes of certification and licensure, I think we've lost touch with the cutting edge of political analysis and criticism that was found in the homebirth movement and in the emergence of homebirth midwifery. I think that there will continue to be a need for midwives who stand outside the system, are critical of it, and who avoid the shadow of fear the system casts (expressed in such things as liability insurance which alters, I think, the very basis of the midwifery relationship—trust, shared responsibility and awareness of life's uncertainties. Expressed also in increased surveillance and medical screening and in the multiplicity of "choices" women are being asked to make that actually diminish real choice). There will be a need for midwives who can respond to women and families who for a myriad of reasons are not at home in that system. Independent midwifery (apprentice-trained, perhaps not even certified by NARM) offers a route for women to become midwives whose conscience and consciousness require that they seek a different way and keep alive a real woman-centered, culturally critical perspective.

I think regulation and professionalization that gains the stamp of approval of institutions totally alien to women-centered birth can make us strangers to ourselves, will create (have already created) conflicting loyalties and obligations and will reduce us to being members of a healthcare team sleuthing for abnormalities and problems and things to fix instead of affirming and guiding and celebrating the power of birth and the uniqueness of each woman and each labor. As my dear friend Norma Swenson says, "we don't call the medical model dominant for nothing." As an institution, certified nurse-midwifery has tied itself to the institution of medicine and relies on that institution for its blessing. While NARM has certainly been willing to jump through a certain number of hoops and dress itself up and speak a language recognizable to the powers that be, it has tried to maintain the autonomy of self-definition and self-regulation. (I think the MANA Statement of Values and Ethics is a shining example of the best independent midwifery thinking.) In many places midwives have watched this integrity eroded by state regulation. I believe that to preserve our perspective and integrity we (or some of us at least) must maintain a distance or else we will be swallowed up. Being an independent midwife allows this distance. I do think that medicine as an institution and midwifery offer diametrically opposed views of women and of childbirth. Independent midwives can chart new waters in ways those in the mainstream cannot.

What I've seen is that licensing and regulation restrict how one practices; adopting the language that goes with regulation constricts our understanding of ourselves and the role we play in normal childbirth and how we stand in relationship to the women we attend. They introduce the hierarchical values of the medical system, its technological tools and risk assessment approaches. This has been well-documented in Sullivan et al's research on licensing in Arizona. (*Labor Pains: Modern Midwives and Home Birth*. New Haven: Yale University Press, 1988.) Language isn't neutral. I choose carefully the words I use; as an independent midwife I try to keep our "mother tongue" alive in the face of the foreign language that often accompanies professionalization, certification and licensing. More often than not, university based educational programs with clinical sites attached to medical institutions alter how midwives view birth and introduce risk management and labor management as central to practice, concepts that are foreign to a midwifery approach. I do not question that there are worlds to learn and discover about normal childbirth, about keeping it normal, about inspiring confidence in women, about correcting or responding to complications in pregnancy and childbirth. I question how we package this knowledge, the language we use, the excess academic baggage we attach to credentials. It is possible to know the name of every part of the human body, of every system and how it works and not "know" our own bodies, not "know" in a way that counts, that our bodies actually work and birth works (check out your local obstetrical practice).

"Patient" and "client," "manage" and "management," and "risk assessment" bring whole institutions and narrow institutional perspectives with them that rob us of the rich narrative that is the midwifery story and midwifery relationship to women and birth. In this culture women are taught to understand their bodies not just in biological terms but in clinical terms, terms that don't begin to accurately convey labor and birth any more than sexology manuals convey a sexual relationship. When I think of birth I think of the lovely unfolding of passionate, relational sexuality—the timing, the texture, the gentle rhythm, the dance, the pulsing, the opening, the flowering, the eruption, the violet that, undamaged, pushes through the concrete. . . . The reality of birth and the reality of sexuality are most aptly conveyed through the language of metaphor, through images and poetry. As lay midwives we can hold on to this language and use it in service of women.

I have just returned from the first-time birth of a young mother who has left me in awe of the wisdom that flows from within, that's almost genetically encoded and unfolds beautifully and powerfully when not obstructed or repressed by cultural messages imbued with fear about pain, inadequacy, risk. I still can hear Candace Whitridge, a California midwife, describing a seventeen year old birthing woman who had shown up for her first prenatal the day before she went into labor: the young woman's self-composure, her bodily awareness, her peacefulness, her power—as she reminded us, in her birthing, that "we've forgotten that we do remember how to give birth."

My assistant and I have seen this scenario played out over and over in the past months—young, first-time mothers steeped in confidence (not books or classes or scientific facts and studies) who trust their bodies to work and their ability to embrace labor with strength and courage moment by moment. With their midwives and with their families and friends, they have created a sacred place of love and support and affirmation in which to give birth. We have supported them simply with our presence and done so very little. (I think of Nikki Leap's powerful talk in Chicago, "Doing More by Doing Less.") They have birthed powerfully, quickly and with ease.

I think of the thirty-four year old with a persistent breech, virtually assured of a cesarean in the hospital, who came to me very late in her pregnancy looking for a midwife who would honor her, what she knew of her capacity, and her right to choose what felt best for her and her child. After seven hours of labor and one hour of squatting to push she gave birth to a beautiful lusty eight pound baby girl. Several months ago a mother came to me pregnant with twins (she had a six and four year old already; her labor with the latter was under three hours). She never felt healthier, more able. She felt violated and disempowered by the fear inducing, mandated clinical intrusion of "high risk" care—monthly ultrasounds, close surveillance, threats of c-section if the first baby were breech, heparin lock requirements, and so on—presented to her by even the best obstetricians around. I had to deal with possible censure from sister midwives: attending this woman was viewed by some as placing all midwifery and homebirth in jeopardy. The day after I met with this woman I woke feeling that if I didn't attend her I wouldn't know who I was as a midwife any longer; that something in me would have died. She carried to term, shopped for food the day she went into labor, had a hemoglobin of 12.8, and after a two-hour labor gave birth to twin girls—the first weighing six pounds, born breech; the second seven pounds, three ounces, born vertex. Six minutes later two huge placentas came. Blood loss was minimal. I feel honored to have been able to attend these women; I want the freedom to continue to be available to work with such women. This is a freedom that comes with finding a non-institutional and perhaps not officially sanctioned route to midwifery.

There are many challenges that come with trying to preserve this kind of midwifery, not least of which are political and economic. The politics surrounding midwifery—the threat of arrest, prosecution or harassment, or constricting regulation—can induce fear. I don't think the only response is to give in and join the club. We need to draw on the power and safety that comes in the numbers of women who choose homebirth and midwives. We need to build that force.

Often I hear women say that they want professional licensing of some sort in order to receive third party payments. They want malpractice coverage in order to work in institutions such as birth centers and to be able to make a living and, in some instances, to be able to be paid by insurance plans. Third party payments benefit both midwives and women, but they often come with a price attached: restrictions on autonomy and regulation. I find something very powerful in negotiating a mutually acceptable fee with a woman for whom payment is a hardship. It is good to acknowledge the circumstances of people's lives but also for a woman and family to recognize the value of what they are choosing and why. I think if more women chose homebirth and more women chose midwives, the economics would be manageable. For this to happen, more and more women—birthing women and midwives—need to share their stories in a public forum. Nothing, I believe, is as powerful as women telling the stories of the power they have found in birthing. These stories embody in their narrative what is being preserved in homebirth and midwifery care and what is being lost and destroyed in medicalized birth. Women empower others through their stories. This is where midwifery begins and ends.

This article was written especially for this book.

Judy Luce, CPM, has been attending women at home as a community midwife for over twenty-two years. She presently attends women in Vermont through Womancare Home Midwifery in Barre. Since the mid-seventies she has been been active in the women's health movement as a writer, speaker and organizer focusing on the task of women defining the birth experience and reclaiming it. She has also written on midwifery and ethical issues involved in reproductive technology and lectured at colleges. She is the primary author of the Childbearing chapter in the newly updated and revised edition of Our Bodies, Ourselves and assisted in the writing and research for the Pregnancy chapter. Her passion is looking critically at language and women's ways of knowing and developing a philosophy and language of birth that embodies a woman's perspective on childbirth and women's embodied experience.

She is past MANA New England regional representative and a member of the editorial board for the MANA News. Active with the Vermont Midwives Alliance, she has been involved with the VMA certification process and in developing and implementing the CPM credential. She is a member of the Women's Institute for Childbearing Policy which authored the collaborative paper, "Childbearing Policy Within a National Health Program: An Evolving Consensus for New Directions."

THE SEARCH FOR AUTONOMY

by Jan Tritten

I once asked author and midwifery advocate Marsden Wagner, who travels extensively, what he perceived to be the most important issue facing midwives around the world. He answered without hesitation, "autonomy." After my midwife friend Barbara Harper attended midwives' meetings in Japan, I asked her what seemed to concern Japanese midwives most. She answered swiftly that they had talked often about how doctors were taking away their power, and that it was difficult to make their voices heard. In short, they were concerned about autonomy.

Autonomy is defined as "the condition or quality of being self governing; self determination; independence; a self-governing state, community or group." When I talk about autonomy, I am not talking about working alone. In the event of serious difficulties, collaboration with physicians who are experts in various specialties is an essential element of good midwifery. But there is no better practitioner than the midwife for recognizing potential complications and safely bringing those situations into the realm of normal birth.

Unfortunately we have been seriously derailed from our long tradition of trusting women and trusting birth. Earlier in this century, midwifery nearly died out, and rather than reclaim its original intent, in many ways we have allowed it to be reborn out of the medical model. We are now faced with the challenge to recreate what midwifery is all about. As London-based midwife Suzanne Colson says, "midwifery is a profession looking for a philosophy."

Another major concern I have on the subject of autonomy is knowing that many, many nurse-midwives are losing their jobs. They are at the mercy of those who hire them and at the same time consider them the competition. I hope that in response more and more nurse-midwives will decide to become entrepreneurs and go into business for themselves. I have known some excellent practices where the nurse-midwife is autonomous simply because she owns her own business.

There was a CNM who had a birth center in southern California for twenty years. When she moved to Michigan a year and a half ago she found a backup doctor and started another birth center. I would encourage midwives who are unhappy with their lack of freedom to try this idea. The National Association of Childbearing Centers (NACC) is a great resource and support organization for those who choose this option. Fortunately for some, there are also excellent hospital-based practices where the midwives have freedom to practice as they see fit.

It is often thought that empirical midwives have more autonomy, and for the most part that is an accurate assumption. More and more frequently, however, state licensing complicates the picture. From what I have observed, as soon as a state gets into the business of regulation, freedom is the cost. I know a midwife in Arizona who gave up her license because she wouldn't compromise her clients. This tells me her bottom line is the pregnant women she serves, and I can't agree with her more. It is ultimately their freedom that is restricted when the midwives' freedom is compromised.

The double-edged sword of "protecting the public" and maintaining one's independence is continually being honed, but the irony is that the public is not really being protected at all. Instead, women are made the sacrificial lambs to the money and power brokers who dictate how and where they will birth. What results is a wholesale selling-out of women and their birth experience.

Giving continuity of care is part of an autonomous practice. To really help women avoid dangerous technology, we have to work with them very early in their pregnancies, and follow through. We make the commitment to nurture the entire birth cycle as we care for a woman's nutrition, emotions and physical well-being, calm her fears and make sure she is well informed. This has to start early and remain consistent.

As we piece the autonomy puzzle together, let's remember before all else that our reason for being midwives is to serve women and their babies and families. Whatever restricts our ability to serve them well should not be tolerated.

This article first appeared as an editorial in Midwifery Today Issue No. 42.

Jan Tritten became a homebirth midwife in 1976, following the homebirth of her second child. Her first was born in the hospital, and the difference between the two births sent her into her midwifery career. She retired from active midwifery in 1989 in order to devote her time to her work as founder and editor of Midwifery Today and The Birthkit. Changing the way birth is done is her calling.

AUTONOMY: USING YOUR FULL POTENTIAL

by Naolí Vinaver

Maria called me one morning to say her waters had broken. She was thirty-five weeks and one day pregnant. During the first half of that day we felt disappointed and somewhat helpless, but during the second half we worked as a team to research, meditate and make decisions that led us to decide to bypass my established protocol of not attending a homebirth before thirty-six weeks gestation.

We reviewed standard medical procedures as well as possible alternatives, and we used midwifery and homeopathic techniques to prevent the risk of infection while we tried to prolong the onset of labor. During our research we were comforted by the discovery that if at least twenty-four hours elapse between rupture of membranes and the birth of a premature baby, the baby has a much greater chance of being born with mature lungs than if he were forced to come out sooner.

I also contacted other midwives whose experienced opinions came from working within alternative communities and autonomous midwifery. Together we decided it was best to sidestep standard protocol in an effort to avoid the senseless interventions that Maria and her child were sure to experience if they put themselves in the hands of the local medical establishment.

Meanwhile, Maria, her husband, their close family and I discussed at length the possibility of death, the meaning of life, and what it could mean to follow one's heart when society as a whole could disapprove of one's choices. We talked about what it could mean to work as a team in a common and ultimate experience such as the giving and receiving of life. We also read together and spoke calmly and carefully about the worst and best possible outcomes if we were to go ahead with the homebirth.

We made a clear and concise plan of action in which each person present had a specific assignment in case anything out of the ordinary had to be done or if we needed to transport to the hospital. If the couple decided to go ahead with the homebirth, I asked them to base their decision on their own sense of "rightness," independent of my own. I urged them to separate their sense of security from the trust they felt in my abilities as their midwife, and to question whether they would be ready to face and accept the worst outcome without feeling they had made their decisions based on a false sense of security. In other words, I asked them to take responsibility for their decisions while I took responsibility for mine.

Any couple who plans a homebirth should go through this process, but Maria's situation helped me see within a new context what autonomous midwifery can come to mean. Our shared research, introspection and decisions established a deep mutual respect based on facts, responsibility and trust. We were ready to face life and encounter what was coming, paving the way for the best possible outcome at the same time we were readying ourselves for the worst, with full grace, responsibility and love—together.

AUTONOMY

An autonomous midwife uses varying kinds of logic that help her make decisions suitable to a specific situation. She respects the woman's ways and is flexible to her needs while together they weigh the clinical, scientific, personal, economic, cultural, political, intuitive and all other possible kinds of logic that may come into play. The kind of logic that does not recognize a midwife's autonomy is wholly concerned with following strict clinical or hospital protocols or regulations, regardless of a client's needs. Midwives in many countries are working within medical or even midwifery systems that do not allow for autonomy.

Sooner or later most midwives are confronted by situations that challenge us and oblige us to search deeply inside for possibilities and answers. We search for ways to continue caring for our clients with honesty of heart and spirit in tandem with what we consider safe, remembering that normalcy and risk are often subjective and depend on what lens we are looking through.

My practice encompasses both rural and urban communities in the state of Veracruz, Mexico. These settings provide me with multiple opportunities to be enriched and challenged daily. I also have a degree in anthropology, which serves as an interesting springboard with which to exercise my mind. The concepts of a good life, death, health, good birth, good care, risk and so forth depend upon personal, cultural, economic and other contextual factors that define reality in a certain situation at any given moment.

I am a devoted and passionate midwife. I am cautious and careful about clinical detail, and at the same time, I respect a client's individual needs. This may seem contradictory, and it is indeed challenging at times to be both cautious and permissive or relaxed while dealing with something new or unusual in my practice. I am deeply committed to respecting and honoring my clients and their families while protecting their well being like an eagle protects her young.

Autonomous midwifery is the most difficult kind of midwifery because it is the midwife who carries most of the weight of the process and who shoulders the social and legal responsibility for the outcome. Ultimately, though, the autonomous midwife will feel the most satisfaction with her work, given that the families are fully aware of all decisions made for their care. And indeed, autonomous midwifery practices should have standards, guidelines and protocols, but in the hands of responsible midwives these should be made of stretchable fabric to suit specific needs of individual women and their unique birth processes.

MARIA'S BIRTH

Maria took excellent care of herself during the three and a half days between the initial rupture of her membranes and the onset of labor. Every four hours, we monitored her temperature, pulse, baby's heart rate, smell of the amniotic fluid on her pads, and her general sense of well being. All the signs were perfect. She drank about five liters of water daily, took Sepia 30x and eight grams of vitamin C every day to support her body's ability to continue in good health. We planned to begin a course of antibiotics on the fourth day, as a way to further prevent a possible infection, and to go to the hospital if we began to see any signs of infection.

That same morning, at thirty-five weeks plus five days gestation, Maria woke with light contractions. The birth process was beginning. Maria got up to walk and welcome the bigger contractions that would bring on her child. Her contractions, though very strong, were irregular and never closer than every eight to twenty minutes apart. I didn't even notice when she went into transition, although in retrospect it probably was when she became ill-mannered with her mother, saying she was going to walk outside in her nightgown and take the bus to the hospital!

When I checked Maria for the first time, she was ten centimeters dilated with a nice head pressing down. She was still having strong contractions about every ten to twenty minutes. I gave her a homeopathic to help establish a rhythmic labor. She pushed eagerly and well. She asked for cup after cup of yogurt, joked and teased with all of us, and stuffed her mouth with handfuls of almonds between contractions and naps. Sometimes she looked at a photograph of her long-dead father and asked him for strength and guidance. The baby's head never failed to move down with each push, even if only a little bit, and his scalp color and heartbeat were always perfect. The baby's cranium had time to slowly mold and slowly crown, which is beneficial because a preterm baby's skull can be softer and could suffer from too fast a delivery.

Three and a half hours passed before the baby was born. The second his head emerged he cried lustily, and was pinker than any pink baby I have ever seen. This baby made it clear to all present that he was determined to breathe and be present and well. This birth was the essence of beauty and perfection, enjoyed by everyone, although in rather slow motion.

WHAT ARE WE WILLING TO NEGOTIATE?

I have worked with women and birth since 1988; seven of those years have been in an independent midwifery practice in Mexico, where midwifery is a-legal. I attend women in their homes, oftentimes far away from roads and hospitals. Some of the women I care for are anemic or not fully healthy in some way, and some already have several children who need their mother to be present to care for their needs. Economic resources are very scarce for most families, yet others receive the university's health coverage plan and have almost everything available to them. I have seen birth as an emotional experience, a physical ordeal and ecstasy, a difficult rite of passage, a feminine task to do and get over with. Birth is an exciting way of claiming independence for a teenage mother, or a frightening bridge made of unsubstantial materials that needs to be crossed.

I take all of these factors into account when I think about my autonomy. Many are the ways of birthing—there are many challenges, many ways of attaining good outcomes, and the opinions on how to do one thing the "best" way are varied. But without autonomy, I would never have the flexibility to serve women in all the ways their lives require.

I am a midwife because there is nothing else I could do better. I was invited through dreams and circumstances to attend women in birth and to help their babies arrive as safely and lovingly as it could be done. I view my work as a midwife not only as a passionate effort to offer my best possible service to women who need midwifery care, but as an opportunity to learn from each of these women about the immensity of birth.

Mexican midwives are trying to define our profession for the future. We are having to face each other, with our differences, just as thousands of midwives have had to do all over the world in order to create organizations, structures and plans of action to ensure the survival of midwifery. We have begun to discuss terminology that could better suit our legislative efforts. At one meeting, some of us decided to adopt the World Health Organization's definition of "midwife," although it requires that a midwife be trained and recognized by her government. If we are to keep this definition, we are also sure to face a threat to the autonomy of the midwifery profession, which we now enjoy to a great degree.

It is important that we Mexican midwives and all midwives around the world think seriously about the true meaning of our labor as midwives. Thinking about it forces us to appreciate what it means to work as autonomous midwives, and to consider the aspects of our practices we are willing to compromise in the name of safety and protocols, and of a midwifery association.

We cannot simply obey rules and guidelines blindly, without regard to the special needs and situations of each of our clients, because that would require us to offer individuals a practice that comes in only one size. Then we cease to learn about birth from birthing women. Autonomy respects the individual and what she has to teach us. It means putting the well being of the mother and her baby before set guidelines and protocols that don't serve her individual needs. It means respecting the desires and needs of the woman and her family while watching out for, preventing and steering clear of possible harm to them.

An autonomous midwife continues to observe, think, ask, learn and expand her parameters and vision, thanks to the opportunities life has to offer. Autonomous midwifery means acting with full awareness and responsibility, which requires the midwife to have her eyes open along with her heart, mind and spirit. This is as challenging as being a midwife itself, as challenging as living life to the fullest every day. I ask myself, would I want to be a midwife if I were not free and able to tap on my full potential as a thinking and feeling human being?

This article first appeared in Midwifery Today Issue No. 42.

Naolí Vinaver is the MANA representative from Mexico. She is also a popular teacher at Midwifery Today conferences.

A GRAND TRIUMPH

by Judy Edmunds

Pregnant with her first child, Michelle planned to deliver at the local hospital since costs were covered by her subsidized insurance. Also, the medical setting provided her with a sense of security she didn't think she'd feel at home. Personal issues led her to require a female attendant, so she found a woman doctor who had been providing care and agreed to handle the birth. Although her pregnancy was normal, Michelle had had just about every prenatal test money can buy. Now, she was past her due date by five days.

Following a routine prenatal exam, the doctor said, "Oh, by the way…" and nonchalantly informed Michelle she'd be out of town for the next few days. Unless she wanted to go to the hospital for a Pitocin induction right then, Michelle was told that a couple of male doctors would be on call in case she went into labor. She closed the door and left Michelle sitting dumbfounded in the office.

When she returned home, Michelle informed Janna, her doula. Janna then called me, to see if I had any advice. The doctor, although still in town, refused to answer Janna's calls. Finally, the doctor's husband, also a physician, called Janna and told her if Michelle had expected someone to be on call twenty-four hours a day, "she should have hired a midwife." He added, however, that he could not recommend that choice for "safety reasons." Further discussion with him proved fruitless; he maintained that as long as competent male doctors were available, the medical obligation was satisfied—even though she'd been promised a female attendant.

We contacted other female doctors in local obstetrical practices, but none would agree to take call. The consensus was that Michelle would just have to obey her doctor, present at the hospital, and take whoever was on call. The system would not bend. While it was probable that Michelle would not begin labor anytime soon due to the stressful situation, it made sense to prepare contingency plans. At last, after a great deal of work, we made arrangements: A midwife with hospital privileges in a neighboring county agreed to be on call. I had spent hours advocating for a woman whom I'd never met. Later, I spent even more time thinking about it. The physicians' actions struck me as callous and abhorrent, although not particularly unusual in our local medical community. Their lack of regard for Michelle's emotional welfare saddened and angered me.

AT A PREMIUM

While shopping the next day, I noticed hand-dipped chocolates, homegrown vegetables, hand-spun wool, homemade preserves, cottage-industry soaps—all at premium prices, since they were made with care, individually, by hand, at home. I reflected, too, on how "old-fashioned" doctors, famous for house calls and compassion, are remembered fondly as part of the "good old days" and praised for their one-on-one caring. I mused how our society honors unique, special, one-of-a-kind items and services.

Yet when it comes to maternity care, it seems the bigger and busier, the better: high-tech procedures, standardized treatment, massive patient loads, in-and-out, assembly-line-style facilities. We are urged to leave the clean peace and quiet of home and go, instead, to a large, centralized center, entrusting ourselves to a system of detached and often distracted institutional workers whom we've never met and may never see again. I find it hard to believe that anyone would consider hospital care preferable if they really thought about it.

High-tech or hands-on? The choice is not new. In many cases, of course, mechanical and technological advances have been just that: improvements. Other advances, as we all know too well, have resulted in lasting harm.

The Luddites became famous for the way they handled the dilemma of "progress." The skilled English weavers lived in villages centered around, and supported by, the cottage production of quality textiles. The work was honorable, clean, sustainable, fulfilling. When the encroaching mechanization of the industrial revolution of the 1800s forced more and more families from their looms and into poverty, the Luddites rose up and began destroying the new machines. Finally, military force crushed the rebellion. For the most part, history remembers Luddites with ridicule: simple people standing in the way of modern progress. But apart from the obvious reasons for revolt was the seldom considered secondary reason: the marked difference in resulting materials. The factories turned out inferior products. The machines were an affront to the Luddites' profession, an insult to their skill.

There are those who smirkingly label midwives as Neo-Luddites, hopeless sentimentalists, backward in their ways, slow to step aside for the advance of technology. We don't run around smashing electronic fetal heart monitors, but we do point to studies verifying what works and what doesn't, what's cost-effective and what's wasteful. Yes, the truth stands unchallenged: run-amok technology tears at the very fabric of society and results in expensive, though inferior, care. On the other hand, a skilled, intuitive, individualized approach leads to superior client satisfaction and outcomes. This is indisputable.

I ruminated on these two very different options: one in which the patient queues up to enter a machine-monitored maternity system, where a patient is often just a passing face, an interesting case, treated more like an inconvenience, an income generator, and the other, an option laced with choices and careful, one-on-one, hands-on, home-based, intimately involved peer care. How can we communicate the nature of this choice to those who haven't thoroughly considered it? It was precisely the nature of this choice that I was trying to communicate to Michelle.

A BIRTH STORY

So, what did Michelle decide?

She didn't begin labor while her doctor was away, so Michelle kept a scheduled exam when her doctor returned. The doctor told Michelle she didn't remember ever promising her she'd actually deliver the baby herself. She then told Michelle that her baby had to be out prior to two weeks past her due date. Because it was nearing that deadline, Michelle said she felt pressured and pleaded for just a couple more days. Her doctor said something terrible would happen, and went so far as offering the phone numbers of women who'd had bad outcomes after the two-week mark. "Why don't I just break your water now?" she asked.

Michelle wanted to discuss it with her husband, so decided to wait. The next day, she was admitted to the hospital for prostaglandin gel, a non-stress test, and another ultrasound, her fourth. She was now eleven days past her due date.

The tests were normal, but the gel immediately caused Michelle a great deal of burning pain, which the doctor dismissed. She was to return the next day for more gel, then a Pitocin induction. Feeling more and more pressured and out of control, she confided to Janna that she felt she might as well just go in and let them do whatever they wanted to her, including a cesarean, just to get it over with. She had severe back pain and incoordinate contractions due to the gel, which made sleep impossible. If labor is worse than this, she told Janna, I know I'll never make it. Janna asked her if she might like to talk to a midwife for suggestions on comfort measures, or for answers to any questions she might have.

Michelle called me the next day and we talked for a long time. I explained ways to ease her back pain and encourage functional contractions, and went into detail about her options. I told her if she went in for the induction, and corresponding epidural, her chances of surgical delivery were greatly increased. Still, she had to decide for herself what to do. She asked how I handled overdue pregnancies. I explained that if it was really time for the baby to come out, I might use a combination of herbs, homeopathy, walking, castor oil, massage, visualization, nipple stimulation, evening primrose oil, warm baths, and cervical stretching, depending on the situation.

She questioned the cervical stretching, so I explained: Once the cervix has softened, either on its own or with the aid of prostaglandin enhancers (such as evening primrose oil), or with actual prostaglandins (semen or the gel she'd already had), I gently pull the cervix forward with one finger and let it relax for a few moments. Then I slowly work another finger into it and gradually, very carefully, allow the cervix to open up more and more, as I apply only the slightest pressure. It often takes a couple of hours, but usually results in dilation of at least six centimeters, although it may shrink down to three or four centimeters without continued contractions. However, the cervical contact, in combination with nipple stimulation, usually produces the required contractions, motivating a sluggish labor to progress quickly. (While one should consider the possibility of accidentally rupturing the membranes with this technique, I have never had that happen. Michelle and I discussed this, too.) Allowing the cervix to open, rather than forcing it, usually makes it painless. This intrigued her. She asked if I would consider doing that if labor still wasn't established by evening. I agreed.

That night, I met her for the first time. She had cancelled her appointment for more gel, and decided to try to hold out for a more natural approach. I stretched her cervix to six or seven centimeters, explained her baby's position, and answered many questions. I felt much more optimistic for her and hoped she would have the baby by morning.

However, she called after another sleepless night. The contractions had slowed, but her back pain kept her awake. Now she was desperate. This kind of pain was more than she had bargained for. We talked, again, for a very long time. Finally, I told her it sounded like she really needed to eat, and suggested a long, warm bath. But she was supposed to go to the hospital for the induction, she told me. And, her doctor was not on call—the physician's husband was! What should she do? I reminded her to eat, to call Janna for support, to bathe, and to try to relax. I could only hope the doctors wouldn't do their surgery voodoo, but it was looking more and more likely. It was a pathetic situation.

That afternoon, returning from a home visit with my next scheduled client, I couldn't stop thinking of Michelle. How was she doing? What was happening? I wanted so much for her to have a good experience, but I tried to convince myself that it was not my concern: She had chosen the doctor/hospital route; I can't rescue everybody; it's just one of those things. I thought of those arguments and more as I tried to distance myself from a woman I cared about, and a situation I felt I could not change.

Early that evening, when I still hadn't heard anything, I called Janna for an update. She hadn't heard anything either, so I encouraged her to call, knowing Michelle could use the support. Janna called back and reported Michelle had remained at home, laboring in the tub, and was feeling pushy. Would I meet Janna there to check her? Wow! Yes! I threw birth supplies into the car and zoomed to her house. There she was, a changed person, working through her contractions, experiencing pressure. A check revealed she was at nine centimeters, +3 station, strong contractions. Great!

Michelle pleaded with us—she didn't want to leave. Couldn't she just stay in the tub? "This isn't bad at all! I've gotten this far!" she said. Yes, I told her, I think that would be lovely. I brought in equipment while she asked her husband what he thought. She could do it, she said, and wasn't scared anymore. A home waterbirth was not at all what they'd planned. It was a new thought to him, but he guessed it would be OK, since she wanted it so badly.

The bathtub was filled to the brim, and we kept refreshing the hot water from kettles boiling on the stove. During contractions, Michelle turned on the overhead shower, so she was immersed in hot water and drenched with a warm rain. The bathroom was like a tropical jungle. It worked for her. As contractions strengthened, we added a fan, and she enlisted her husband's aid in pulling on a towel wrapped around her hips. He sat on the toilet seat, an awkward, back-twisting spot, to give her his strength. What a team!

After a time, the energy changed, and she got out to utilize gravity. She sat on a rocking chair, working with the towel, sometimes leaping up to plunge back into the tub, until she settled down to push in earnest. She pushed mightily, and the head got closer. After a time, however, it was apparent she would need the extra room afforded by a squat. When she was ready to meet the challenge, she sank down into a deep, wide squat. Instantly, the head was there, and soon the perineum bulged over it. At the peak of the stretch, she paused for several long minutes—the head halfway out, the perineum pulled tight, birth imminent. She was savoring the moment. No scalpels, orders to push, or frantic staff. The baby, doing fine, was patient, too. When she was ready, she pushed again, and her plump, eight pound, ten ounce, Apgar 10-10 girl came kicking and hollering out over her intact perineum. Right at home.

Well, the doctor was none too happy, and some colleagues like to venture their worries of "what if, what if?" But I know a triumph when I see it, and we had a grand one that night. Sometimes, you just have to stand up and take back what's rightfully yours. Ignore the threats and scare tactics and give birth at home, hands-on, with dignity. It's only natural.

This article first appeared in Midwifery Today Issue No. 37.

Judy Edmunds has been an active traditional community midwife in northwest Washington since 1981. She is a chartered herbalist, registered nutritional consultant, community health educator and cervical cap fitter. She integrates all her training into whole-woman care. Judy is a contributing editor at Midwifery Today.

DIRECT-ENTRY MIDWIFERY EDUCATION:
CAUGHT IN THE MIDDLE

by Sharon Wells, LM, CPM

> "There is no such thing as a neutral educational process. Education either functions as an instrument which is used to facilitate the integration of a person into the logic of the present system and brings about the conformity to it, or it becomes 'the practice of freedom,' the means by which men and women deal critically and creatively with reality and discover how to participate in the transformation of their world. The development of an educational methodology that facilitates this process will inevitably lead to tension and conflict within our society."
>
> — Paolo Freire, *Pedagogy of the Oppressed*

Midwives are caught in a vise between this nation's maternity care crisis and the political-educational debate that surrounds midwifery education. At the same time that maternity care needs of women and babies are not being met because of the acute shortage of care providers, a readily available pool of direct-entry midwives who have been trained through a variety of educational routes stands ready to help alleviate the maternity care crisis. They are being prevented from contributing to the solution by lack of legal recognition, however, which essentially hinges on the question of their education. This quandary requires that we work quickly to solve the midwifery education dilemma. In doing so, however, prevailing attitudes about the means and ends of education have to be examined and addressed in order to understand the impasse direct-entry midwives are locked in.

An educational master plan developed in the early 1900s and discussed in the essay "Gospel of Wealth" by Andrew Carnegie was designed to promote societal management through public education in the United States. This plan was intended to reinforce conformity and standardization and produce automatons with pre-thought ideas for a safe, non-revolutionary world. It is aimed at molding the student into measurable behaviors and fostering loyalty to the state rather than strengthening family ties, promoting community involvement and encouraging spirituality and culture. According to John Gatto, author of *Dumbing Us Down*, schools are where modern scientific stupidity masquerades as real knowledge, whereas real knowledge is learned through self-questioning and individuality. He refers to the institution of public education as "government factory schools" and "government monopoly schools."

Behavioral psychologist and educator B.F. Skinner, who advocated the use of predetermined, measurable outcomes called behavioral objectives, once wrote that "we must accept that some kind of control of human affairs is inevitable." On the other hand, experiential psychologist and educator Carl Rogers put forth that "there are two types of learning: meaningless rote and significant, meaningful, experiential learning that is self-motivated." To him, knowledge is cumulative; everyone needs the freedom to learn and choose self-direction.

Looking at the history of American education in these conflicting terms, we have to ask ourselves which philosophy of education underlies present-day midwifery education. As many states and national organizations explore direct-entry midwifery education, significant issues are being raised: Does direct-entry midwifery education have a curriculum or educational format? Can it fit into a specified time frame? What test format will be used; how will apprentice education be validated; do schools need to be university-based or affiliated; do they need to be accredited and if so, by whom? In what setting will this midwife work? Just what kind of midwife are we aiming to produce? And after all is said and done, who gets the final say-so?

THE EVOLUTION OF MIDWIFERY EDUCATION

In the colonial and pioneer days of this country, most babies were delivered by midwives or family members. Prior to World War II in the rural South, the poor were delivered by midwives trained through midwifery apprenticeships, the local health department and local doctors. The methods of training were apprenticeship, self-study and short term midwifery intensive courses. These midwives delivered babies at home. In the North in the early 1900s, the frequent subject of debate within the medical community was the "midwife problem"— immigrant midwives who were attending births at home within their own ethnic groups.

In 1925, Mary Breckinridge, an American-trained nurse and British-trained midwife, brought other British-trained midwives to the Kentucky Appalachian Mountains and started the Frontier Nursing Service. Aspiring midwives first trained as nurses in the United States, next went to Great Britain for midwifery training, then returned to Frontier Nursing Service to attend homebirths in rural Appalachia. With the onset of World War II it became necessary to develop a school to train nurses to become midwives without sending them overseas.

In 1939, The Frontier School of Midwifery graduated its first two American-trained nurse-midwives. At the same time in New York City the Association for the Promotion and the Standardization of Midwifery Education was created. Its educational model was the British midwifery curricula, and this started the attempt to standardize midwifery education in the United States.

Meanwhile obstetrics had become an established medical specialty. According to Helen Varney, author of *Nurse-Midwifery*, "obstetric care began a mass movement out of the home into the hospital, and laws were passed to regulate the practice of the indigenous midwife." In the 1940s obstetrical care was offered free for low-income women if they would go to a teaching hospital to be delivered by a student doctor. At this point, many of the rural poor were duped into thinking that a hospital birth that had previously been unavailable to them was superior to the services of their community midwife.

Except for Frontier Nursing Service, midwifery almost died out in the United States.

It was restored during the resurgence of homebirths in the 1960s and 1970s among women who taught themselves to be midwives through their own experiences, self study and apprenticeships with a few willing doctors, midwives and health departments.

Both educational routes of entry into midwifery—formal and informal—began to grow in the United States. Certified nurse-midwives became recognized and licensed in all fifty states. Jessica Mitford, author of *The American Way of Birth*, described CNMs as "adjuncts to obstetrical personnel in hospitals, subordinate to physicians in charge. In general they do not officiate at homebirths, which are frowned on by their medical superiors." In contrast, Mitford explains, the underlying philosophy of direct-entry midwifery is that in more than 98 percent of cases child-birth is a natural procedure in which medical intervention is not only unnecessary, but often harmful. The direct-entry midwife attends family-centered homebirths and "her clients are for the most part well-educated women . . . determined to avoid the male-dominated world of the hospital."

THE EDUCATION SPECTRUM

One of the educational movements within the medical community has been to produce a standardized midwife through an accredited educational institution. The programs provide for a prescribed course of study with specific behavioral objectives and a predetermined time frame according to each institution of education. Nursing is the prerequisite for these midwifery programs. Hospitals and clinics are the prima-ry clinical sites. Within this structure, midwifery educators promote critical thinking and provide experiential learning in the clinical sites available to them. Students in some programs report that even though they are taught to handle many complica-tions independently, often they are required to call the doctor at signs of anything abnormal. The standard of normality is usually adopted from a white, male-idealized concept of the female body and the birth process.

This midwifery student has been taught to approach complications allopathically because of the practice environment. The student often has a difficult time working in a manner that incorporates continuity of care in such a setting. Nurse-midwifery educators fight to avoid the dangers pointed out by Carl Rogers when he discusses institutionally based education. Writes one, "We are locked into a traditional and conventional approach which makes significant learning improbable if not impossi-ble. When we are put together in one scheme, such elements as a prescribed cur-riculum, similar assignments for all students, lecturing as the major mode of instruc-tion, standard tests by which all students are externally evaluated, and instructor-chosen grades as the measure of learning can almost guarantee that meaningful learn-ing will be at an absolute minimum."

Midwifery educators are affecting change within the existing institutions, but it comes slowly in the pathology-oriented environment of the hospital. There mid-wifery remains under the surveillance of the American College of Obstetrics and Gynecology (ACOG) and the American Medical Association (AMA) who think they are at the top of the power and educational hierarchy.

In many states, medical legislation is indirectly controlled by medical coalitions that give large contributions to legislators and legislative campaigns. Can we logically deduce that the subtle message being sent is that the medical cartel aims to control the educational process for midwifery, and that they wish to turn out "factory-educated" obstetrical technicians who are called nurse-midwives or professional midwives working in institutional settings—clinics and hospitals—under physician supervision?

The apprenticeship model of education is at the opposite end of the midwifery educational spectrum. Many direct-entry midwives are trained by apprenticeship. This student is in an experientially based educational setting that is client centered, where education is self paced, self motivated and community oriented. Learning occurs within the setting of the midwifery practice and is not a separate clinical site. Most learning is experiential and/or problem solving in nature. Didactic learning occurs by self study, guided study courses or workshops. The educational focus is upon normal pregnancy, labor, delivery, postpartum and the newborn. The student learns continuity of care, counseling skills and to trust her intuition as well as her skills. The length of this educational process depends upon the apprentice and the midwife, but usually lasts from two to four years. The mentor may suggest using core competencies and a skills check list if they are available. "Graduation" occurs when the senior midwife and the apprentice think the apprentice is ready to function as a midwife safely on her own. Most births occur at home.

Neither educational route into midwifery is perfect. Direct-entry midwifery educators do not want to mass produce a medical model "obstetrical technician" or mini doctor who bears the title of midwife but who has limited experiential learning. Nor do midwifery educators want to promote birth attendants who call themselves midwives but who have inadequate knowledge and skills and threaten the safety of the public.

The fact remains, however, that the United States finds itself in the midst of a maternity care crisis with an inadequate number of maternity care providers. It also finds itself in the middle of an educational dilemma where the medical monopoly's primary concern is the institutional standardization of midwifery education and practice.

INSTRUMENT FOR CHANGE

Why is the medical monopoly so opposed to the experientially based learning approach to midwifery called apprenticeship? Why does the medical monopoly insist that education occur within or be affiliated with an institution? Has the apprentice-trained, community midwife who is doing homebirths become a threat to the medical monopoly?

The midwife is often the instrument for change within a family because the family members are empowered by the prenatal and birth experiences, and they begin to believe in their own bodies and intuitions. Is the medical monopoly fearful that these families will start investigating alternatives to the medical model? When people in a community begin to take care of their own healthcare needs, the medical monopoly loses money and power. It can be deduced that the push for standardized, institutionalized midwifery education is an effort to stop the growth of the homebirth movement in the United States.

It is vastly important to the total picture of the healthcare revolution whether or not we mass produce midwives out of a medical mold with pre-thought concepts or whether we experientially train midwives who will develop problem solving, thinking skills that may include alternative healthcare. The educational philosophy that we adopt for midwifery education programs is very important because it is how we shape the future of midwifery in the United States. An educational philosophy that is based in experiential learning through the apprenticeship model is the essential choice for the continuation of community midwifery and homebirth.

American midwifery is at the brink of an educational revolution. Direct-entry midwifery educators must be brave and careful that they do not fall into any bureaucratic traps set up with the pretense of "acceptability" and monetary benefits. Direct-entry midwifery education cannot allow itself to be shaped into an image that does not reflect an experiential educational philosophy. Manipulation can only occur if we give our consent. Midwifery educators cannot allow themselves to be coerced into rubber stamping an educational philosophy that does not include apprenticeship—a valid, experientially-based educational model. Midwifery educators must not support an educational model that propagates more "government monopoly schools" that will mass produce more institutionalized midwives under the guise of direct-entry midwifery education.

If a new midwifery educational route is to be created, it must have a strong apprenticeship foundation within a loose educational framework called Core Competencies adopted by the Midwives Alliance of North America (MANA). In the existing educational forum, there are a variety of community based, post-secondary educational models that have mechanisms for validating life experiences and competency-based education for adult learners. Many of these innovative models can be adapted to meet the needs of midwifery education. Educators need to be inclusive rather than exclusive as we look at the variety of educational models. A primary factor in the success of these direct-entry programs, however, is that direct-entry midwives must maintain control and leadership of this educational process.

There is a need for midwives in all settings—hospitals, birth centers and homes. To meet that need, midwifery educators must unite in the primary goal of increasing the number of midwives in a timely fashion. It is not a competition of whether midwives should be nurse-midwives or direct-entry midwives or work in hospitals or homes. Every midwife is necessary, and all routes of entry into midwifery must be validated quickly if we are to make a timely difference in America's maternity care crisis.

References

Davis, E. & Richardson, T. (1992). "The Apprenticeship Route to Midwifery Education–Working Draft." *MANA News.* X(4), 14-15.

Freire, Paolo. (1990). *Pedagogy of the Oppressed.* New York: The Continuum Publishing Co.

Gatto, J. (1992). *Dumbing Us Down.* Philadelphia: New Society Publishers.

Gatto, J. (1992). *The Future of Education: What a School Should Deliver, a Teacher's Views and Ideas.* (Video). New York: Shelter Island Association.

Gatto, J. (1992). *You Won't Get an Education from School Books*. (Video). Hamilton, New York: Alliance for Parental Involvement in Education.

McCallister, W.J. (1971). "The Growth of Freedom and Education." A Crucial Interpretation of Some Historical Views. New York: Kennikat Press. Vol 11.

Mitford, J. (1992). *The American Way of Birth*. New York: Penguin Books.

Proceedings from International Seminar: Philosophy and Education. (1967). Ontario: The Ontario Institute of Studies in Education.

Rogers, C. (1989). *Dialogues*. Boston: Houghton Mifflin Co.

Rogers, C. (1902). *Freedom to Learn: A View of What Education Might Become*. New York: Merrill Publishing Co.

Rogers, C. (1964). "The Place of the Person in the New World of Behavioral Sciences." *Readings in Learning and Human Abilities*.

Skinner, B. F. (1971). *Beyond Freedom and Dignity*. New York: Random House, Inc.

Skinner, B.F. (1955). "Freedom and Control of Men." American Scholar. New York: Random House. 47-65.

Steinberg, I.S. (1980). *Behaviorism and Schooling*. New York: St. Martin.

Varney, H. (1983). *Nurse-Midwifery*. Boston: Blackwell Scientific Publications Inc.

This article was written especially for this book.

Sharon Wells, MS, LM, CPM, is the homebirth mother of two daughters. Sharon has been a practicing midwife for seventeen years and has assisted moms in the birth process of over 400 babies, including her granddaughter. Sharon graduated from the University of Tennessee with her BS in education in 1966, and her MS in educational psychology with a specialization in reading in 1972. She became an emergency medical technician in 1976, and then graduated from the North Florida School of Midwifery and was licensed by the state of Florida in 1988. She became a certified professional midwife (CPM) in 1995.

Sharon was one of the founding mothers and administrator of The North Florida School of Midwifery. She was a founding mother and the first president of the Midwives Alliance of New York (MANY), was a representative from MANA to the Interorganizational Workgroup on Midwifery Education sponsored by the Carnegie Foundation, was one of the original board members and founding mothers of the Midwifery Education Accreditation Council (MEAC), and is listed in Who's Who of American Women. Sharon is presently a member of the North American Registry of Midwives (NARM) board and serves in the capacity as coordinator of certification for the certified professional midwife (CPM).

START WITH THE SMALL CIRCLE:

AN INTERVIEW WITH ELIZABETH DAVIS

by Cher Mikkola

Staff editors Cher Mikkola and Joel Southern met with author, educator, lecturer and midwife Elizabeth Davis during the Sixth Annual West Coast Midwifery Today Conference in June, 1997 to talk about her role in birth change. Elizabeth emphasized education as one of the most telling forces in changing childbirth and the arena in which she has accomplished the most work. The following is an interview Elizabeth shared with Cher Mikkola for Midwifery Today:

In 1972, at age twenty-one, Elizabeth Davis was in labor with her first child. Because she started labor a month early and the woman she planned to have attend her birth was out of town, she was in a hospital, facing the routines and interventions common during that time. They included buccal Pitocin, lateral episiotomy and painkillers after delivery that led to a seven-hour separation from her son, even though she'd pleaded to have him brought to her. Once he was finally in her arms, combed, bathed and groomed, she fought the rejective behaviors that all mammals—humans included—display if their young are taken from them at birth and later reintroduced.

"As I began the postpartum attempt to reconstruct myself and my intimacy with my son, to breastfeed and cope with the miserable pain in my bottom, to deal with the Amazon complex that led me to wash diapers in my wringer washer and hang them up on the line two days after I gave birth, to make bread and can peaches and God knows what, I called my mom for assistance. I said to her, 'Why didn't you tell me what birth would be like?' She said, 'As my doctor told me after your sister's difficult birth, if the cake is good, eat it'—meaning that a healthy baby is the important thing. That was the point when something in me said, 'No! I'm worth more than that. Women are worth more than that. I am not going down that road.' If I had bought that line, my whole identity would have funneled down, with me emotionally disabled. Even though I didn't at the time connect that 'no' to the 'yes' of midwifery, that was the turning point."

In the years that followed, Elizabeth completed her training as a midwife, and later became an educator, lecturer, political activist, and author of numerous books on midwifery, birth and women's issues. Driven by her desire to help other women have satisfying births, and by her passion to secure the future of midwifery, she now concentrates much of her attention on radicalizing the nature of midwifery education.

"My journey in midwifery had taken me increasingly into areas of women's psychology, specifically into the study of how women learn. I discovered that women tend to learn differently than men. In general, men are more comfortable learning in a linear fashion, acquiring chunks of knowledge and more or less stacking them bricklayer style until a conclusion can be drawn. In contrast, women prefer to learn by encircling their area of inquiry. They cast as large a net as possible around the subject at hand, and will often deliberately solicit conflicting viewpoints, just to consider things from all angles. Once they have a complete package of information, they move to the center, or the heart of the matter, for a solution.

"This connects to recent research on the neurophysiology of men and women cited in my book, *Women, Sex and Desire: Exploring Your Sexuality at Every Stage of Life*, on the basic differences in male and female brain structure. In the female brain, verbal and emotional centers are replicated in both hemispheres, with a very broad corpus callosum uniting both hemispheres. Thus, women are adept at verbalizing a multiplicity of factors, at handling complexity, at juggling four or five activities at a time.

"In the male brain, the verbal center is in one hemisphere, the emotional center in the other, with a much narrower corpus callosum connecting the two. So if we wonder why it is that men sometimes have trouble articulating feelings, perhaps the reason is not as much cultural as biological. My concern here is that, as regards midwifery education, we stop trying to utilize educational models unsuited to women's ways of knowing and learning.

"In conventional midwifery training courses, students are expected to tackle an entire anatomy course and know everything there is to know about the subject without any idea of its relevance to midwifery. They must obediently learn, memorize, and spit this information back to their instructor. They go on the same way with physiology, microbiology, genetics, nutrition. After all this, someone on the faculty may tie it all together for them if they are lucky."

In contrast, Elizabeth's beginning course, Heart and Hands Midwifery Intensives, provides an integrated overview of the subject in which all aspects of midwifery care are presented in context. "Beyond details, students want meaning, relevance, connection of one subject area to another." After the beginning course, students wishing to enroll in her three year program, The Midwifery Institute of California, progress to in-depth study in specific subject areas. Elizabeth has observed that most students want the big picture at the beginning, so they know where they stand, and can realistically assess their strengths and weaknesses both personally and academically. "I think it's best to start with the small circle—like you're making a clay pot," Elizabeth mused. "Make the circle complete in the beginning, for a good, strong base. Hit all the points on the spectrum, cover all the basic areas. Then make a larger circle, and in this larger sweep, go more in-depth. As this occurs, give the student clinical experience so that each time she comes around to a specific subject area again, her questions and her application of knowledge will be ever more profound."

MIDWIFERY TRAINING

In harmonious concert with women's learning style is the apprenticeship training model, which Elizabeth considers to be the best method for preparing midwives. The advantages are many—not only does the student experience continuity of care in her training, but she experiences continuity of caregiver, and thus has opportunity to explore and develop her own capacity for intimate relationship. Elizabeth considers these to be linchpins of the midwifery model.

"The ability to form profound intimate relationships is one of the most essential requisites of the aspiring midwife," Elizabeth said quietly. "As midwifery goes mainstream, we're beginning to see that you really can't substitute for this ability. A student may learn 'X' number of skills and demonstrate great technical competence, but if she doesn't have the ability to form deep intimate relationships, she will not be able to hear and understand what her clients want, and provide care that is truly woman-centered. There are larger issues in the future of midwifery than what I commonly refer to as our ability to jump through an endless series of legitimacy hoops."

Having recognized the medical profession's and ACNM's growing interest in direct-entry midwifery as a demonstration of its increasing power, Elizabeth has given much thought to the questions of what direct-entry midwifery will look like in the future and what kind of work direct-entry midwives will be doing. She concluded that it is important to offer the women who wish to become direct-entry midwives a flexible yet structured way in which to be trained. Take for example her Midwifery Institute of California, which became the first MEAC-accredited program in the country based on the apprenticeship model. Students take the Heart and Hands, and other program course work, either on-site in San Francisco or at-a-distance via modules. They then apprentice with a midwife in their own community, or wherever they choose. Both she and co-founder Shannon Anton believe this to be better than centralized, university-based training, in which students are often out of touch with the populations they serve.

Current apprehension about ACNM's proposal to accredit direct-entry programs has inspired Elizabeth to take a much longer view. "The fact that the ACNM has become concerned with our growing power is basically a good sign, and all the more reason for us to hold ever more strongly to what we know. This is a time for midwives who believe in autonomous, woman-centered care to pull together and refine their models of education and practice, because such is our springboard for the future. We're now at a crossroads where what we hold dear, and how firmly we hold it, will affect our profession for generations to come. We must seek to be as inclusive as possible in the institutional structures that we will inevitably create."

Not to say that underground midwifery won't continue, even if exclusion is minimized. "There will always be an underground," Elizabeth said calmly, "because of our tendency to ostracize those who don't participate. Once the underground gets organized and articulates itself, it chinks away at the established structure and creates a new wave. And that new wave will engender yet another underground. That's the process of social change. We can keep our eyes open as we move along this trail, and know that behind us will be another generation that will shake us down, that we are wise not to exclude or censor."

THE NEW WAVE

Every beginning midwife needs a foundation of self-awareness, according to Elizabeth. After years of being a midwifery educator and seeing changes in the backgrounds of women who were coming to her for training, she wondered what might suit these women for the work of being a midwife. She found that they all had some experience of meeting their demons, encountering grief, engaging in struggle or being pushed to the edge of their capabilities to transcend hardship. "That's what it takes to make a good midwife. You've got to have guts, humility and openness. I have some extremely brazen and challenging students. I try to make myself available to them to take me down, because I really believe that's a necessary part of their training. AND I give them not just my most glorious success stories, but my big, fat mistakes. I tell them, 'Boy, I blew it because I overestimated my strength,' or 'I was self-serving in this case,' etc. . . . I know those are the cases they learn the most from. I do my best not to teach in a hierarchical way." She continually tries to bring out qualities of self-awareness, fair play and courage in her students. In addition, she believes it is crucial to establish midwifery curriculum that takes these concerns to heart. In other words, how well-rounded and how deeply informed "on a myriad of levels" will a new midwife be after she's completed her training?

Fortunately, many contemporary midwifery students have the advantage of beginning their training at a different starting point than midwives of the recent past. "My students in their twenties are much more sure of their basic rights as women, and much more acknowledging of their sexual power. They're coming to me ready to study midwifery, not needing as extensive an overhaul in the areas of womancraft. I love this generation because as much as they have forced me to acknowledge my age, to reckon with the fact that I am of another era, they are going to go places that I can hardly envision. What could be better than being with the next generation of midwives who honor not only the work, but who honor my work? It's a completion for me; I am indeed passing on that which I need to transmit in my life."

Elizabeth cautions all midwives to remember that the ultimate focus is not the advancement of the profession, but healthy mothers and babies. When she teaches or works politically with other midwives, she tries to make a heart connection in this regard. "Especially if I'm speaking to midwives outside this country who are just beginning to organize, I always try to reassure them that it's normal to feel afraid, it is okay to feel afraid. Fear is genetically encoded in midwives. We know it well—we have a long history of persecution. However, we must try not to be frightened by our fear. If we react to fear with more fear, all those legitimacy hoops begin to look like the best and safest way to go. I think far too many of us have fallen prey to the seductive nature of those hoops. We need to acknowledge our fear; we need to say, 'Wherever we live and work, certain ones of us have been and will be persecuted for our wisdom and knowledge. It takes courage to hold it up. We can't do it alone, in isolation, so let's stick together, let's really get down to the heart and the soul of what it is we want to put forth and let's expand our model. Let's not worry about how medicine defines us anymore."

Elizabeth is quick to confirm how satisfied she feels with her life. Increasingly, she is concerned that midwives reclaim their traditional scope of practice, that of care 'from womb to tomb,' which she explores in depth in her most recent book, *The Women's Wheel of Life: Thirteen Archetypes of Woman at Her Fullest Power.* She feels we must re-sacralize the entirety of women's lives, and begin teaching our daughters much sooner about birth, love and sexuality. "There have been times when I've been tired, and I've wished that things were a little easier for me. But I'm living the life I want to live, and I have a voice in society, and a strong one with my peers. I'm surrounded by young women whom I respect and who respect me. I think that because of my experience of having heard my mother advise me as she did after my first birth, if any young woman looks me in the eye and says, 'Help me. Tell me there's hope for me as a woman, that I can be free and powerful, tell me it's true,' I'll do anything, anything for her. That's my fate, my destiny."

This article first appeared in Midwifery Today Issue No. 43.

Cher Mikkola has been an editor at Midwifery Today for twelve years and is also a freelance writer, editor and proofreader. She lives in Eugene, Oregon with her family.

Elizabeth Davis, BA, CPM, has been a midwife, women's healthcare specialist, author, educator and consultant for more than twenty years. She is active at national and international levels in issues of midwifery education and self-regulation, and is co-founder of the Midwifery Institute of California, a three year, MEAC accredited program. She is the author of five books, including the classic midwifery text, Heart & Hands: A Midwife's Guide to Pregnancy and Birth, now in its 3rd edition.

An Excerpt from *Heart and Hands*

BECOMING A MIDWIFE

by Elizabeth Davis, CPM

It is one thing to decide to become a midwife, and another to face the realities of acquiring the necessary training. Current educational pathways are often circuitous and may require much determination and endurance of the student. But what more appropriate introduction to the diligence and dedication required of the midwife? Although many women are attracted to midwifery for glory and glamour, it is probably one of the most challenging and personally rending professions in existence. Even as a student, the aspiring midwife must endure long hours, intense personal interactions and repeated sacrifice of personal and/or family time. Thus it is best if midwifery is less a career choice, and more a calling.

Should you choose to go through training to become a nurse-midwife, your course of study will be fairly well mapped out for you. A central advantage of becoming a nurse-midwife is legal practice anywhere in the country, and reciprocity state to state. Having utilized the political infrastructure of nursing to advance as a profession, nurse-midwifery is fairly well-positioned in our current healthcare system. But changes in this system may render certain perks of being a nurse-midwife obsolete. As HMOs seek cost-containment by using midwives in high-volume clinics or L & D units with little or no continuity of care, the midwifery model is subsumed by profit margins and institutional efficiency, and midwives are reduced to obstetrical technicians. In addition, CNMs are losing their collective bargaining power as HMOs systematically fire them, only to rehire them for longer hours at less pay, and without benefits. After so many years of struggling within the system and resisting the urge to relax and become complacent, will nurse-midwives have the strength to fight for autonomy of practice as their apprenticeship-trained, direct-entry sisters are now doing? Who is really ahead in this game, and who is behind? And who's running the game in the first place?

It may take some years before we have the answers to these questions. Meanwhile, we must recognize that at the root of how and what we practice, how we define ourselves both professionally and politically, is the manner in which we are educated. Most nurse-midwifery programs are housed within complex medical care delivery systems; instructor and student alike are subject to highly restrictive practice protocols. These programs are heavily weighted with theoretical instruction, but have minimal hands-on training, little or no continuity of care, and limited scope of practice. Students consequently suffer an overdevelopment of their analytical faculties at the expense of intuitive, compassionate qualities so necessary to humane caregiving. In my experience, the most common complaint of a nurse-midwifery graduate is fear—fear of the responsibility of private practice, fear of being inadequately prepared to work out of hospital. These fears are quite reasonable, considering what nurse-midwifery training does, and does not, accomplish.

The challenge to midwifery education today is to create a curriculum that develops the student as a human being, while providing supportively supervised clinical experience. All too often, the nurse-midwifery graduate has done countless rotations in clinical settings, but has never known primary responsibility for a single client from start to finish. When life-threatening complications of shoulder dystocia or hemorrhage occurred in her training, she was obligated by protocol to call for help, and then step aside. Predictably, she feels ill equipped to practice "on her own responsibility."

In contrast, the midwife trained by apprenticeship is one-on-one with her senior midwife's clients throughout the entire perinatal cycle. She is also one-on-one with her preceptor, requiring her to develop and refine not only technical skills, but equally important abilities to communicate assertively and listen effectively. Learning takes place in context, as the senior midwife debriefs the day's events and suggests sources for further study. Student evaluation is done as much for appropriate clinical application of knowledge as for the ability to commit facts to paper. Continuity of both care and instruction force the student to put herself into her learning process, as is the case in any long-term relationship. She is more likely to be confronted with her technical and personal shortcomings when she has been involved in a case from start to finish, and when her interactions with her preceptor are ongoing.

Nurse-midwifery programs may come and go as funding dictates, but training by apprenticeship will endure because it is community-based, cost-effective, and perfect for women with small children who require a program with elastic time, i.e., one which allows students as much time as necessary to complete program requirements. If you are considering the apprenticeship route, check first to see if your state has any provisions for qualifying midwives. Some states require that students attend formal, on-site academic programs in conjunction with apprenticeship; others have course work requirements that can be met at-a-distance (similar to external degree programs or independent study provisions offered by many universities). Still other states have licensing or certifying mechanisms entirely competency-based, with the usual requisites of documented experience, skills verification and comprehensive exam. Several states have incorporated NARM certification requirements. Consult MANA for a list of representatives that can familiarize you with their respective states' educational and practice requirements; consult NARM for an updated listing of all states that recognize CPMs. Consult the Midwifery Education Accreditation Council (MEAC) for a list of accredited direct-entry programs.

If your state has no mechanism for regulating midwifery, you may wish to investigate the guidelines established by NARM for becoming a CPM, and on that basis, create your own framework for learning. Once you know the experience you must acquire, and the clinical skills and general knowledge you must be able to demonstrate, you will have some idea of how to structure your learning. Your initial efforts will probably involve: 1) studying midwifery texts; 2) participating in a group learning situation or midwifery study group; and 3) attending births as a birth assistant or labor coach.

In less formal situations, the backbone of apprenticeship training is skills acquisition and evaluation. In 1995, NARM conducted a survey of midwives throughout North America to determine entry-level skills for direct-entry midwifery. The resulting practical skills list is utilized by NARM in its certification process. Acquisition of these skills is outlined step-by-step in the *Practical Skills Guide* by Sharon Evans and Pam Weaver. These tools can provide needed structure for senior midwife and apprentice alike. Together, they can formulate a plan to see that both skills and the experience necessary for certification or licensure are acquired by the apprentice in a reasonable amount of time.

What about cost? Apprenticeship is traditionally a relationship of exchange, whereby a master of a given trade exchanges knowledge for labor. But if part of a formal program leads directly to licensure or certification, the student can expect to pay for apprenticeship. In less structured situations, the apprentice may receive a nominal sum to cover transportation and childcare, and if the midwife intends to incorporate the apprentice as a partner, she may increase her pay over time to full partnership level.

How will an apprentice know when she is ready to practice independently? Meeting minimum standards for skills and experience is just one aspect of her preparedness. Some students are by nature over-eager and need to be repeatedly instructed in the art of caregiving; others are timid and must be given unexpected responsibilities to appreciate their competence. If their relationship is good, an apprentice can trust her teacher's judgment regarding her readiness to practice. However, some students feel the need for experience beyond that offered by their preceptor. Senior apprentices sometimes practice briefly with other preceptors, or undertake brief internships at high-volume midwifery practices or out-of-hospital birth centers in order to complete their training.

For students wishing a little more structure, midwifery programs offering academic preparation and formalized apprenticeship have recently been developed. An example is the Midwifery Institute of California, which combines Heart & Hands and Study Group course work (available on-site or at-a-distance) with apprenticeship. The intention of this program is to provide the student a solid theoretical foundation in midwifery while helping her find apprenticeship opportunities in her own locale. She can take advantage of community-based, community-sensitive training and be spared the considerable cost of having to relocate for schooling.

This article was excerpted from Heart & Hands: A Midwife's Guide to Pregnancy and Birth.

Elizabeth Davis, BA, CPM, has been a midwife, women's healthcare specialist, author, educator and consultant for more than twenty years. She is active at national and international levels in issues of midwifery education and self-regulation, and is co-founder of the Midwifery Institute of California, a three year, MEAC accredited program. She is the author of five books, including the classic midwifery text, Heart & Hands: A Midwife's Guide to Pregnancy and Birth, now in its 3rd edition.

THOUGHTS ON THE APPRENTICE'S PATH

by Alison Parra

Naomi recently attended her close friend's birth. She now wants to study midwifery so she can begin to help other birthing women in her rural area. Anne is completing a one year internship at a maternity clinic. Sara is trained as an obstetrical nurse but would like to get out of the hospital and attend births at home.

At some point, all of these women may find themselves in the role of apprentice, one of the oldest forms of education. For an aspiring midwife, it is often the turning point in her study. The midwife-apprentice relationship is only acknowledged in a few midwifery texts, and curiously, never examined in much detail. Yet it should be, because apprenticeship is a key element in the evolution of a midwife's education, and plays a major role in shaping how she will approach her practice and her people. There is ample material on the acquisition of technical knowledge, but we need to become aware of the psychological and spiritual processes involved in apprenticing as well. This article will look at seven "stumbling blocks" on the apprentice's path.

THE HEROINE

In some cases, when a woman finds a mentor, she may adopt a style that is something just short of worship. A Bradley teacher I once knew explained it this way: "I observed Anne X's classes as part of my training. When I started teaching on my own, I just did everything she did—she was such a good midwife and teacher, I figured if I just did everything like her, I would be great, too. As I gained more experience, I eventually found my own voice and my own opinions."

I meet apprentices and midwives all the time who swear they are learning or have learned from the BEST midwife ever. Such enthusiastic role modeling has positive value in the initial total-absorption phase of learning. Normally, like the woman above, it is followed by individuation, when one separates the Heroine from one's own sense of self.

The trouble comes when separation does not occur and you have a woman who cannot consider doing things any way but THE WAY that her mentor did. Sometimes it is a way for an apprentice to gain esteem or power: "MY midwife was So and So," which doesn't necessarily mean she herself is as qualified and caring as her mentor, but implies as much.

At a prenatal exam, I asked a midwife who was just starting out to check a woman's pulse. "Oh, MY midwife never did that," she told me, and would not take the pulse. The issue here is not the pulse, but the assumption that if her Heroine didn't do it, there was no need to explore the idea further. By seeing one's mentor as infallible or setting ourselves up as such, we are seeing neither her nor ourselves as whole. We also run the risk of giving our own or the birthing couple's power over to our Heroine's undeniable rightness.

Empowerment

A skilled midwife is one who directs the responsibilities of pregnancy and birth back to the parents and offers herself as guide, support and resource person. I am wary of women who, in the course of their work, draw the focus to themselves (or their mentor), dominate the energy and claim their knowledge as personal domain or personal power. A wise woman will not hesitate to say "I don't know" when she doesn't, then share in the search to find out. Couples used to authoritarian-style healthcare may initially react: "She doesn't even know? Perhaps she's not any good, then." But the goal is to break the illusion of omnipotence. We are here to work WITH couples, not FOR them.

Desire

This is an issue particular to the empirically trained midwife, who must create her opportunities and guidelines as she goes along. A woman who wants to apprentice so badly may join others who are unable to give her the skills she needs. Or she may over-assess her abilities. She may take clients other midwives have turned down, not because she feels qualified to do so, but because she so desperately wants to "be at a birth."

Letting Go

The early stages of apprenticing involve a crucial letting go of ego, a taking in, a quiet observing. Letting go implies release. Release requires opening, and in opening we become ready to receive. Accept that you may not be at every birth. A couple's choice to have or not have you present is not a personal ego judgment. You may know as much as the next woman, but nothing is gained by talking the most or the loudest. Pregnant intuition will see who you are, anyway. Letting go of fervent desires to "be at the birth" doesn't imply apathy. It does mean an emotional letting go of your ego involvement. Keep yourself directed—study, learn, teach, share—with all your heart, but not your ego.

Judging

Judging is inevitable. We naturally appraise new methods or ideas against our own beliefs and values. But again, problems arise when we can't let go. When a conflict arises, acknowledge the fact that you would have done differently. If there are steps you wish to take to improve the situation or if there is more research you can do for future options, then do it. And let go.

There is no one way a "real" midwife dresses, talks, raises her children or attends births. It is especially hard at times to let go of judgments about a birthing couple's choices. There is a fine line between offering information and offering "shoulds." You may really "know" a couple's birth would be "better" if only they would do this or that. But the ultimate, informed choice is theirs alone. When you present information in a non-judgmental way and acknowledge your own opinions yet accept that the couple may choose differently, you create an emotional environment where the couple can feel safe to explore new ideas that may have previously seemed threatening.

It is unrealistic to think all midwives are "holy" in the sense that we never judge, gossip or have competitive feelings. We need to be gentle with ourselves, let go of our own "shoulds" of perfection so that we can relate to one another more humanely.

SPIRITUAL CONSUMERISM

"How many births have you attended?" This is a very valid question at times, but it tends to promote a consumer mentality—chalking up births like notches in a belt. The birthing woman is thus depersonalized as an objective to be "won."

I am uncomfortable when midwives speak in numerical or possessive terms about their experiences: "All MY ladies do this and that." "After my seventh birth I was . . ." Note the possessive pronoun popping up. My ladies. My births. Once, while I was labor coaching in a hospital, the nurse-midwife greeted a laboring woman cheerily with: "Oh-ho! You're number seven today!" She may have been the seventh delivery for the midwife that day, but to the birthing woman, it is her one and only time birthing this unique and special baby—hers. Her birth is not the midwife's to claim.

The numbers game is also misleading. Most obstetricians have attended hundreds or thousands of births but that doesn't mean I would want one at my birth. It means they have rushed in for the last five or ten minutes of labor of fifteen women a day for the past ten years. A midwife who has attended only fifteen or twenty births may not have the exposure to all the variations and complications labor can present, but I would prefer the intensity and quality of care she may offer.

SHARING AND BALANCING

Some midwives and apprentices don't "click" right away. Maybe a midwife is "holding back" to maintain her authority. Maybe an apprentice is overly eager to take on responsibilities for which she isn't ready.

We need to find balance in terms of time, energy and priorities. If you find that you are resentful, anxious, pressured or martyred as you attend a long, slow labor, you need to reexamine your priorities. For those of us with young children, that is a very tough balance. On one hand, we feel incredibly connected to that baby-energy; on the other, we want to be directing it toward our own babies as well. We need time to love our families, and time to be alone, too. We may find that no one, including the birthing couple, is getting the quality of attention they need.

Often, the more experienced we become, the more likely we are to overextend ourselves, attending many births back to back. The more births we attend, the less likely it is that we can be "there" emotionally and physically. We end up spending less time with each couple, until we resemble the classic obstetrician who rushes in at the last push to catch the baby, then hurries off. This can be advantageous for the apprentice, but bewildering to the couple, who may feel "abandoned." The parents may also feel that their emotional and monetary investment in the midwife's services was misplaced, since the apprentice "did all the work."

In conclusion, there are numerous potential problems that apprentices and midwives themselves may encounter, but still, in most cases, the joys and rewards of midwifery far outweigh the disadvantages.

It is hardly likely that we would ever hear the head obstetrician at a large teaching hospital say, "So, gentlemen, strive to be unimportant, let go, and try not to get too busy." But that is why I love midwifery.

This article first appeared in Midwifery Today Issue No. 4.

Alison Parra, originally from the United States, taught prepared childbirth and attended births in central Mexico, and was writing a book in Spanish on alternatives in pregnancy and birth when she wrote this article.

A MODEL FOR POLICY MAKING:

SEATTLE MIDWIFERY SCHOOL

by Therese Charvet LM, CPM & Jo Anne Myers-Ciecko, MPH

The Seattle Midwifery School (SMS) was founded in 1978 with the aim of providing high-quality midwifery education as one way to improve the health and well-being of childbearing women and their families. By 1998, more than 120 midwives will have completed the basic program, and hundreds have participated in conferences and continuing education programs sponsored by the school. Most recently, the school has offered a popular four-day labor support course. Thousands of women and their families benefit each year from the care and support provided by the ever-growing cadre of SMS graduates.

TO BEGIN WITH

The women who first organized the Seattle Midwifery School worked in the grass-roots Women's Health Centers that were active in the Seattle area in the early 1970s. Because of their work with women and the fact that many of their friends were having babies, they were inspired to expand their services to include pregnancy and birth. With encouragement from the young physicians who worked with them in the clinics, these women began learning midwifery by studying in the University of Washington's health science library and by apprenticing with these doctors. For several years they practiced midwifery as part of a health collective.

In 1978, the director of the Washington State Department of Licensing suggested that these midwives might meet the requirements of the midwifery law (passed in 1917) if they could formally articulate their course of study. The 1917 law required a midwife seeking licensure to graduate from an "incorporated school in good standing." Although the midwives struggled with the decision to pursue licensing, they decided to act on it, believing that midwifery care would be accessible to more women if midwifery were legally recognized. Thus, the Seattle Midwifery School was born and the "founding mothers" became the pilot class—the first direct-entry, U.S.-trained midwives to become licensed in Washington state.

LICENSURE CROSSES SOME STATE LINES

Midwives from Denmark, Chile and Australia were practicing in the area during this same period and encouraged the school founders to draw upon the well-established international models of direct-entry midwifery education. Other American health professional training programs and the experiential learning of the founding mothers also helped shape the school. Presently, the program meets standards for midwifery education established by the International Confederation of Midwives (ICM) and new guidelines adopted by the European community. SMS is accredited by the Washington State Department of Health and has been recognized as a path to licensure by the Arizona Department of Health and the California Board of Nursing. Graduates are also eligible for licensure in several other states.

THE PROGRAM OF LEARNING

The basic midwifery educational program is designed to establish a theoretical knowledge base in all of the components of midwifery practice (antepartum, intra-partum, postpartum, newborn, and gynecology/family planning) and to develop the clinical skills, judgment and intuition necessary for entry level midwifery practice. The program is three academic years (twenty-seven months) in length.

In the first part of the program, nearly 600 hours are spent in the classroom and skills lab to build a theoretical foundation. The classroom curriculum is composed of the following core courses: assessment of women, gynecology/women's health, pro-fessional issues in midwifery, midwifery seminar, perinatal care series, nursing skills. These courses include instruction in the physical, emotional, sexual, psychosocial and political aspects of midwifery care. They emphasize normal physiologic process-es, but also teach students to identify disease, manage emergencies and seek consul-tation when appropriate.

Other courses are provided which supplement the core curriculum and expand the theoretical knowledge base to encompass related subjects. These courses are: sta-tistics and epidemiology, embryology/fetal development, genetics, women's health and nutrition, midwife as educator and pharmacology.

Instructors come from the community and include midwives and others with expertise in their field. Approximately fifteen different teachers provide instruction in the courses, with numerous "guest lecturers" enhancing course content. Two of the founding mothers are presently core faculty members and many others have been involved with SMS for years.

CLINICAL EXPERIENCE

The practical or clinical component of the program consists of two different phas-es. The first phase is interwoven with classroom work and provides students with exposure to many different styles and sites of practice. Students participate in rota-tions in prenatal, postpartum, gynecology and primary care clinics. They have some experience being "on call" with a midwife and can participate in a newborn nursery rotation with a clinical nurse specialist. Students begin to integrate the theoretical material they are learning in the classroom with real clinical situations, have expo-sure to a variety of role models, and begin to develop their hands-on skills.

The second phase of clinical training consists of "external preceptorships," a model akin to apprenticeship, and follows the classroom part of the program. During this phase, students are working intensively with midwives who provide full-spec-trum maternity care. They participate in clinics, home visits and births with the mid-wife. These preceptorships are located all over the country and are provided by mid-wives and nurse-midwives, although occasionally physicians are used as preceptors as well. Another option during this phase is an overseas clinical internship. SMS has ongoing relationships with hospitals in Jamaica and St. Lucia, where our students participate in high volume birth settings staffed by midwives.

During their training, students participate in at least a hundred births, fifty of which must be managed under supervision, over 800 hours of clinical time in addition to these births, and over 700 client contacts. In addition to the clinical work done during this time, students also participate in monthly seminars at the school and other activities that enhance their experiential learning and reinforce their theoretical learning. By the end of their preceptorships, students are ready for entry-level midwifery practice.

FUNDING AND OUTREACH

Seattle Midwifery School supporters contribute approximately one-fourth of all operating funds and new sources are being sought to create an at-a-distance learning option, to implement the nurse-midwifery pathway that has already been approved by the American College of Nurse-Midwives/Division of Accreditation, and to purchase computer equipment needed to access new information systems and facilitate new learning modes. In the meantime, SMS continues to serve as a model for direct-entry midwifery education for various legislative efforts across North America. SMS staff provides support to numerous midwifery groups and policy makers requesting information about midwifery education and practice. Representatives also participate in a variety of organizations and forums serving to promote the development and expansion of the midwifery profession, for we remain firmly dedicated to the principles underlying midwifery practice and to the improvement of women's health and well-being.

This article first appeared in Midwifery Today Issue No. 20.

Therese Charvet, LM, CPM, is currently the midwifery program director of Seattle Midwifery School. She operated a homebirth service in rural Kitsap County in Washington state from 1981–1988 before taking on her current position at SMS. She was the founding president of the Midwives Alliance of North America (MANA), has been on the board for the Midwives Association of Washington State, and is currently the president of the Midwifery Education Accreditation Council (MEAC). In addition to her work in midwifery, Therese is also involved in the Women's Spirituality Movement, offering her workshop "Women's Rite for Healing and Empowerment" in a variety of Northwest venues.

Jo Anne Myers-Ciecko, MPH, executive director and faculty member at Seattle Midwifery School, is a long-time ally and activist on behalf of midwifery. Over the past two decades she has contributed her expertise in health policy, reimbursement for midwives, midwifery education and regulation, the history and politics of midwifery on national, state, local and international committees, boards and work groups.

SEATTLE MIDWIFERY SCHOOL

by Jo Anne Myers-Ciecko, executive director

> It has often been said that educate means "to draw out" a person's talents as opposed to putting in knowledge or instruction. This is an interesting idea, but it is not quite true in terms of the etymology of the word. Educate comes from the Latin word *educare*, "to educate," which is derived from a specialized use of Latin *educere* (from *e-*, "out," and *decere*, "to lead," meaning "to assist at the birth of a child.)"
>
> —Webster's II New Riverside University Dictionary (1988)

I first came across this little gem in the dictionary after I had been facilitating a course in professional issues for midwifery students for several years. It was thrilling to discover words supported my growing sense that "teaching" and "mid-wifing" are very similar processes. I was beginning to think that you could no more *teach* anyone anything than you can *deliver* their baby for them. You might think that's an odd statement from someone so involved in formal education, but I assert that our emphasis must be on what the student wants and is able to learn, just as the midwife supports the woman making choices in her pregnancy and birth. And, similarly, those who want to become midwives should examine their options for education carefully and make choices based on their own values and expecting. Twenty years ago, I was a consumer supporting the creation of the Seattle Midwifery School (SMS) with the hope that my children and their generation, unlike my own, would have access to midwives no matter what state they were in, what insurance plan they had, or where they wanted to give birth. As a consumer activist, I was also involved in the development of MANA and our state midwifery association. With that background and perspective, I began teaching at SMS and focused my energy on creating a course that no one else in the country seemed to be offering. I wanted to combine midwifery history, economic, political, ethical and healthcare system curriculum with practical experiences in lobbying and the business of midwifery.

At first, I lacked teaching experience and confidence in public speaking. I was preoccupied with my own performance. It took every bit of courage I had to stand up in front of these wonderful midwifery students and hold myself out as an expert on this subject matter. That was, after all, what I expected of a teacher. But as time went by, my concern reality shifted to the students, to what they were learning and not what I was teaching. Midwifery students generally bring a vast wealth of knowledge and experience to their study of midwifery. Given the right context and the opportunity to share what they know, these highly motivated students will dig into any relevant new information with enthusiasm. What a joy to discover that I don't need to be the expert, because the students are each experts in their own right and will make their own choices about learning.

Which isn't to say that my colleagues and I don't have a responsibility to create a context and opportunities for learning. In fact, articulating the expected outcomes of learning is an important function of any educational program. Core competencies described by the professional association should be evident in the learning objectives of the program. Once everyone knows where she is headed, then begins the process of sorting out how best to get there. Students should be given the opportunity to increase their own self-awareness regarding learning styles and special needs. Educators must be prepared to support a variety of learning activities and students should play a role in determining what activities will best meet their needs. Other resources are also critical in fostering an effective learning environment, including mentors and role models; library and online services, the physical setting; clinic, lab and AV equipment, and connections to the surrounding community, both professional and birthing. Relationships of trust, mutual respect and partnership are also key to the success of educational programs serving midwifery students. It can be a challenge to cultivate relationships with these qualities when there is necessarily a power differential between the student and the teacher or program officials who hold the key to her future as a midwife. Nevertheless, it is both learning and evaluation which the student requires of the educational program. And if evaluations are made fairly, based on clearly established criteria, and feedback is communicated effectively to the student, this aspect of the relationship should not interfere with trust building.

When making a decision about what program best meets the needs and expectations of the learner, prospective students should examine the program's philosophy, learning objectives and curriculum carefully to determine whether or not these are clearly stated and are a good fit with their own. They should also find out about the resources available to support their learning and optional learning activities. If a prospective student is most interested in working with women who experience high-risk pregnancies, does the program provide classes and clinical training sites that will prepare her for this kind of practice? How does the program address conflicts between the medical and midwifery model of care? What about the student who wants to build her own birth center? Or the one who envisions a career in international health? What are their options? Does coursework address these interests? Ask to see sample course outlines and learning activities. Find out where students complete their clinical training. Are there options? What are the restrictions? What are graduates doing?

Prospective students should also inquire whether or not prior experience is recognized and valued by teachers and program officials. How much credit, if any, can the student earn for prior learning? Can assignments be modified to better meet the individual's background and interests? Are the criteria for evaluation clearly stated and fairly applied? How is communication between students and instructors or administrators encouraged and supported? These may be questions that are best asked of current students or recent graduates of the program. Find out if you will have an opportunity to meet students or visit graduates. As an educator, I look forward to meeting students who have made well-informed, thoughtful decisions about their midwifery education. They are more likely to be active participants in their learning and able to share their valuable knowledge and experience with their colleagues—student, instructors and preceptors alike. And in the end, they will become midwives who understand the importance of self-awareness and informed choice when caring for women and their families.

This article was written especially for this book.

Jo Anne Myers-Ciecko, MPH, executive director and faculty member at Seattle Midwifery School, is a long-time ally and activist on behalf of midwifery. Over the past two decades she has contributed her expertise in health policy, reimbursement for midwives, midwifery education and regulation, the history and politics of midwifery on national, state, local and international committees, boards and work groups.

Maternidad La Luz: The Birth Place

by Cindy Lara Haag

It is the first of September and thirty women are snuggled into the upstairs classroom at Maternidad La Luz: The Birth Place. The bright El Paso sun streams through the skylights and heightens the radiance in their faces. This circle holds the resounding energy of many journeys. Some women are beginning their midwifery journeys this morning as they join our community. Their anticipation and excitement are palpable as they take in the sights and sounds of their new home of the next months. Other women are leaving our circle to continue their midwifery paths all over the world. The sense of pride of completion, fatigue from all their hard work and love for each other is obvious on their faces. Some of those students are also staying on for advanced study. Other women in the circle are teachers and practicing staff midwives who daily share their knowledge of and passion for birth with the students. Their dedication and strength permeate every corner of the birth center. Finally, other women who support the students and center in myriad ways lend their smiles and wisdom to the circle. Everyone sits together, cries and laughs and tells their stories. It is a powerful sharing of women's lives that never ceases to move and teach.

In the coming months the students learn at an accelerated pace. The one year program which satisfies NARM requirements covers everything from basic skills, to normal and complicated prenatal, intrapartum and postpartum issues, to advanced concepts in midwifery. It follows a natural progression, building upon the expanding knowledge base of the students.

One aspect that makes this midwifery education so unique and profound is the hands-on experience that at the same time solidifies and stimulates the academic learning. Concepts learned in class are often immediately put to use in the clinic and questions from issues that arose during appointments and births are explored and answered in class. Besides the constant contact with staff and teachers, the easy access to the center's library, the curiosity of fellow students and ensuing discussions, there are formal times to link academics and clinical experience. Every week at birth talks, births and transports are discussed in detail, providing many valuable insights.

Our clientele make up another group of inspiring women. They are mostly Mexican Nationals and Mexican-Americans. These women are the student's most valuable teachers. Even across the language and cultural differences, students and clients form close, loving bonds, some that last a long time. Many clients have returned to have their second, third and even fourth babies with us.

Traditional education seeks to cultivate support for midwifery goals while advocating for the preservation of midwifery practice in its broadest sense.

Often it is the connection with the client, along with the support of fellow students, that helps one through a long labor or challenging birth.

Often it is the connection with the client, along with the support of fellow students, that helps one through a long labor or challenging birth.

The student community forms the core support network. Students work about two and a half to three twenty-four hour shifts every week and attend nine hours of class a week. Amidst an atmosphere of mutual encouragement, we all work toward a common goal of learning, teaching and providing superb midwifery care.

I came here as a student in September of 1989. After school and working with a midwife in Vermont attending homebirths, I returned to El Paso to continue my training. I trained to be a staff midwife and have been practicing here (and briefly in Xalapa, Vera Cruz) ever since. I also teach classes and help as clinical director. My love for this place and for all the amazing women who have shared a piece of their lives here is unshakable.

Courses begin September and March. The following options are now available: short term (one week or more), three month and six month programs, the one year MEAC accredited program, and a three year pilot project. Interested students are invited to spend a twenty-four hour shift with us to get to know the center and school.

For information, contact: Maternidad La Luz: The Birth Place, 1308 Magoffin Ave., El Paso, TX 79901 (915) 532-5895.

This article was written especially for this book.

Cindy Lara Haag is the clinical director of Maternidad La Luz: The Birth Place and has worked there since 1989.

A STUDENT'S JOURNEY

by Karen Shaw

Early in my first year at the Seattle Midwifery School (SMS), my teachers reassured my classmates and me that "each of you will be able to integrate all the skills and knowledge that you need." With a leap of faith, I believed them. Now, as a full-fledged midwife with three years at SMS behind me, I find that my life is full, demanding, exciting and satisfying. SMS provided a good midwifery education and laid a solid groundwork for my current practice.

My classmates came from all parts of the country and our individual approaches and motivations for choosing midwifery as a profession were as varied as our personalities. Some of us had human service or healthcare experience, some were practicing lay midwives, most had children. There was richness, conflict, laughter and frustration among us.

During our first three months, we adjusted to the academic demands of gynecology reading assignments, genetics papers, pregnancy presentations and nutrition exams. The next nine months combined classroom study and clinic work. Clinics and practices in the greater Seattle area accept SMS students for short gynecology/prenatal rotations. Each clinic is different and presents its own unique opportunities and limitations. Some allow much time for a student to become accustomed to "hands on" work while other clinics emphasize observation. I worked in a gynecology clinic one day a week for three months and by the end of that time I was proficient in well-woman care, birth control counseling, diaphragm fitting and problem solving.

In the next six months I began to sharpen my midwifery skills in a prenatal/postpartum clinic, assisting a CNM with a homebirth practice. I learned to take fundal height measurements, palpate for position, locate fetal heart tones, determine many variations of "normal," conduct lab tests and communicate with the backup MD. With no prior midwifery experience, I required much procedural practice to learn to link hand knowledge to mind knowledge. As I became more comfortable with the skills, I began to understand the concerns of the woman or family I was serving. I was learning to integrate hands, heart and mind.

Most of us assisted at births during our first year of study. Some students responded to requests for labor support, others worked as OB/postpartum nurses, assisted friends or made connections in their prenatal clinic placements. I assisted at births through a prenatal clinic, and the experience was invaluable. Questions and perplexing situations were fresh in my mind, and I could present them for class discussion, enjoying regular access to the advice of midwives and midwives-in-training.

To graduate, an aspiring midwife has to attend a hundred births, fifty observed and fifty managed, so during the second term, we worked in midwifery practices as student midwives. Because I was present at their prenatal visits and births, I had an opportunity to get to know each client. My role with each family varied depending on their personalities, needs and labor.

Each student worked in at least two midwifery practices. These preceptor arrangements were made primarily by the student, and most of us had to relocate. Some went with their families, some went alone.

I worked in one rural and two urban practices, and in a St. Lucian hospital with midwives who used all styles and approaches. I became familiar with the creative aspect of midwifery—a problem arises, a solution evolves, and the needs of a particular labor, family and midwife are met. I attended births seeing many variations of normal, as well as births in crisis situations. I got scared a lot. Birth is a momentous event, and I was there, in the moment, over and over again, doing what was needed. In talks with practicing midwives, I learned how one enjoys, copes, and grows while doing this work. I got an idea of what comes after graduation when one has a practice and a family life.

During my first year at Seattle Midwifery School I had said "I'm studying midwifery." During my second year I had said "I'm a student midwife." When graduation came, I was ready to call myself a midwife. I felt trained, educated and supported enough to take on the responsibility of being in my own practice. My training at SMS was a long, hard, exciting and satisfying experience, and my work as a midwife is the joyous fulfillment of that three-year journey.

This article first appeared in Midwifery Today Issue No. 4.

Karen Shaw lived in New England and planned a move to New York state when she wrote this article.

Chapter

4

Certified Nurse-Midwifery

"I'm helping women I would not have helped birth at home—they either wouldn't have chosen such a birth or would have been considered too risky. I'm using technology appropriately, for the benefit of mothers and babies. While yesterday two mothers chose Pitocin and epidurals, one chose cohosh tincture, enemas and castor oil. Another birthed without any medication. And I had the privilege of serving them all."

— *Sharon Glass Jonquil, CNM*

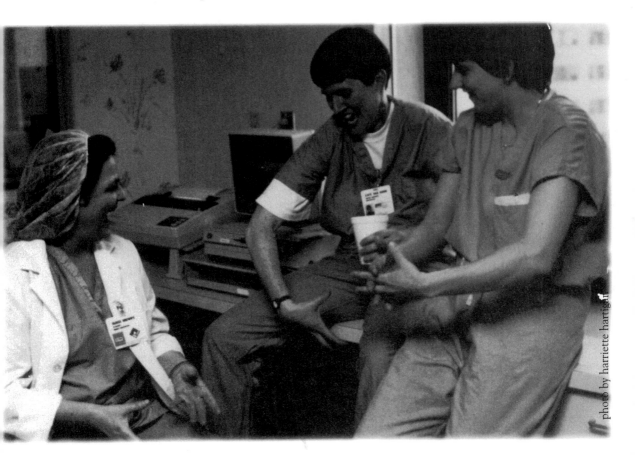

photo by harriette hartigan

A Midwife to All

by Virginia Jackson, CNM

The hospital is in a very big city. The place itself is very big—one of the largest employers in the area. More than three thousand women go there each year to have their babies. Many more come to the hospital for healthcare for themselves and their families. The hospital is a public institution owned by the city. It belongs to the people.

The women come from all over the world: Mexico, Colombia, Dominican Republic, Somalia, Ghana, Nigeria, Bangladesh, India, America. They are not wealthy, not even financially stable. Their lives are difficult. They struggle to provide security, shelter and food for themselves and their families. Some of them go through life with the daily, nonchalant bravery of legendary heroines. Some of them break with thundering finality, some in a multitude of little chips. Some have, with pain, pulled all the shards back together.

Do we do well by them? Do we welcome them, honor their wishes, abide by their traditions, consider their varying individual needs and styles? Do we meet their minimal requirements for comfort and safety? Well, yes and no.

Hospitals, ours included, are specifically designed for the provision of a minimal standard of care to the maximum number of patients. As such, it is quite an inflexible entity. Yes, vegetarians get vegetables and Moslems don't find pork on their plates. Usually. However, everyone must wear a hospital gown, everyone has an IV, everyone has continuous electronic fetal monitoring, everyone is confined to a bed or stretcher for the duration of labor and no one gets to eat or drink. Informed consent consists of "sign here." The women sign papers whether they can read or not, whether they can understand the language or not. They give themselves over to our care.

We midwives work in shifts and are not on call for our own clinic patients. It is not usual to know the laboring woman prior to her admission. The women don't usually choose a midwife. Although they often prefer a female provider and are comfortable with a midwife, they have not done extensive research on their options. Attending prepared childbirth classes, even though they are free, does not rank high in their priorities. Some of the women do not have homes. Some are shunted from shelter to shelter; some make their way on the streets. Some have a roof over them but no water, heat or electricity. Some don't have enough food. Some use illegal drugs. Some have no prenatal care. Some don't want their babies. Some have severe medical or psychiatric problems. Some of them are abused; some are abusers. They are all our patients.

The day-to-day protocols challenge us constantly. We cannot waste energy being upset about not being respected. The doctors with whom we work have, themselves, worked very hard over many years to achieve their professional standing. The residents have just traded the difficulties of medical school for the opportunity to work at least eighty hours a week, study and adapt to their new role as doctors. These people are not going to hand out respect. Additionally, they have very little understanding of midwives and midwifery. They tend to view us as "mid-level providers" or "physician extenders." This error in perception is something we must, and do, correct. We correct it by reading books and clinical literature. We have the obligation to know better than the medical staff what the latest studies are. We have the obligation to maintain a calm, professional attitude. We have the obligation to raise our voices and be heard in committees and during rounds. We have the obligation to teach those who think we have nothing to teach.

The nurses with whom we work offer a related challenge. Their attitude toward midwifery ranges from hostile to enthusiastically supportive. Their jobs are not the same as ours. They have rules and charting and multiple patients. At times, our ways of doing things are seen as making more work and in some ways that may be true. A nurse who devotes herself to the failure of a midwife not only ruins a single midwife, but she harms our entire service. How can one deflect or avoid such conflicts? Again, respect must be earned. If a midwife gives consistently good care she will eventually convert the skeptical. Good care includes management that is safe and supported by published literature; individualizing plans for the patient; hands-on care of the patient; and respect for the patient. To some this is self-evident. However, many nurses have seen bad care and many have felt powerless to do anything about it. Many have good reason to be suspicious. Nurses have a large impact on the patient and the success of any plan of care. The midwife would do well to include the nurse in making decisions, acknowledging that it is essential to solicit the nurse's opinions, observations and suggestions. This is an opportunity for exchange so the midwife should not feel offended if the nurse requests explanations. Because the nurses watch us all the time, they are well able to evaluate the clinical skills and mode of practice of the midwife. Prove yourself and gain an important ally.

> We have the obligation to raise our voices and be heard in committees and during rounds. We have the obligation to teach those who think we have nothing to teach.

Too often the nurses are the enforcers of hospital rules and policies. Although it is impolitic to declare the hospital rules ridiculous, it is vital to remember that rules can be changed. If you want a patient up and walking in labor, then discuss it with the patient, write an order for ambulation, remove the monitor belts, get the patient foot coverings and some covering for her back and walk with her as long as you can. Show her support person how to help her. Don't just complain that the nurse won't get the patient up.

If you want to offer physical support to a woman who is pushing and you think her support person should sit behind her on the bed but there is an objection that the support person may be "non-sterile," invent a barrier. Explain why you think this position would help. Enlist the agreement of the support person. Place Chux all over the parts of the bed which the support person might touch, creating a "clean" area. If this strikes you as silly, consider that it is no sillier than the idea that birth is sterile. Remember, the staff of hospitals are encouraged to come to work when they are ill. Also, studies have shown that hospital staff are very noncompliant about handwashing. These points can be made quietly and reasonably at meetings. Interdisciplinary, of course.

The midwife is a midwife to all in our environment. We are in a position to offer our care, our intelligence, our skills and our respect to all. We not only protect our patients but what is and should be normal. We never lose sight of the fact that birth is normal and that a baby will result. We may need to call in all sorts of fancy consults, but the entire patient is someone we will not forget. Doctors and nurses are our colleagues. We do not benefit and neither do our patients benefit from a dysfunctional relationship. We hold to the essence, the soul of midwifery and we are models for others. Because we are open to new information, we bring information to others. We can bring in articles, encourage reading and discussion. We strive to make change that will aid our patients. This cannot happen during a shouting fight in the hallway. We give of our time and ideas in the grinding work of consensus building and protocol updating. We show, by our own actions, the positive effects of midwifery care by the direct physical care of the patient. Our hands, voices and eyes are our tools of service we offer to all we work with.

This article first appeared in Midwifery Today Issue No. 45.

Virginia Jackson, CNM, works in New York City. She is also a presenter at Midwifery Today conferences.

FROM FETOSCOPE TO DOPPLER

. . . AND BACK AGAIN?

by Sharon Glass Jonquil, CNM

When I first began to think of becoming a certified nurse-midwife, I felt great resistance from within—guilt for even entertaining such thoughts, and a sense of betrayal to my roots and to my sister lay midwives. Much to my dismay, the ancient path of midwifery is caught up in the nuclear age. How can a CNM protect the ideal of "heart and hands" while working in a time when people know the sex of their baby prior to birth, where the ultrasound record and electronic fetal heart monitor tracing are nestled in the baby book, and women birth in rooms that look like hotel suites?

Yet I continue to pursue licensing. In retrospect I trace the tracks of my lay midwifery career as they follow a broader pathway toward a CNM practice. Some of the steps I take are still halting, unsure. I review the reasons, decisions, issues and steps taken. Other lay midwives as well are dealing with those issues, making choices which are right for them, for their families and for the times and the areas in which they live. Some are taking the same path as I am; others are diverging.

I was brought to midwifery on the gentle wings of Raven Lang's School of Feminine Arts and Womencare in California's Santa Cruz Mountains. There I formed my strongest, most deeply held beliefs about the nature of birth and the power of birthing women. From there, I was bombarded by the bootcamp atmosphere of a maternity center in Texas, where I received valuable experience at the expense of my self-esteem and Blessingway approach.

When I returned to California, I worked in a migrant farm workers' prenatal clinic, where I helped women birth with dignity amidst the squalor of poverty. Following the homebirth of my daughter, my family moved to Oregon where I slowly became part of the community and the local circle of midwives. I was hungry to learn. I accumulated a personal library, attended conferences, enrolled in classes. I taught childbirth classes, ovulation method, prenatal yoga and infant massage. And I attended births. My circle of experience widened as I became more and more involved in the politics of midwifery on the local level, then the statewide level, and when I joined Midwives Alliance of North America, on the national level. I was beginning to get a sense of midwifery on a larger scale.

I chose to work in a low-income prenatal clinic which served a lot of street women, prostitutes, drug addicts, battered women, teens, women with no money, no resources, no home. I rolled up sleeves to measure blood pressure and saw first the scarred wrists, then the needle tracks. I felt overwhelmed, impotent, yet fascinated by the sudden unlooked-for moments of joy, the smile with the sound of the baby's heartbeat, the appreciation for being treated as a worthwhile person, for being given free Nystatin, vitamins, help in finding shelter and the gift of a layette.

I enrolled in prerequisite classes for nursing school, assuring myself and my lay midwife friends that I was only keeping my options open. I agonized over what to do while I felt the ambition rise in me, yet was frightened by its implications. I wrote "pro" and "con" lists; months went by and the pro list got longer and the con list stabilized. I discussed the issue with friends and got a lot of support. I also got mixed messages—some midwives told me they would never go to nursing school but if I wanted to, they understood.

I also confronted my stereotypes of nurses as pill pushers and bed pan changers, and "Yes sir, Dr. Omnipotent, I'll crank up that Pitocin right away, sir." There was so much non-midwifery related learning to do, and sizable investments of time, money and energy to make. I contemplated the scenario of ceasing to do births, teaching, attending midwifery meetings, all the things with which I identified myself "professionally." My identity hung in a sort of symbolic limbo between fetoscope midwife and Doppler midwife.

Perhaps not too coincidentally, I became pregnant right after I found out that I had been accepted to nursing school. What a relief! Now I could just deal with having a baby for awhile. As time passed, I felt an easing inside myself. "I can do this," I assured myself. "I can live through, even benefit from, nursing school." I made an effort to meet and get to know some nurse-midwives in my area whom I respected and admired, and viewed them as positive role models.

> I needed the assurance that I could support myself and my family if the need ever arose, and I knew of very few lay midwives who could do that and maintain a decent lifestyle.

I thought about which I would rather be at age thirty-five—a lay midwife or a nurse-midwife. The answer became clearer as the advantages of being licensed became more apparent. I wanted to reach more people, a greater variety of women. I wanted to assist higher-risk women in the hospital as well as lower-risk women who chose home, birth center or hospital births. I realized that licensure might make my practice more legitimate in the eyes of an individual seeking a practitioner, and in the eyes of the public at large.

I also wanted to be paid reasonably for what I do. Midwifery, much as it is my breath and soul, is very stressful. Being well-paid helps compensate. I needed the assurance that I could support myself and my family if the need ever arose, and I knew of very few lay midwives who could do that and maintain a decent lifestyle.

I wanted to be legal. Whereas CNMs are legal in all states, lay midwives are often either working undercover, harassed or even prosecuted. Restrictive legislation always seems to be around the corner in my at-present liberal state.

Various other reasons to pursue licensing came to mind. I wanted to learn more. I wanted to be able to conduct a comprehensive physical exam, to do well-woman gynecology, to write prescriptions, to master suturing, to administer IVs. I had never felt I knew quite enough to gracefully handle all the possibilities inherent in birth. I have been intensely one-sided in my life—I eat, breathe and sleep birth. Becoming a CNM offered an opportunity to expand, to round out, to learn microbiology, care of the elderly, mental health, nursing skills, pharmacology. I also looked forward to experiencing the interfaces between other disciplines and midwifery as well as learning purely for the sake of knowing more about this world and my possible places within it.

However, certified nurse-midwifery is certainly not a panacea for all midwifery ills, and actually carries many of its own sets of problems. The issue of malpractice has really frightened a lot of people, although less than 10 percent of CNMs have been sued. I am also very aware of the problems CNMs have in obtaining backup for homebirths, and even in gaining hospital privileges. CNMs are often considered second-rate practitioners by the medical community, and can face harassment over infringement on what physicians perceive as their territory.

> The hippie midwife in my secret soul is engaged in a battle of ideologies with the budding yuppie midwife who is opening Pandora's box.

Furthermore, the sad truth is that once a CNM is licensed, she must toe the party line or face having her license revoked. So why should I pursue licensure, only to end up, in a sense, where I began? Why spend three years in a nursing school when I don't consider nursing a necessary prerequisite to midwifery? Why work for a year as an L & D nurse when the prospect somewhat appalls and frightens me? Why complete graduate work, struggle through two more oppressive years as the perpetual student when what I really want to do is palpate bellies and coo with babies?

The actual torment is fairly ludicrous. The hippie midwife in my secret soul is engaged in a battle of ideologies with the budding yuppie midwife who is opening Pandora's box. Since I have always been on the outside looking in with distaste and distrust, how do I reconcile my subversive tendencies with a desire to belong, make changes from within the system, be accepted and promote social change simultaneously? Will I cop out of the battle, be brainwashed, lose sight of the "whys" in pursuit of the "hows"? Will I begin to see pathology where before I saw normal variations?

So today I wonder if I will still "fit in" with my direct-entry friends, and if I will feel comfortable in a room full of CNMs. I feel as if I am between two worlds and am unsure how to balance and bridge them. Can I follow the wise woman traditions with the scent of a hospital in my nostrils?

This article first appeared in Midwifery Today Issue No. 4.

Sharon Glass Jonquil is a CNM in practice at Emanuel Hospital in Portland, Oregon in their nurse-midwifery service. She still enjoys writing as well as raising six children: her own three and her three stepchildren. She was just embarking on the transition from direct-entry midwifery to certified nurse-midwifery when she wrote this article.

FROM FETOSCOPE TO DOPPLER

. . . AND NOT YET BACK AGAIN

by Sharon Glass Jonquil, CNM

In 1987, I wrote an article for *Midwifery Today* about being a midwife on the CNM path. I spoke of my decision-making process based upon my experiences and ambitions. When I wrote that article five years ago, I was seriously concerned with how difficult it might be to remain true to my personal integrity while undergoing an about-face in practicing birth work.

I joined the existing power structure and majority rule of modern obstetrics as an RN, making the switch from homebirth to hospital, from client-centered control to hospital and physician-based protocol. My journey has been interesting, with unexpected rewards and pleasures, changes in rigid opinions, some ongoing ambivalence and occasional fury, as I participate in the "Great American Birth Scene."

I entered the hospital for the first time feeling like some kind of undercover agent. I was on a subversive mission with the hidden agenda of infiltrating behind enemy lines to foment needed revolution. Hardly anyone at the Labor and Delivery, Recovery and Postpartum (LDRP) unit knew my background. I didn't want to be prejudged and labeled before I had a chance to prove and make a place for myself, unhindered by any lurking stereotypes about a former lay midwife turned nurse.

It pretty much blew my cover when I realized I was pregnant with my third baby the month I started work. People started asking me who my doctor was and what hospital I was going to deliver at. I smiled and said hesitantly, "Well, my midwives are Mary and Evie and I'm planning a homebirth." The responses ranged from polite incredulity to warm support, much the same as you'd find anywhere.

I found, to my delight, that the RNs I worked with were caring, compassionate women who would go the extra mile for their patients. While many didn't share my commitment to noninterventive birth, they happily supported women in their individual birth experiences.

It was rather shocking to go from attending nearly all unmedicated deliveries to a seventy-five percent epidural rate, plus frequent use of IV narcotics in labor. I slowly realized that obstetric med use wasn't some terrible scam being foisted on unsuspecting women, but that women themselves often demanded interventions and medications. Some of the time, though, physicians and nurses applied well-meaning pressure due to their own agendas to move things along as rapidly and painlessly as possible.

There were times when I have felt, as a labor and delivery nurse, that I was participating in some mass hallucination that everybody but me was having; that birth was inherently dangerous and required total intervention and control for baby and mother to come out OK. Of course, my perspective was colored by previous homebirths and midwife experience that my colleagues had not had.

I was flabbergasted by the readiness of doctors and nurses to determine a course of action based on the clock rather than on individual circumstances. I wonder what would happen to the cesarean epidemic if clocks were abolished on maternity wards.

It became clear to me that the type of birth experience a woman has is very much determined by her physician. I have worked with awful doctors who truly hated women and completely mistrusted birth. In my opinion, they performed birth rape, just as I did my level best to protect women and babies. I have also worked with physicians who I would not hesitate to term midwives, who gently remind me to "chill out" when I get caught up in some notion of a birth ideal. Some of my ambivalence and anger has come from having to work with, and surreptitiously undermine, the horrid doctors who mistreat women's births, then take as their due women saying, "Oh, thank you, Dr. So-and-So, I couldn't have done it without you."

I have to remind myself that these women have chosen this path, and it is my place to aid them in whatever works best for them. There have been times when I have talked women into having an epidural, satisfied that I was giving the best possible care. It has been an important part of my growth as a birth worker to come to terms with women who choose doctors I wouldn't let deliver my gerbil and who permit interventions that I know often lead to unnecessary problems, when I know the end result will be their complete satisfaction and acceptance.

I like the variety of people I work with in the hospital. We serve primarily a white middle class insurance-covered population, but we also care for people from different racial and ethnic backgrounds, ages and income levels. Sometimes, attending home-births felt very insular. I now enjoy the mainstream feel to my work.

I'm happy with the skills I've acquired as a maternity nurse, particularly IV use. I used to think if a woman needed an IV she ought to be in the hospital—now I think IVs can be great for hydrating women and that midwives would really benefit from using them.

Fetal heart rate interpretation is another useful skill I have attained, but I am frustrated by routine monitoring and think it's overvalued in light of the lack of supporting evidence and the restriction of activity and increased pain. Another routine that I have trouble with is elective induction. I have to restrain myself from inappropriate comments when I ask women why they are being induced and they say, "Because the doctor told me to." Oy vay.

I'm very comfortable with much of our postpartum activity. My unit does not limit visitors or visiting hours, family togetherness, rooming in, or breastfeeding support. I disagree with other procedures, such as mandating checking babies for hypoglycemia—too many pokes for too little gain. And I am seriously considering refusing to assist at circumcisions when the dinosaur docs won't use local anesthesia, even

> I was flabbergasted by the readiness of doctors and nurses to determine a course of action based on the clock rather than on individual circumstances.

though I will get in big time hot water.

I like my job much of the time. Sometimes I really like it a lot: the camaraderie with the other nurses and some of the doctors, the feeling of satisfaction when making a positive difference in people's birth experiences. I can still feel the midwife in me reaching out, lending a healing hand. I feel comfortable as the "granola" nurse on the unit and have come to terms with most of the compromises I have made. There's truth to the phrase, "If you can't beat 'em, join 'em."

I have no regrets. I am looking forward to CNM school next fall with a combination of excitement and dread (over jumping through grad school hoops). And while there are times when I miss the feeling of being "called" that lay midwifery gave me, I feel I am doing important birth work that can make a crucial difference for many women and their families. And for me, it is still important to be "with women," just like a real midwife.

This article first appeared in Midwifery Today Issue No. 21.

Sharon Glass Jonquil is a CNM in practice at Emanuel Hospital in Portland, Oregon in their nurse-midwifery service. She still enjoys writing as well as raising six children: her own three and her three stepchildren. She was just embarking on the transition from direct-entry midwifery to certified nurse-midwifery when she wrote this article.

FOUR IN TWENTY-FOUR IS PART OF WHY . . .

by Sharon Glass Jonquil, CNM

I arrived yesterday at a goal set twelve years ago. Having been a lay midwife for a number of years, I had decided to become a certified nurse-midwife. My decision was influenced by a number of factors: a desire to reach more people, to be able to work in any setting, to learn more, to have a more dependable income and less stressful lifestyle, and a desire to still do what I knew was my right livelihood.

I took the nursing prerequisites, enjoying anatomy and struggling through chemistry. I went to nursing school, appreciating the broadening experience, yet at times despairing over the circuitous, time-consuming, expensive process. I remember finding myself debriding a wound dressing over an 80-year-old diabetic veteran's gangrenous stump, thinking, "Help! I'm stuck in someone else's movie! I'm supposed to be measuring fundal heights, not assessing depth of dead tissue on an old man's leg!"

Microbiology caused me to go through a spell of compulsive hand washing and feverish cleaning of the fridge, throwing away leftovers, sure the lasagna was breeding some malignant bacteria. I recall determinedly typing on the word processor, trying to meet class deadlines as my children came in every few minutes, wanting to know when Mommy was going to come play.

Three years passed as a maternity nurse, learning helpful skills like IVs and interpreting fetal monitor strips. There were days I felt like a midwife, that I made a positive difference in someone else's birth experience, and there were also days of frustration as I carried out orders for routine elective inductions or assisting while a doctor cut an unnecessary episiotomy. I was relieved and excited to finally begin nurse-midwifery school.

Midwifery school was wonderful in numerous ways. I adored many of my instructors, enjoyed all my midwifery classes, and some of the research classes, and I learned volumes in clinical classes. Gynecology was particularly rewarding: to be able to provide full-scope women's healthcare was a dream come true.

It helped a lot in school that I immediately bonded with a fellow student who had previously been a lay midwife, and we spent two years together "joined at the hip." We would call each other after each birth and yakkity-yak every detail, commiserating over the difficult ones, rejoicing over the positive ones. (Thank you, Karen Parker—I love you all up.)

I resented and resisted a few of my classes that were general "master's in nursing" type classes. It was hard when a few experiences as a student left me feeling woefully inadequate as a midwife. It took me forever to feel like I sort of knew what I was doing when I sutured a perineum. (That goes where?!)

I was definitely ready when graduation came around. Such celebration! We had a big jolly party and all the students roasted the faculty (we made them play Women's Healthcare Jeopardy: "Intrapartum for 200 please, Alex"). We left with warm hugs and lots of support as fledgling nurse-midwives.

The next hurdle was passing national boards. A very intense month of focused study helped draw together the previous years, distilling a lot of knowledge into practical assimilation. The actual Boards were almost anticlimactic, but a major relief to have done. After taking the rest of the summer off, I got serious about job hunting. I was truly grateful and pleased when I was hired (on-call but hopefully to become part-time) into a midwifery practice that I had been around as a graduate research assistant collecting data for a low birth weight study.

> I'm helping women I would not have helped birth at home—they either wouldn't have chosen such a birth or would have been considered too risky.

This brings me to yesterday. It's the fourth week of six weeks of full-time orientation. The first two weeks were all in clinic—doing prenatals, postpartums, some gyn and annual exams. I then began to do labor checks, attend deliveries and do hospital rounds. The teeter-totter of role assimilation was underway. Yesterday I came on shift to find two women being induced (one elective at forty plus weeks due to severe social stressors including her mother just dying, the other a postdates lady with a non-reactive non-stress test). A third woman was in early latent phase with SROM from the day before.

Another woman awaited in postpartum to be discharged with her baby. Catherine (my backup midwife) and I also got beeped to come evaluate Z.M., who was writhing in pain and screaming from either pyelonephritis or kidney stones. We got her settled with some morphine and transferred to physician care. We then had time to labor sit. A.G. was the first to birth, a lovely delivery with a tired but pleased mom. A.S. was next, with the resuscitation team standing by due to increasingly worrisome heart tones—minimal variability, advancing tachycardia, variable decelerations with many pushes. The baby had a tight cord body wrap and nuchal hand, but Apgars of 8 and 9 and the team quickly and quietly disappeared.

Meanwhile, E.M. went active, and her son was born into a party of five sisters and friends with babies and toddlers on hips, dancing to pounding rap music, yelling "Hurry up girl, come on, get it on!" I thankfully went home to bed, and miraculously got six hours of uninterrupted sleep.

The beeper went off at 4:30 in the morning. "Hello, it's P.W. and I've been contracting for a half hour."

"What number baby is this?"

"My fifth."

"Well, come on in!"

Two hours later her daughter came flying into the world through copious meconium after a two minute second stage. Following suctioning and evaluation she nursed contentedly on her mother's breast.

After giving a report to the incoming midwife, I came home and first told my husband about my work experiences. Then I called Karen. I told her how I finally feel that I have "arrived"—that I feel steady and ready and right doing what I am doing. It's not just midwifing the four labors and births in twenty-four hours, although that is part of it. It has more to do with the fact that I'm doing what I set out to do twelve years ago. I'm helping women I would not have helped birth at home—they either wouldn't have chosen such a birth or would have been considered too risky. I'm using technology appropriately, for the benefit of mothers and babies. While yesterday two mothers chose Pitocin and epidurals, one chose cohosh tincture, enemas and castor oil. Another birthed without any medication. And I had the privilege of serving them all.

Quality of care can certainly suffer with *quantity* of care service. Numbers don't tell the whole story—just one important part. I can't give the kind of ideal time and energy to each woman I see in the hospital, that I used to have available in home-birth practice. But, on the other hand, my family sure appreciates that when I'm on, I'm on, and when I'm off, I'm off, on a weekly basis.

I caught a homebirth baby about a month ago. It was so beautiful! And afterward I said to Mary, my highly experienced direct-entry partner, "You know, most hospital births can't touch this." Yet the reality is, I want to be where more women are that need me: where women of color are. Where teens are. Where poor women are. Abused women, drug-using women, homeless women facing hard times. Women with medical problems. Illiterate women. Middle class alternative women who want in-hospital midwifery care. Women who don't speak English. Many different kinds of women, all in need of midwifery care. And for now, I've found it. And although I've gone from fetoscope to Doppler, and not back again, I am at intermittent monitoring. And that's the right place for me to be.

This article was written especially for this book.

Sharon Glass Jonquil is a CNM in practice at Emanuel Hospital in Portland, Oregon in their nurse-midwifery service. She still enjoys writing as well as raising six children: her own three and her three stepchildren.

BAND-AID MIDWIFERY

by Sharon Glass Jonquil, CNM

Latoya calls at midnight. Her headache is back and she can't sleep. Tanisha calls at three a.m. She has sharp pains going down the side of her abdomen and into her groin. Lori phones in at seven-thirty a.m.; she's been throwing up, she has diarrhea and she is miserable. All of these women are pregnant, they want relief and they are relying on me. I can and do offer simple comfort measures, I give words of encouragement, and I have people come in when I don't feel triaging them over the phone suffices. But what if Latoya's headache means the onset of toxemia? She is a fifteen year old primip at term. I'd better check her blood pressure.

The personal and social contexts of many of these women I cannot impact. For example: Latoya was sexually abused from age five to eleven by her stepfather. This baby is the result of a rape. Tanisha and her boyfriend are about to be evicted. She doesn't know where they will go with their toddler—maybe back to living in their car. Lori has three other children (two of whom are sick) by three different men, none of whom are around.

Sometimes, we talk and visit with the same woman several times daily, day after day; her aches and pains seem to flow up one side of her body and down the other, with us no sooner fixing one problem before two more spring forth. Many of these women have chaotic lives, dysfunctional families with rampant abuse of all kinds. Many face a daily barrage of poverty, lack of options, racism and sexism. Often they know very little about their bodies and how they work. Their diets are highly processed, with few healthy foods. Many smoke—many drink and do drugs.

These women often live in the inner city in unsafe neighborhoods and have little contact with nature. Their lives have taught them many lessons about being victims. They are hopeless and cynical, depressed and angry, their present life a misery and their future an unknowable burden. When they are pregnant, they are scared and they aren't getting enough love and nourishment on all levels—body, mind and spirit.

I try my best to be a good midwife but I can't fix their real problems—like dead-end jobs because they are high school dropouts or having a boyfriend who beats them up but whom they won't leave. I can sometimes fix their constipation or their back pain, or even get them into drug treatment programs or help them succeed at breast-feeding instead of putting their baby to bottle. Sometimes I go home and I feel good that I made a difference. But sometimes I spend my days and nights putting Band-Aids over gaping wounds and I have a terrible and profound sense of helplessness.

Irina came in last week for a labor check. She had called me several times that shift and insisted that despite my various suggestions, she was hurting worse and needed to be seen in labor and delivery.

When I walked into her room she was in bed on the monitor. Her room reeked of alcohol, her anorexic looking mother was mumbling and stumbling around. The television was blaring and her boyfriend was cuffing their screaming snotty nosed toddler for doing things like trying to climb up on the bed with her. She was not in labor; she was in a world of pain that is real and to my thinking is about her life.

What can I do that will work in this woman's reality? I tell her how beautiful her baby looks on the monitor and then take her off it. I hold her hand, I rub her belly, I get her some juice. I tell her boyfriend it's just fine with me for the little guy to clamber up to snuggle mama. I turn the television down, cheerfully apologizing for not being able to hear what they are telling me. She wants to know why I can't induce her. I commiserate with her about how tough late pregnancy is and I give her a sleeping pill to take home. After they leave, I do a referral to our social worker regarding her living with her alcoholic mom. I put a Band-Aid on her life for a small moment in time.

The manifold opportunities and gifts of pregnancy, birth, and babies are frequently lost, drowned under a flood of suffering. Subtleties and delicate possibilities go by unexamined and untouched because a stomping elephant—like not enough food stamps to get through the end of the month—is what gets the attention. When you are focused on survival, it is difficult to make space for and have patience with that which is not apparent or immediately pertinent. The changes of this life passage become obstacles in your path, hurdles to struggle over and more defeats to endure rather than being anything positive. Street smarts and how to work the system serve you better than abstract notions of blessings in disguise or opportunities for personal growth.

> Midwifery is about loving these women and acknowledging that what is in them is also in me.

I wonder about my job description as a midwife when their pain becomes my pain, and when I find myself acting more like a combination social worker, therapist and mother. I wonder when I find myself happier over someone getting a tubal ligation than when I caught their baby because I know that family and I know that there are generations of ill people passing the disease of lack of love from grandparent on to baby. It is hard to keep addressing the symptoms and offering Band-Aids when I feel a desire and even need to touch the root problems.

My personal story of being a midwife is a journey. From a young, earnest, alternative-oriented lay midwife to a tertiary care, writing a prescription nurse-midwife, I have learned to synthesize, to step outside the bounds of all systems and trust in a higher spirit to guide me in truly being a healer. Many of my patients' problems are simply too big for me to fix—even with the wonderful support of my sister midwives and all the books I keep reading. Knowledge is only a part of wisdom. And while sometimes heartburn is just truly heartburn, I need to be able to tune in when it is not; when it is about being a neglected human being, I can offer something beyond Tums and papaya enzyme tablets.

In all practicality, what does this mean? If I have only a twenty minute time slot to spend with a patient, what can I really do? If she wants me to give her Terazol because she knows it makes her chronic yeast infection go away for awhile and I want her to stop drinking a liter of Dr. Pepper a day and talk to me about her philandering boyfriend who won't use condoms, where do we meet?

I'm guessing and hoping and trying to meet them in a place that gives them an immediate sense of being helped by my simply listening—really listening to them, with both my ears and my inner knowing so I can pick up on both verbal and nonverbal clues—using my experience and knowledge and prayer and intuition. Sometimes what isn't said is as important as what is. Being with them in a way that facilitates trust, being a respectful detective is vital. A shift in perspective allows a paradigm shift to take place. Mind-body-spirit stuff.

Midwifery is about service, and the longer I am doing this service, the more I allow it to take me to where I am not afraid to be uncomfortable, stretch and feel my connections to people who are living constricted lives. Midwifery is about being okay with not being able to please all the people all the time. It is about not allowing my judgments, blaming thoughts and opinions (why doesn't she just get a life and stop waking me at three a.m.) to stop me from a truly compassionate response. Midwifery is about loving these women and acknowledging that what is in them is also in me. Someone asked Bernie Siegal how he deals with people who are really difficult to be with and he said, "Act like you love them." By that effort, love will be made manifest. Through this effort, I know I can truly be a healing change agent, and not merely practicing Band-Aid midwifery.

This article first appeared in Midwifery Today Issue No. 45.

Sharon Glass Jonquil is a CNM in practice at Emanuel Hospital in Portland, Oregon in their nurse-midwifery service. She still enjoys writing as well as raising six children: her own three and her three stepchildren.

DIVERSITY IN PRACTICE SETTINGS

by Ida Laserson, CNM

Educational routes which lead to nurse-midwifery provide great diversity of employment opportunity. Certified nurse-midwives, currently licensed in all fifty of the United States, are increasingly recognized as valuable and cost-effective providers of high quality prenatal, intrapartum, postpartum and well-woman/family planning care. This recognition is evidenced by the steady increase in the number of job offerings posted in publications such as the ACNM newsletter, *Quickening*, and the *Journal of Nurse-Midwifery*. Almost weekly, private mailings to ACNM members offer a variety of new job openings.

Today's nurse-midwife may choose from a wide variety of job settings which serve diverse populations of women. Agencies in the public sector such as the United States Public Health Service, The Bureau of Indian Affairs, local county health departments, county hospitals and the branches of the military all actively seek to employ certified nurse-midwives. These positions offer the CNM the opportunity to assist economically and traditionally underserved populations such as migrant farm workers, low income inner city and rural populations.

The Public Health Service Corps funds the educational costs for nurse-midwives who contract to serve an underserved area such as an Indian reservation. There are many geographical areas within the scope of the United States Public Health Service Corps. All branches of the military employ nurse-midwives to care for military dependents. The military CNM is commissioned as an officer and often will have all her (his) educational debts and continuing education fees paid for by the military. There are military bases throughout the United States and the world—so again, there is wide geographical diversity.

The nurse-midwife with a desire to travel to exotic places can accept a position with the United States Agency for International Development in a Third World nation. As a teacher, the midwife will design and implement curriculum to educate traditional village midwives to bring safer basic maternity care to their village women. The American College of Nurse-Midwives sponsors and coordinates many nurse-midwifery projects in Asian, African and South American countries. Nurse-midwives are hired to staff these projects.

Turning to the private sector, there are again many job options. Large prepaid health maintenance organizations (such as Kaiser-Permanente) employ many nurse-midwives on their obstetrical staffs. There are positions with physician/midwife group practices, and private hospital midwifery services in all areas of the United States. Freestanding birth centers operated by CNMs with backup obstetrical consultants offer practice in a non-hospital setting. Developing or joining an established home-birth service is an available option for serving low risk women who want to give birth at home. Colleges, universities, certificate nurse-midwifery programs and non-nurse direct-entry midwife educational programs offer academic positions in which the

CNM can disseminate her clinical expertise and knowledge to many new aspiring midwives.

Looking at the economic/financial aspects of nurse-midwife practice, there are excellent incentives. Malpractice insurance is almost always funded by the employer or practice group. The average starting yearly salary for new graduates (in 1993) was $32,000. Depending upon geographical location and years of experience, salaries can exceed $75,000 per year. The median salary in 1991 was between $40,000 and $50,000 per year. Benefits such as paid vacations, paid continuing education, paid health and dental insurance and subsidized retirement pension plans further enhance CNM practice.

In summary, the CNM of the 1990s has the very good fortune to be well paid to do what she really loves doing, with a population she chooses, in a location of her choosing. Nurse-midwives as described in the above job settings generally work in groups with set time on call and time off. This allows the CNM a respite from the continual tension of being "on call" all the time, as experienced by the solo midwife. This helps us avoid burnout and allows the nurse-midwife time to relax, enjoy her family and pursue other interests.

This article first appeared in Midwifery Today Issue No. 20.

Ida Laserson, CNM, has been practicing in the Sacred Heart Hospital Prenatal Clinic in Eugene, Oregon for the past ten years. She has been a CNM since 1977.

NURSE-MIDWIFERY IN THE '90S

by Barbara Hughes, CNM, MS

The nursing profession is doing a lot of growing these days. Nursing theory, nursing research, and nursing practice are all areas in which nurses are blossoming to bring their profession to the foreground. Nursing is caring. To provide the special caring that nurses bring to many settings, not the least of which is childbearing, nurses need a significant knowledge base, clinical judgment and a positive framework in which to practice.

I am seeing nurses grow from the stereotypical "handmaiden" to leaders in many innovative areas in healthcare today. Nurse-midwifery is one of those areas. Nurses with a specialized knowledge base and clinical experience in obstetrics are pursuing additional education to allow them to provide complete care to healthy women and their newborns. Nurses entering nurse-midwifery schools are highly motivated to obtain additional knowledge and skills to meet the needs of women. They embrace the new knowledge and incorporate not only traditional medical values but many alternative approaches to providing healthcare services to their clients.

Certainly, practice situations vary around the country. Some nurse-midwifery services are small, single practitioner sites with care being provided in the home, while others are large services in a tertiary care setting. The theme is still the same, providing quality care to women in a nurturing environment and involving the woman and her family in care and decision making.

I have been practicing nurse-midwifery since 1985 and have had the pleasure to work in two very different practice sites. One was a private nurse-midwifery/MD practice at a private Level II hospital, and my current position is with a faculty practice in a tertiary care center. In both settings there has been a wonderful working relationship between the CNMs and the physicians. I have always felt that my physician colleagues and consultants have been very supportive of my role as an obstetrical care provider and of my clinical judgment. I have rarely had a situation involving disagreement about a management decision, and in all cases the wishes of the family were respected. The physicians I have worked with have voiced appreciation, respect and admiration of nurse-midwives, and many have stated that in a medical school setting, nurse-midwives should teach normal obstetrics to all medical students since we are the experts in healthy pregnancy care. Being part of the healthcare team provides me and my clients with a rich resource of knowledge and skills. I am happy to be part of that healthcare team.

The American College of Nurse-Midwives (ACNM) document *Standards for the Practice of Nurse-Midwifery* states:

> Nurse-Midwifery care occurs interdependently within the health care system of the community, using appropriate resources for referrals that meet psychosocial, economic, and cultural, or family needs. The certified nurse-midwife . . . demonstrates an agreement with a physician for a safe mechanism of obtaining medical consultation, collaboration, and referral.

This "agreement" can be negotiated in many ways. There are practices in which a physician or group of physicians hires a nurse-midwife. The practice pays the CNM's salary; pays for her benefits, malpractice insurance and professional needs; and provides a mechanism for physician consultation. This does not mean that the practice dictates the scope of nurse-midwifery care. Other nurse-midwives establish an independent practice and contract with a physician for consultation services. The reality is that all hospitals and malpractice insurance companies also require proof of a relationship with a physician consultant. Therefore, in order for a CNM to provide continuity of care to her clients, this agreement serves a dual purpose. Finally, the CNMs I work with and others I have spoken with on the national level feel an ethical obligation to meet this criterion so that the full realm of obstetrical services is available to each client.

> This "agreement" can be negotiated in many ways. . . . This does not mean that the practice dictates the scope of nurse-midwifery care.

I find that working with physicians has been very positive. I am the director of a seven-CNM faculty practice. We have developed our own protocols for what we consider safe practice. Our physician consultations provide us with a mechanism for consultation, co-management and referral as we as a team see appropriate. I acknowledge the limits of my professional skills and knowledge and am happy to be in an environment where my clients can be provided with care by my physician colleagues when their skills are needed.

As the scientific body of knowledge about obstetrics grows, it impresses on me one big point: We don't know as much as we think we do. For every study supporting a new management protocol, there is another in opposition to that same protocol.

One of the things I enjoy about nurse-midwifery is the critical thinking skills that were nurtured in graduate school that help me seek out the literature and look for answers to my questions. When I am with a client in labor who has "fallen off the curve" (Friedman's), I have the freedom to use my knowledge about the physiology of labor, add in the individual factors surrounding this woman and family, involve the client in the decision making, and come up with a number of potential courses of action. If I am able to state a reasonable rationale for our course of action, it is wholeheartedly supported. In fact, the resident physicians I work with have been heard to say, "Well, if I were a nurse-midwife I might, so maybe I'll try that."

Nurse-midwives from all over the country have shared with me anecdotes about changes in hospital practices and physician practices that were influenced by nurse-midwives. Yes, there are some "rules" and "protocols" in any institution, but I believe that some of these are there for the safety and protection of mothers and babies. As to the others, well, we need to keep working on increasing our knowledge base about normal pregnancy and childbirth and educate our nurse and physician colleagues about these.

Certainly, there are challenging days being a nurse-midwife. But, I am very proud of my profession and pleased to be able to offer such a special service to families. I see the profession of nurse-midwifery growing in numbers and strength in the years to come. One of ACNM's goals is to have "10,000 CNMs by the year 2001." Nationally, there are hundreds of job openings for CNMs. National health policy organizations, such as the Institute of Medicine, have recognized the importance of nurse-midwifery care and are encouraging increased utilization of nurse-midwives in many settings. Most of all, the special contribution a nurse-midwife makes to each birthing family she attends makes me excited to be a part of this profession.

This article first appeared in Midwifery Today Issue No. 21.

Barbara Hughes has been a CNM since 1984, and was practice director of the nurse-midwifery faculty practice at University Hospital in Denver, Colorado when she wrote this article.

Philosophy and Approach
to Midwifery Education

by Katherine Camacho Carr, CNM

Introduction

Each nurse-midwifery and midwifery education program develops its own philosophy that must be congruent with the overall philosophy of the American College of Nurse-Midwives (ACNM), as required by the Division of Accreditation (DOA), the accrediting body. Program objectives and the entire curriculum flow from this philosophy. Each educational program is affiliated with or resides within an institution of higher learning, such as a university or college, and must also establish philosophical congruency with that institution. Within those parameters programs can establish their own unique philosophy and approach pertaining to midwifery education and midwifery practice. While the philosophical underpinnings of midwifery education have changed very little with regard to practice, a new philosophy and approach to education has developed in the past five to seven years. Nurse-midwifery education has undergone a curricular revolution, reflective of current trends in other fields.

In the past most of us were educated through grade school, high school and college in a directed, teacher led kind of education, called the pedagogic style (meaning "leading the child"). This approach is still appropriate in midwifery education when teaching precise tasks with little room for error, such as insertion of a Norplant or incubation of the newborn. In pedagogical teaching and learning the student contributes little to the situation and is dependent upon the teacher to learn the correct way to do things or get the correct message. The teacher is responsible for "depositing" knowledge into students and must appear all-knowing, hiding her/his imperfections or inadequacies. Lecture is the predominant teaching style. This type of traditional education is called "the banking style" by Belenky in *Women's Ways of Knowing* (1986). Currently, many nurse-midwifery education programs have implemented a different approach—androgogical teaching/learning styles. Androgogical teaching and learning, based on the work of Malcolm Knowles (1980), is student centered with the teacher acting as midwife-teacher, assisting the student to expand and articulate her own latent knowledge. The midwife teacher draws out knowledge and assists the students to "give birth" to their own ideas (Belenky, 1986). This type of learning is called "yogurt teaching and learning," and provides the right culture and the correct growing environment for the development of student midwives. Guided self-study is the predominant learning style.

Transactional Education

Educational theorists have also described this kind of learning environment as transactional education, where a dialogue takes place between teachers and learners and no one member has a monopoly on insight or knowledge. This philosophical approach works well in adult education where learners have a variety of professional and life experiences to integrate with new learning. Knowles identified four principles of adult learning that typify the needs of the adult learners. Transactional education is designed to meet these needs:

- The adult learner has the need to move toward self-direction.

- The adult learner has a reservoir of life experience to use as a resource during learning.

- The adult learner has a particular desire to learn how to solve real-life problems.

- The adult learner is oriented toward immediate application of knowledge that is performance-centered.

TRANSACTIONAL EDUCATION IN ACTION

Educational theories which emphasize these principles of adult education and transactional learning between teacher and learner are most evident in the newly developed community-based, distance education programs, including the Frontier School of Midwifery & Family Nursing, Community-based Nurse-midwifery Education Program (CNEP), the Institute of Midwifery, Women & Health Nurse-Midwifery Education Program (IMWAH) and the State University of New York, Stony Brook Nurse-Midwifery Education Program (SUNY-S) and several others. In the above educational programs teachers and students are separated by distance (for the academic components of the educational program) and each program is based on a philosophy of transactional education. In these educational programs the interaction between student and teacher mirrors the respect and support that midwives give to women during labor. Students are treated as adult peers and are responsible for self-directed learning. The faculty provide structure, such as a written or electronic course syllabus, and guidance/evaluation through discussion (when on campus, via telephone or electronic means), feedback on learning activities/exams and during on-campus sessions. Faculty are not abdicating their responsibility in such a model, they are assuming the role of midwife-teacher—encouraging and validating progress, recognizing problems, intervening only when necessary, and most importantly acting as supportive resources. This Chinese proverb summarizes the role of faculty: Teachers open the door, but you must enter yourself.

CURRICULAR STRUCTURE

Each curriculum is rigorous and is structured so that students proceed through several levels of learning, from basic underlying theory and knowledge to application in clinical practice. Courses are developed based upon the core competencies and whatever unique curricular threads faculty have identified that they wish to add. Modules or courses, including objectives, learning activities, methods of evaluation and required readings, are developed by faculty and are continuously updated and revised based on student feedback and new information. Modified mastery learning forms the foundation for course and program evaluation. Students must meet the

This Chinese proverb summarizes the role of faculty: Teachers open the door, but you must enter yourself.

course objectives and are evaluated through closed book exams, papers, case studies and other required learning activities. If a student "fails," she or he is encouraged to remediate and retake an exam or redo a learning activity until the material is mastered. Policies have been established in each program describing the modifications or limitations applied to this practice.

The student's own community is used as the classroom. Learning activities throughout the curriculum are designed to focus on community assessment and intervention, as well as the use of community resources. Students also spend a large portion of their educational program in a clinical setting in or near their own community with qualified midwifery faculty. Library facilities within their own community or via electronic access are also utilized by students.

Communication is also an important aspect of these programs. With students and faculty geographically separated, some system of asynchronous electronic communication has been used successfully for communication and teaching/learning by each of these educational programs. In addition, faculty have established office hours when they are available by telephone. Mail and facsimile are also used for communication between faculty and students.

A strong education and service linkage is inherent in each of these education programs. Applicants must interview with community midwives, qualified to be faculty, and be accepted by them for a clinical preceptorship or they will not be admitted to the educational program. Community midwives and academic faculty form a partnership from Day One to educate the student midwife. These preceptors are also provided with information about transactional education, clinical teaching techniques, performance evaluation and problem-solving mechanisms so that they are working cooperatively with students and academic faculty. Community site visits are conducted by the academic program to assist preceptors, as well as to evaluate students and clinical sites. These programs do not view practice and education as separate entities but part of a continuum. Curricula must be reflective of "real" practice and practice must be academically sound.

LEARNING ACTIVITIES

Learning activities that reflect transactional education are many and varied, facilitating the variety of learning styles that students have. The mystique surrounding distance education also revolves around the teaching/learning activities. Some educators have questioned the ability to transmit complex, multidimensional, non-linear information using very limited lecture, seminar or other personal interaction. Lecture and face-to-face seminar meetings are reserved for the few on-campus sessions integrated into these programs. Teaching/learning methods primarily include case studies, guided teaching and information search. And as usual, texts and journal articles provide an important source of information. Computerized interactive programs provide the framework for several of the educational programs. These programs may also provide graphics, video clips and hypertext techniques to aid student learning.

The case study format is used frequently in midwifery and nurse practitioner education. In the case study, faculty give a real life or fictitious account of a clinical situation with questions to assist the student in analyzing the problem. Content information that would normally be given in a lecture format can be embedded within the case study and supporting materials that the student must use for reference. The student can be guided through a critical decision-making process utilizing case studies. It can be used in a course syllabus, on-line or in a group presentation on-campus.

Guided teaching uses a Socratic-like teaching strategy where faculty ask the student a series of questions at the end of a module or section of a module/course. This allows the student to use prior knowledge as well as new knowledge obtained in readings. Students can also "discuss" their conclusions and rationale for any clinical decision-making. When these learning activities are evaluated/graded, faculty can easily identify areas of knowledge deficit, misconception or failure to arrive at the appropriate clinical decision. Group inquiry is also used by faculty when a topic is presented on-line and the group "discusses" it.

When using information search, course faculty carefully design worksheets to be completed or questions to be answered by students. A worksheet may include a diagram, fill-in-the-blanks, true/false items, matching and short answers. Students must use texts and other reference materials to complete the worksheets or questions. Students can also be asked to write a position paper on a controversial issue in clinical practice, which requires information search to document one's position.

Demonstration and role modeling are also useful techniques and can still be provided at a distance through video and audiotape. Faculty are also investigating the utilization of problem-based learning, a framework for the development of deductive problem-solving using small groups (live or asynchronous electronic communication). Problem-based learning has been applied to medical education with good results (Berkson, 1993).

SUMMARY

Midwifery education has made some significant changes; however, the current and anticipated changes in education and the healthcare system demand further reform. The programs cited incorporate a philosophical approach to education and many structural elements that are in line with current trends and future direction toward community-based education, integration of appropriate technology, flexibility for adult learners and ability to operate large education programs without federal or state funding, which is on the decline. This shift toward student centered education in schools "without walls" requires a creative, dedicated and highly qualified faculty, who set the stage for student learning and safe beginning level practice in a variety of settings. These faculty are committed to moving ahead with a variety of options, articulations and affiliations to facilitate the further development of quality midwifery education.

References

Belenky, M., et al. (1986). *Women's Ways of Knowing: The Development of Self, Voice and Mind*. New York: Basic Books.

Berkson, L. (1993). "Problem-based learning: have expectations been met?" *Academic Medicine*, 68(10) s79-s88.

Camacho Carr, K. (1995). Community-based education and strategies for distance teaching and learning. *Marketing and Teaching Strategies for Advanced Practice Nursing*. San Antonio, Texas: American Association of Colleges of Nursing.

Henderson, V. (1990). *Curriculum revolution: a review*. NLN Publications (15-2351).

Knowles, M. (1980). *The Modern Practice of Adult Education*. Englewood Cliffs, NJ: Cambridge Adult Education.

McHugh, K., & Armstrong, P. (1991). *CNEP/FSMFN Preceptor Training Manual*. Hyden, KY: FSMFN.

Piskurich, G. (1993). *Self-Directed Learning*. San Francisco: Jossey-Bass Publishers.

Silberman, M. (1992). *Active Training: A Handbook of Techniques, Designs, Case Examples and Tips*. New York: Lexington Books (Macmillan, Inc.).

FOR MORE INFORMATION:

Frontier School of Midwifery & Family Nursing Community-based Nurse-midwifery Education Program, P.O. Box 528, Hyden, KY 41749, 606-672-2312

Institute of Midwifery, Women & Health Nurse-Midwifery Education Program, c/o Philadelphia College of Textiles & Science, Schoolhouse Lane & Henry Avenue, Philadelphia, PA 19144, 215-951-2525, IMWAH@bbs.acnm.org

State University of New York Stony Brook Nurse-Midwifery Education Program, School of Nursing Health Sciences Center, Stony Brook, NY 11794-8240, 516-444-2879, <judith.treistman@sunysb.edu>.

This article was written especially for this book.

Katherine Camacho Carr, CNM, PhD, formerly served as the director of special projects, Institute of Midwifery, Women and Health where she is involved in the development of the master of science in midwifery curriculum and Internet access to the Institute's program. She maintains a part-time clinical practice, has served on the faculty of the Seattle Midwifery School, the University of Washington School of Nursing and the School of Medicine, the Pacific Lutheran University School of Nursing, and as the director of research and development for the Frontier School of Midwifery and Family Nursing, Community-based Nurse-midwifery Education Program (CNEP). Dr. Carr has won numerous awards for her pioneering work in primary healthcare policy. She is currently vice-president of the ACNM, and on the faculty of State University of New York (SUNY) Health Sciences Center at Brooklyn, where she teaches graduate courses in distance learning for the State University.

CHOOSING A

CERTIFIED NURSE-MIDWIFERY PROGRAM

by Natasha Beauchamp

Are you a lay midwife who wants more legitimacy, but you're not sure how to get it or where? The local junior college offers an RN program, but there is no school nearby for the midwifery component of a CNM degree. Is nursing even what you want to do? What are your options? How do you choose a school?

Those considering mainstream licensure with no prior degree are often faced with such questions. Fortunately, there are educational options available.

PHILOSOPHIES

The philosophy statements of many schools are inspiring; they speak of the integrity of birth, a commitment to wellness and the need to balance both the art and science of midwifery. Many schools are affiliated with high volume hospitals in large urban centers and multicultural sensitivity is high, as is a strong political consciousness concerning racism, sexism and classicism in the American medical model. While homebirth is often not a part of a program's official structure, many maintain an encouraging and respectful attitude toward it. Graduates from several of these programs feel well-received and are impressed with the compassion, patient advocacy and high level of awareness of their teachers. They say that learning how effective they could be as a member of the "healthcare team" is one of the best surprises of their training.

With no previous license (LPN, RN, etc.) there are three options to choose from:

1. Become an RN through a local junior college program, then apply to a CNM program;

2. Apply to a school that integrates a nursing degree into its CNM program, which allows non-nurses to gain their RN in the process of gaining their CNM;

3. Become a physician's assistant to expand into more family and general medicine, and take an enrichment program that will allow you to practice as a certified midwife.

OPTION 1: JUNIOR COLLEGE/CNM

The advantage of the first option, the two-step junior college/CNM route, is that nursing schools are usually near community colleges, and part of your schooling can be accomplished without a long commute or relocation. Since many CNM programs require a year or two of nursing experience before you are accepted, studying locally followed by work at a local hospital allows you three to five years before turning your attention to the midwifery component of your training.

This option also provides a natural breaking point, giving you a chance to stop and take a breather after nursing school. Maybe the strain becomes too hard on your kids, or it is too hard financially. Getting your RN first, with the option of saving the CNM part for later, allows your family to regroup and benefit from your working for a few years with better wages as an RN.

OPTION 2: RN ON THE WAY TO CNM

Some people prefer to consolidate their studies and enroll in a program where they can enter as a non-nurse and get their RN along the way. Generally, a combined RN-CNM program requires a bachelor's degree and takes longer than a CNM program for experienced RNs; on the other hand, if you already have a bachelor's, it doesn't take as long to complete as the junior college/CNM route. (The RN component of these programs adds only an additional year. The junior college route takes two additional years of schooling for the RN, once you have taken about a year of biology, anatomy and physiology. Then, you must usually work for a few years before you do your CNM training.)

For some families, minimizing the amount of time that mom is in school and not earning money is a high priority, thus the combined RN/CNM program can be ideal. RN programs integrated into the CNM program will generally teach you methods of nursing practice that conform to the overall philosophy of the CNM school. From our survey of philosophy statements, it was clear that many midwifery schools emphasize wellness and take a stand against unnecessary intervention. The nursing profession, along with public opinion, is generally moving more in this direction, but there are thousands of nursing schools nationwide and not all of them will have such an orientation.

OPTION 3: PHYSICIAN'S ASSISTANT

The third option is not as common as the other two. Physician's assistants (PAs) are mid-level practitioners in the medical hierarchy. Unlike RNs, they are given specific training and licensing to diagnose and treat routine conditions in family medicine. (RNs can elect to go to further schooling and become Nurse Practitioners [NPs] gaining similar direct care rights and skills, but the PA route is generally shorter than the NP path.) The advantage to becoming a PA is that you learn many skills pertaining to general medicine, so you can maintain a holistic approach. It also allows for more flexibility as you can work in family medical clinics, pediatrics and so forth.

As with the junior college/CNM route, becoming a PA first gives you a natural break in your training should you want it. It also gives you a license with more autonomy than an RN alone. Your training is very firmly based in being able to diagnose and treat, not simply on facilitating the diagnostic and treatment methods of physicians, so it has these advantages.

Unfortunately, the schooling is a bit longer for a PA, and PA programs are not as readily available as RN programs are. Several CNM schools allow PAs and NPs to challenge parts of their programs and some already have an established shorter track for those who already possess these licenses. PAs with the extra midwifery training are licensed to practice much as CNMs—they can bill insurance companies, work in hospitals, birth centers and homebirth settings—but as a group they are very small nationally and they tend to be a political anomaly in the healthcare system. Again, as with each route, there are advantages and disadvantages, but the PA path is one that is not often discussed and deserves serious consideration.

IF YOU ALREADY HAVE AN RN . . .

Suppose you already have your RN; what CNM program is best for you? Why not consider the possibility of a master's degree or Ph.D.? Many schools offer a graduate degree in conjunction with a CNM licensure program, and the extra classes needed to make up the degree turn out to be minimal. Also, if you think you might ever practice in the field of public health as a CNM, the government often bases its pay scale on the level of an employee's education—the higher the degree, the higher the salary. (On the other hand, this can sometimes work against you if you are perceived as overqualified.) A graduate degree can also enable you to teach. You can teach in a junior college or nursing school, expanding opportunities later in your career. If any of these considerations are important to you, you might want to seriously look at a school that would allow you to apply your CNM credits toward an MSN or ND.

FINANCIAL AND LOGISTICAL CONSIDERATIONS

Many of us decide to seek licensure because we are financially strapped and need the legitimacy of a license to do what we do best and get paid a living wage for it. How can we possibly take time from our income-earning ability and pay tuition on top of that? It isn't easy, but there are programs that will help. Student loans are available and you become eligible for an even broader range of student loan programs if you are going for a graduate degree in conjunction with a CNM. There are also state, federal and even individual hospital grants that will pay your tuition in exchange for your working in underserved areas for a few years after you graduate.

If you are like many of us—you became a midwife as a result of being pregnant and becoming a mom yourself—classrooms, labs and lectures seem very distant, far from diapers, childcare, soccer games and orthodontia bills. Even if there is school support for the issues you have as a "reentry" student, how can you begin to consider a program if there are none close by?

Some women have been able to relocate their families. Others find creative solutions. One woman I know had her mom take care of her kids during the week, her husband care for them on the weekends and she came to visit when she could. She essentially took a few years off from motherhood and moved from California to Connecticut to attend Yale, which was one of the only CNM programs around at the time. For most of us, an arrangement like this is nowhere near possible, or even desirable. So what can you do?

Is further schooling simply out of the picture, at least until your kids are grown?

TECHNOLOGY AND COLLEGE WITHOUT WALLS

Thankfully, no. One of the most innovative uses of technology in education has been applied to midwifery training. The Frontier Nursing School, a pioneer of midwifery education in the United States, developed a CNM program called Community-based Nurse-midwifery Education Program (CNEP). [See the article "Community-Based Nurse-Midwifery Education Program: Distance Learning in Nurse-Midwifery Education" at the end of this chapter.]

To do the CNEP program, you need a budget for regularly scheduled phone calls to program faculty, a computer to communicate via the Electronic Bulletin Board, and travel expenses for two trips—one for Midwifery Bound Orientation, five days, and one for Level III preclinical which is two weeks. These trips meet over a two year span and give you the chance to meet with the other students in your "class" at the program headquarters in Kentucky. Much more than limited financial aid is available. In fact, our students qualify for more than double (in Guaranteed Student Loans) what our tuition is. Many state and federal student grant and loan programs are also available, depending upon your family income and expenses. As an added plus, Case Western Reserve University in Cleveland, Ohio, will let you apply your CNEP classes toward a master's degree or a Nursing Doctorate (ND) in their nursing school.

A direct-entry midwife, who went to nursing school and then chose CNEP as her path to a CNM, was shocked at her first class meeting to realize how many of her fellow students were direct-entry midwives, like herself, seeking accreditation. Rather than walking into "foreign territory" as she had feared, she described it as "coming home." Concerns she had about hostility toward her homebirth experience were quickly allayed.

Of course, there are drawbacks. You must be extremely self-directed and self-motivated to complete the program. There is a strong sense of community between the students, but not in the same way that meeting daily in a specific location would naturally engender, thus peer support is a bit diffused. While homebirth experience is respected in a student's past, a CNM license means you are experienced and qualified in birth center and hospital work, thus preceptor arrangements are made accordingly. You can, of course, go on and develop a homebirth practice once you are licensed, but homebirth is not a specific option in your training.

Lastly, as with any preceptor-based program, finding and keeping a preceptor, getting the support you need and getting her the support she needs, are not that easy. It involves perseverance. The CNEP program has a workshop and support system for preceptors to address this issue.

Midwifery is an ancient profession developed by women to serve women. We have practiced in many settings and in many contexts over the years. Sadly, with increased medical misunderstanding of birth, a schism has developed which appears to separate one midwife from the other. CNMs developed their area of expertise while direct-entry midwives developed theirs. The division has weakened all midwives.

Mary Breckenridge, who founded Frontier Nursing Service in 1939, used a beautiful analogy of the banyan tree in her vision of midwifery education. This ancient tree has a typical trunk, branches and root system, but as it spreads it periodically drops a root from an overhanging branch back down into the ground. This provides enough support to allow the tree to branch out even farther, drop another root and so on.

> Like the banyan tree, CNEP starts with the roots of midwifery, utilizing self-study and the apprenticeship method along with a student's own community base.

While not the only way to learn midwifery, the Frontier Nursing Service offers a CNM model that begins to bring us all together. Like the banyan tree, CNEP starts with the roots of midwifery, utilizing self-study and the apprenticeship method along with a student's own community base. By integrating the modern technologies of the telephone, computer and airplane, CNEP brings the two worlds of the certified nurse-midwife and the direct-entry midwife closer together than they have ever been before, expanding and securing the roots for the profession to grow.

Seven years ago, the American College of Nurse-Midwifery (ACNM), the national accreditation board for all CNM schools, set a goal to double the number of practicing nurse-midwives by the year 2000. We at Midwifery Today applaud and support the goal as it means more and more women and babies will receive the benefits of "with-woman" birth care. A survey completed several years ago showed that numerous CNM programs are responding with flexibility and creativity to the needs of direct-entry midwives and women with children. Becoming a CNM is one of the many roads to serving the birthing community and we are delighted to report that there are now several ways to pursue this dream.

This article first appeared in Midwifery Today Issue No. 21.

Natasha Beauchamp is a wife and mother, and has been involved in making interactive health education videotapes since she stopped attending births.

FRONTIER SCHOOL OF MIDWIFERY

AND FAMILY NURSING

by Kitty Ernst, CNM

People think I have strong opinions about nurse-midwifery vs. direct-entry midwifery partly because I was educated into both nursing and midwifery. My only strong opinion, however, is that, for a variety of reasons in the United States, midwifery falls short in delivering care to childbearing families. We have not been able to educate enough midwives to make midwifery a viable part of the healthcare system. At a high-level policy meeting addressing the need to reduce the nation's embarrassing infant mortality, it was suggested that nurse-midwives had demonstrated their ability to reduce infant mortality even in the most disadvantaged populations. Despite this acknowledgement, however, it was clear that we needed to figure out how to exponentially increase the numbers of nurse-midwives.

When the Community-based Nurse-midwifery Program (CNEP) was first announced in the Childbirth Graphics Catalog, a few of the 2,000 women who responded in the first year asked why we were not developing a direct-entry program. I had not thought about the direct-entry approach to midwifery because it was not where my roots were. I was thinking about the many closet midwives in nursing who had told me over the years they "always wanted to be a midwife" but due to circumstances in their lives, couldn't realize their dream. Either they were unable to relocate to study in the few existing programs, or the enrollment was so limited they were wait-listed past the time of possibility in their lives. Many had gone into nursing to become midwives but were sidetracked by marriage and rearing a family or other career choices. This was the market I instinctively felt was ready to be tapped to expand the number of midwives to make midwifery a more viable force in the care of childbearing women. The announcement of the CNEP—a distance-learning program which would enable students to remain in their own communities—rekindled old flames of passion for being "with woman" in thousands of nurses and brought their dream closer to the realm of possibility than ever before.

My instinct about nurses wanting to be midwives has proven to be right. Since the first class was admitted to the pilot program in Perkiomenville, Pennsylvania in the spring of 1989, over five hundred nurses have completed the two-year, graduate-level program offered by the Frontier School of Midwifery and Family Nursing. We also offer a master's degree option from Case Western Reserve University. A large percentage of the graduates have broken new ground for services in rural and underserved urban areas where midwifery care has never been available before. The distance learning program has been replicated at the State University of New York at Stony Brook, Ohio State University, and most recently at the Midwifery Institute in Philadelphia.

Over the past several decades a dedicated group of nurse-midwives has labored to bring midwifery into the mainstream of maternity care to:

- publish research that documented the effectiveness of adding midwifery to the delivery of maternity care services—from the first experiences of the Frontier Nursing Service to the recent National Birth Center Study;

- establish an organization to develop the benchmarks for the profession;

- lay down the standards for quality education through accreditation of programs;

- define core competency requirements for entry into practice;

- develop a national certifying examination;

- define standards for practice and make them part of the requirements for licensing regulations in all fifty states;

- publish a respected refereed journal on midwifery and a newsletter for their members;

- create programs for continuing education and mandated peer review;

- obtain statements of policy for joint practice with obstetrician colleagues;

- obtain direct access to hospitals by hospital staff privileges;

- obtain direct reimbursement for midwifery services; and

- obtain professional liability insurance for members of the professional association.

All these accomplishments were achieved by volunteers committed to constructing a foundation needed to make midwifery viable in the United States. The window of opportunity for that growth has come with the paradigm shift from fee for service to managed care. I felt that this window might be closed by the time we restructured the foundation to accommodate non nurse-midwives, however. As it was, it took six years of planning and negotiation to implement the program, relying on support from nursing for program funding and student support. This is why I chose only to tap into the known market of closet midwives in nursing. Throughout this long journey, the leadership in nursing, specifically the dean of the Frances Payne Bolton School of Nursing, the director of the Frontier Nursing Service, the director of Maternity Center Association, and the Division of Nursing at the federal level, has been a strong advocate and ally.

Does this mean I am opposed to "direct-entry" midwifery? Not at all. I applaud the pioneer efforts to establish quality education by the Seattle School of Midwifery and more recently at the State University of New York at Brooklyn. We all must develop quality midwifery education programs, regardless of how a nurse, doctor or other individual or group enters that education program.

Some colleagues have questioned the need for exponential growth in midwifery in the United States. They say that there are not enough jobs. If you believe, as I do, every woman should have the choice of a midwife or obstetrician team, and that midwifery is not a replacement for obstetrics but an addition to obstetrics, it follows that if we match the needs of those we serve, we will work to reverse the ratio of midwives to obstetricians. Instead of four obstetricians to one midwife we will have five or six midwives to one obstetrician. This goal will require tens of thousands of midwives to be trained over the next two or three generations.

If midwifery is to become a viable part of the system for care of women and child-bearing families, we have to demonstrate how it is different from obstetrics and from obstetrical nursing. More of the same is not a solution to the myriad problems we face in the delivery of care today. The journey will continue to be long and difficult. But I am confident that if we put the needs of those we serve first, midwifery will come into its own in ways that we cannot even contemplate today.

This article was written especially for this book.

Kitty Ernst, CNM, MPH, holds the Mary Breckinridge Chair of Midwifery and is the director of the National Association of Childbearing Centers Consulting Group (NACC). She is past president of ACNM, past director of the Pilot CNEP program and is currently on the faculty of CNEP.

COMMUNITY-BASED NURSE-MIDWIFERY EDUCATION PROGRAM:

DISTANCE LEARNING IN NURSE-MIDWIFERY EDUCATION

by Judith M. Treistman, CNM, PhD, Katherine Camacho Carr, CNM, PhD, & Mary Kate McHugh, CNM

ABSTRACT: This article describes the Community-based Nurse-midwifery Education Program (CNEP) of the Frontier School of Midwifery and Family Nursing. The organization structure and curriculum of CNEP combines apprenticeship learning with academic rigor, permitting students who cannot relocate to the university to pursue graduate education. New technology, such as an interactive electronic bulletin board, networks students and faculty. The program emphasizes theories of independent, adult learning. There is a master's completion option available through affiliation with Case Western Reserve University.

The Community-based Nurse-midwifery Education Program (CNEP) of the Frontier School of Midwifery and Family Nursing admitted its first class in the spring of 1989, and graduated over one hundred students by the end of 1993. The purpose of CNEP is to increase significantly the number of practicing nurse-midwives to meet the needs of families residing in rural or other underserved areas as well as those choosing birth-center care.

ADULT EDUCATION

The educational philosophy of CNEP assumes that the student and instructor are active partners in a common enterprise and that the student is an adult who brings to the learning process all the accumulated knowledge and experience of her life. The theoretical content of the curriculum is largely delivered in the familiar "modules" that lay out the objectives that must be mastered to achieve clinical competency in nurse-midwifery. These modules are written by the faculty and are continuously updated and revised. The student complements and meets these objectives by designing her own learning plan, identifying and confronting barriers to successful learning, and maximizing potential resources, including family, colleagues, and friends. Treating the community as the "university," students learn to draw upon these resources rather than build dependence on faculty. They are also compelled to engage in continuous self-evaluation and not become distracted by judging success in terms of others. The clinical component of the curriculum is treated in much the same way, providing an apprenticeship experience guided by a master teacher.

THE SERVICE-EDUCATION LINK

In CNEP, the student is intimately involved with faculty who are actively providing clinical care to clients. This is an apprenticeship with a master midwife, and the student has the opportunity to learn from the expert. Because the student is often "sponsored" by the clinical site and retains her ties to the community as a healthcare professional, she is looked upon as a potential colleague and builds upon her previous experience with that community.

How CNEP Works

The CNEP curriculum is structured so that students progress through several "levels" of learning, expanding the theoretical foundation for clinical practice through a series of courses taught by academic faculty and expert practitioners. There are four levels in the CNEP curriculum. After coming together for a three-day orientation to the program, students return home and begin their studies. Levels I and II concentrate on the theoretical basis for practice; level III is a two-week intensive workshop during which faculty and students come together in small groups to work on the primary clinical skills necessary for practice; level IV is an extended practicum during which the student develops these basic skills and expands her theoretical knowledge base under the tutelage of a clinical preceptor. As the student moves through the levels of learning, she is in constant electronic contact with her instructors, preceptors and fellow students. Upon completion of level IV, the student takes a comprehensive exam and is declared to be a safe beginning practitioner. She is then eligible to sit for the American College of Nurse-Midwives National Examination and will become a CNM.

THE FACULTY

ACADEMIC

Courses comprising the theoretical foundations for practice are each taught by a faculty team led by a course coordinator. The course coordinator has overall responsibility for curriculum design, development and revision in the area of specialty, and for ensuring the smooth functioning of the team. Large courses have additional faculty and teaching associates who grade examinations and learning activities, and share level III teaching responsibilities. A student advisor assists the academic director and monitors the progress of students through the levels. There are approximately twenty-five part-time academic faculty, although this number fluctuates during the year as students move in and out of courses. The academic director is responsible for curriculum planning, management of course production and faculty evaluation.

CLINICAL

The clinical director manages the clinical component of the curriculum. She directs and supervises the regional clinical coordinators and works closely with the quality-assurance officer to maintain a rigorous risk-assessment program. There are eighteen regional coordinators who work with the clinical director. The regional coordinators are the "eyes and ears" of CNEP in the field. They are responsible for clinical site identification and development, making preliminary visits to assure that each site is appropriate for student learning and meets CNEP's quality-assurance criteria. While the student is in the clinical practicum, which averages between six to eight months, the regional coordinator monitors her progress through performance evaluations and observation, and confers with the clinical preceptor. The regional coordinator is available for problem identification during the clinical practicum and facilitates resolution through a system of learning plans and contracts. All clinical preceptors must attend the CNEP preceptor training workshop prior to teaching. Sixty-five percent of clinical training sites utilized by CNEP have accepted their first nurse-midwifery student; in large part this is due to the supportive infrastructure CNEP offers the clinical preceptor. Clinical sites include: hospital in-patient (about 34 percent of placements), physician/CNM practices (about 16 percent), birth centers (about 13 percent), community health facilities (about 11 percent), CNM practices (about 10 percent), university health facilities (about 6 percent), public health facilities (about 4 percent), HMOs (about 2 percent), and hospital out-patient facilities (about 1 percent of placements).

FACULTY-STUDENT LINKAGES: TELECOMMUNICATIONS

Communication and information flow between faculty and students is the major challenge of distance education programs. Because the CNEP model has few face-to-face meetings between faculty and students, communication in many other forms becomes critical. A bimonthly newsletter is an important channel for program-wide communication. Students communicate with faculty and CNEP Central by telephone, mail, facsimile and the electronic bulletin board system. Papers can be mailed or transmitted electronically through the system. Some exams will be given by computer. Faculty have also established office hours when they are available on the voice line for student consultations.

More than three hundred CNEP faculty and students utilize the bulletin board system. This includes approximately forty faculty and staff (course coordinators, course faculty, regional clinical coordinators and CNEP Central staff) and 280 students in various levels of the curriculum.

Many thanks to the *Journal of Nurse-Midwifery* for permitting the use of this article. Contact the school if you have questions not answered in this and other articles in this book.

This article was first published in the Journal of Nurse-Midwifery, Volume 38, No. 6, November/December, 1993.

Katherine Camacho Carr, CNM, PhD, formerly served as the director of special projects, Institute of Midwifery, Women and Health where she is involved in the development of the master of science in midwifery curriculum and Internet access to the Institute's program. She maintains a part-time clinical practice, has served on the faculty of the Seattle Midwifery School, the University of Washington School of Nursing and the School of Medicine, the Pacific Lutheran University School of Nursing, and as the director of research and development for the Frontier School of Midwifery and Family Nursing, Community-based Nurse-midwifery Education Program (CNEP). Dr. Carr has won numerous awards for her pioneering work in primary healthcare policy. She is currently vice-president of the ACNM, and on the faculty of State University of New York (SUNY) Health Sciences Center at Brooklyn, where she teaches graduate courses in distance learning for the State University.

Judith M. Treistman, CNM, PhD, is the former director of the Community-Based Nurse-Midwifery Program (CNEP). She is involved in planning a statewide distance-learning program in nurse-midwifery with the State University of New York at Stony Brook.

Mary Kate McHugh, CNM, is academic director of CNEP. She received her nurse-midwifery education at St. Louis School of Nursing. She has taught midwifery at Yale University and the University of Pennsylvania.

See the Resource section for contact information on CNEP.

Chapter 5

Childbirth Education, Labor Support, & Postpartum Care

"Every woman deserves a doula. Notice the word 'deserves.' This does not
imply that every woman must have a doula in order to have a positive birth
or postpartum experience, but that each and every woman deserves to be
nurtured and cared for in this way."

— *Jennifer Rosenberg, ICCE, CD(DONA)*

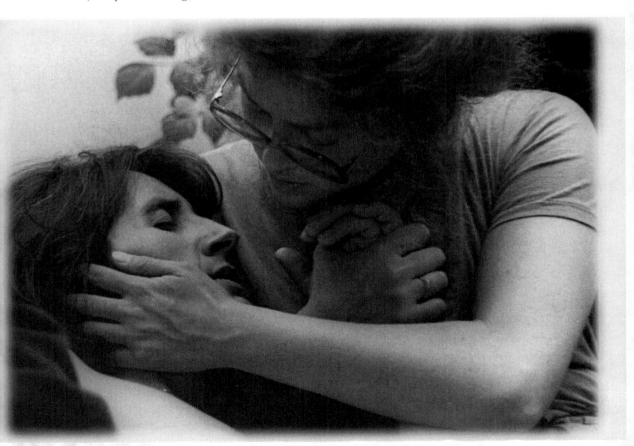

EDUCATION FROM THE INSIDE OUT

by Jennifer Rosenberg, ICCE, CD(DONA)

I started my birth education when I was seven years old. I was camping with relatives when a stray cat wandered in and adopted us during our stay. We kids assumed it was a boy because the cat was so big. One afternoon, my cousin looked over at the cat, lying on my sleeping bag, and shrieked "It's pooping and peeing on your bed!" I looked over, curious, and realized it wasn't either; it was having kittens. We realized then that it must be a girl cat. I watched, fascinated, as she delivered her second kitten and licked both of them clean. My cousin was grossed out. I was thoroughly intrigued. Five years later my mother became pregnant, and I grew completely involved in learning about her pregnancy and the coming birth. I went with my parents to most of their childbirth classes, and read every book they brought home from the library. I learned several important lessons from my mom that summer. I learned that:

1. Medications have risks, and should not be used unless there's a good reason. My mother's birth plan said, "Don't ask me if I want drugs. I'll ask you if I think I need them."

2. Cesareans are not the easy way out. Her birth plan also stated "Don't even suggest a cesarean to me unless it's an emergency and needs to be performed in the next five minutes."

3. Babies are people too, and deserve to be handled gently and lovingly in the moments after birth. My dad and I got to do the Leboyer bath for my sister a few minutes after her birth. Rosie was a calm and happy baby.

4. Breastfeeding isn't optional, it's a necessity. Mother's milk is vital for babies even if you don't find breastfeeding the most enjoyable thing you've ever done. My mom nursed both my sister and me for seven or eight months with no support, bad information and bad latches. It hurt the whole time she nursed. She even pumped for my sister when she felt her afternoon supply was inadequate.

5. You can't spoil a baby by holding it too much in the first six months. Damage is done by not holding a baby enough.

These lessons put me a huge step ahead as I began researching my options when I became pregnant unexpectedly at age twenty. I didn't consider midwifery an option because I considered myself high risk, though I was very aware that I had an obligation to my child to approach childbirth as a consumer rather than a patient. I was my own best advocate, finding childbirth classes I could pay for on a sliding scale, and reading every book I could. I haunted the library through my whole pregnancy, and asked tons of questions. When I realized at seven months along that I was having fantasies of hiding in the bathroom and not coming out until my baby was born, I realized I needed more support than my doctor or partner were giving me. I called several midwives in the area, and was connected to a direct-entry midwife who agreed to be my monitrice. At that point I still associated the word doula exclusively with postpartum care.

By checking me when I was having contractions five minutes apart for an hour and discovering I was only 2 cm (at thirty-six weeks), my midwife kept me from an unnecessary jaunt to the hospital and the hazards of early augmentation of prodromal labor. I went in and out of labor over the next four weeks, until she told me how to do a castor oil induction. The induction failed; however, her threat that I'd have to do castor oil again if I didn't go into labor worked like a charm and I went into labor within two hours.

My labor was everything I hoped for, but traumatic still. It was wonderful in that I took no medications and got through it actively. It was difficult in that I had a nasty doctor until twenty minutes before my daughter was born, and the delivery was not handled the way I wanted—I had no perineal support, a fairly deep second degree tear, and rapid cord cutting due to tea-colored amniotic fluid. Breastfeeding got off to a rough start since I began in a bad position (lying on my back) and my daughter put blisters on my nipples by the time she was forty-five minutes old. Breastfeeding was agony for the first week, compounded by the disintegration of my relationship with her father. I called my midwife to ask about breast pumps because I was hurting so much. She came over, corrected our latch, and breastfeeding has gone well ever since. My mom almost cried when she saw how simple it had been to fix the problem, as she'd had the same difficulty with latch and nursed through it for seven and eight months respectively.

I started sharing my birth story with childbirth education classes taught by the same woman who'd taught mine, and one evening she asked me if I would consider teaching classes myself. I dismissed the idea at first, but when she explained the schedule, training and requirements, I realized this would be a good way to earn money as a single mom. So I sent away for information from ICEA and began studying. When my daughter was ten months old, I attended my first single-day conference. An open and diverse discussion of active management of labor woke me up to some of the broader issues in this field. I actually stood up and asked an obstetrician with a 75 percent induction rate and a 99 percent epidural rate why people should use his method when it was so much cheaper and safer to hire someone to sit with the mother and hold her hand. When he asked me for studies to back it up, three midwives jumped up and said, "I have them!"

A month or two later I attended a teacher training workshop, and a month after that, the first DONA (Doulas of North America) conference, titled "The Warmest Welcome." At that point I was observing an independently taught childbirth class, and still thought of doulas as postpartum helpers only. That conference, which included Penny Simkin, John Marshall, and the Klauses, was a turning point for me. I realized that I was a doula. Not that I wanted to be one, but that I was one, from the top of my head to the tips of my fingers to the soles of my feet. I attended my first birth about a month later.

My first mom-to-be and her husband had been in the class I was observing. Her labor appeared more difficult and scarier than my own, but at the same time, she integrated the experience with less trauma than I had. The fundamental difference? She knew exactly what was happening, and she trusted her caregivers. She was attended by a nurse midwife, and had a doula to explain moment by moment all that happened when the midwife was too busy handling a baby born in thick meconium. This birth made me realize that it was not the "what" of my daughter's birth that bothered me, but the "how." I let go of trauma I'd held for more than a year. That fall I concentrated on my daughter, learned about slings, sewed nursing clothing, and learned more about childbirth. Then my welfare worker told me I needed to start looking for work. I panicked, fearing I would have to take a low-wage job and not be able to concentrate on my chosen profession. Yet I was able to work with the system to turn my interviews into networking in the childbirth field, and use a work experience position through a hospital to observe births, work with moms, and understand the systems of the local hospital. I volunteered my time and worked with low income women and families. I began this process within the welfare system in November 1994. The following year I completed all the requirements for ICEA certification as a childbirth educator and most of the requirements for certification as a doula through DONA. My parents were a vital support for me and my daughter, letting me rent a room from them at low cost, providing free childcare, transportation and moral support. I was able to save enough money to buy a car so that I could guarantee my presence with my clients, and was able to find the energy to start rebuilding my life. I saw many babies born at the local hospital and had four or five clients of my own, ranging from young married couples to single moms to developmentally disabled moms. In September 1995, my mom and dad bought a computer, and a whole new avenue of experience and education opened up for me. On CompuServe, I became an "online childbirth educator," providing support, education and an alternative perspective for the hundreds of moms going through pregnancy together on the forum.

I completed my certification for ICEA in late 1995, and began working for a local agency which specialized in offering in-home postpartum and antenatal home care for moms. I delivered breast pumps and cleaned houses and counseled the families I worked with. I took my first paying doula client in June 1997, and the birth went very well. My second paying client was that fall, and I was able to combine all my skills— childbirth classes, labor support and postpartum/breastfeeding support. When my welfare grant closed that month my income dropped precipitously. But I trusted that what I needed would come along. At the end of that month, Jan Tritten called to ask me to come to Midwifery Today as their advertising director. I am finally in a role which combines many of my skills and much of knowledge. I continue to help women online find the support and information they need and am proud to be making a difference. My presence helps these women use their strength and have positive birth experiences.

Through my training and education, I followed my heart and made myself open to the opportunities and lessons that came my way. The three most important parts of my education:

- The moms themselves. Each woman, each birth taught me to be humble and showed me how important the work I do is.
- Conferences and other networking with midwives and doulas. I attended several conferences put on by Midwifery Today, and one by DONA. These conferences

helped bolster my faith in birth as a natural process, and gave me skills and techniques to use with every client.

- Being open to learn from criticism. This was the hardest part of my education.

Being open to constructive criticism is difficult. Our natural reaction is to get defensive. Sometimes we cry. Sometimes we get angry. But these things work to shut down communication, to shut down the learning process.

Here's my general policy for learning from criticism.

If someone offers criticism:

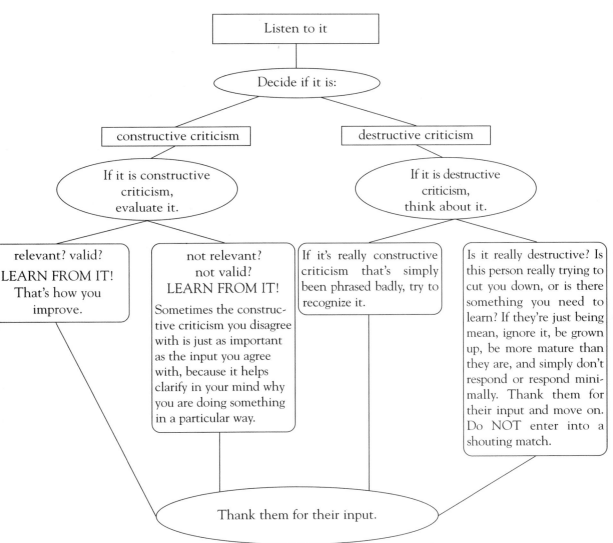

I was working with a "homebirth heart" in a hospital environment. Some of the nurses sat me down and forced me to look at the fact that my ideal birth and my clients' ideal births were not the same. From them I learned to "put my own preferences in an envelope" and leave them outside the birth room. This allowed, and allows, me to truly serve women as they ask to be served. When I was able to meet my clients on their turf, some magical things happened. Labors got shorter. They didn't ask for as much medication. They were happier about their births, even when things went "wrong." If I had not been able to humble myself, to pay attention to WHY the nurses were saying what they were saying, I would not have learned this valuable lesson. Sometimes the best results are had not from fighting the system, but from working within its limits and demonstrating the alternatives rather than proselytizing about them. Learning from criticism does not mean automatically changing my mind about the way I do things simply because someone says, "I don't like the way you did that." Learning from criticism means listening to what people say, thinking about it, and deciding then which parts of the criticism need to cause change.

The biggest advantage I had in my educational process is that I opened myself to change. I opened myself to learning in every situation, and did not dismiss wisdom simply because it came from sources that did not share my ideals. By keeping an open mind and an open heart, I've been able to influence medical professionals to change what they do, not by arguing with them, but by listening to them and asking questions that made them think without making them angry. I've had my moments, times when I was so angry after a birth that I went home and cried, but I learned from those births, too.

My education started from the inside, from the calling, from my own experiences. But it has been the shaping of the outside, learning from the moms, learning from criticism, learning from those with more experience that has allowed me to grow to become the kind of person I'd want helping me at my own birth, at my daughter's birth, at a friend's.

This article was written especially for this book.

Jennifer Rosenberg is an ICEA certified childbirth educator and a DONA certified doula. She is also a single mom, and works at Midwifery Today.

THE ASSOCIATION OF LABOR ASSISTANTS AND CHILDBIRTH EDUCATORS (ALACE):
SUPPORTING WOMAN-CENTERED CHILDBIRTH

by Ananda Lowe

The Association of Labor Assistants and Childbirth Educators, or ALACE (pronounced "Alice"), is an international nonprofit organization dedicated to supporting women's choices in childbirth. ALACE accomplishes this goal by providing training, certification and continuing education for childbirth educators and labor assistants/doulas. ALACE childbirth educators and labor assistants seek to help all women experience birth's transforming power with respect and dignity in safety, support and confidence.

The ALACE training programs are based on the philosophy that midwifery care should be the standard of care for women and families giving birth in every setting: in the home, hospital and birth center. Both the ALACE Childbirth Educator and Labor Assistant Certification programs were designed and developed by midwives, women, mothers and natural birth advocates, and were formerly offered by the organization Informed Homebirth/Informed Birth and Parenting (IH/IBP), founded in 1983. ALACE also offers information and referrals to expectant parents, as well as a mail-order bookstore which carries hard to find books and videos on pregnancy and birth.

LABOR ASSISTING AND CHILDBIRTH EDUCATION AS STEPS TO MIDWIFERY

Many aspiring midwives begin by training as labor assistants and/or childbirth educators with great success. They find that working within these professions is an excellent step on the pathway to becoming a midwife. By becoming a childbirth educator or labor assistant, aspiring midwives develop a strong foundation of knowledge about pregnancy, birth and postpartum care. They also gain direct experience working with women in the childbearing year, and, in the case of labor assistants, they gain valuable experience as well.

Midwifery programs often give preference to candidates who have prior experience. We often hear that a woman's experience as a labor assistant was integral to her admission into a midwifery program or in her receiving an apprenticeship. In addition, attending births as a labor assistant is a good introduction to some of the realities of midwifery—being on call, unusual hours and so forth—and provides experience in balancing the needs of clients with meeting the needs of your family.

Finally, teaching childbirth classes or providing labor support is a great way to earn money to support yourself while you explore midwifery during your training. In fact, we know of many homebirth midwives who offer hospital labor support in order to supplement their income as midwives. Many midwives also continue to offer childbirth preparation classes long after their midwifery practice takes off, as a service to their clients.

ABOUT THE ALACE LABOR ASSISTANT CERTIFICATION PROGRAM

"Labor assistant," "birth doula," "childbirth assistant" and "birth assistant" are just a few of the titles used by professional labor support providers. Each of these refers to an individual who provides continuous emotional and physical support to women during labor and birth. Numerous studies show that having labor support results in shorter, easier labors with better outcomes for mothers and babies.

Usually the labor assistant provides support in early labor at the family's home, accompanies them to the birth center or hospital at the appropriate time, and remains with them for a few hours after the birth. Most labor assistants also meet with their clients once or twice prenatally and provide a few postpartum follow-up visits. While most often labor assistants are hired to work in hospitals or birth centers, many do specialize in attending homebirths or use the training to become a midwife's assistant.

The program originally began as a midwife's assistant course, which evolved into a labor assistant training as more and more women began to provide labor support as a career in itself. In 1994 ALACE was founded to continue the IH/IBP program and expand its outreach. Over 3,000 women have taken the training since its inception, making it the most experienced training program in North America.

The training consists of a three-day weekend workshop which ALACE offers across the United States, Canada and six other countries. To earn certification, candidates must also complete a required reading list, attend six births, complete a written exam and become certified in adult-infant CPR. Our training philosophy is expressed by the following quote:

> *I hear and I forget*
> *I see and I remember*
> *I do and I understand.*
> *— Lao Tse*

ALACE training emphasizes how to provide emotional support, and our workshop is designed with a focus on experiential learning. We provide hands-on experience practicing comfort measures such as positions for labor, breathing and relaxation techniques, and using labor support tools such as the birth ball, aromatherapy and massage. Other topics covered in the workshop include designing your scope of practice, history taking, working with the birth team, ethical standards for labor support providers, avoiding unnecessary intervention and providing support when interventions are in place.

The ALACE workshop also provides an introduction to physical assessments such as palpation, fetal heart tones and pelvic exam. ALACE workshops are distinguished by the inclusion of these exercises, and our graduates constantly rate this aspect of the training very highly. The main objective of these exercises is to help ALACE students understand the procedures that midwives, doctors and nurses use to assess the health of mothers and babies during labor, in order to provide educated, comprehensive support to laboring women and their families. In addition, since so many women who take the workshops are aspiring midwives, they appreciate having a hands-on introduction to these midwifery skills.

After taking the workshop, some women decide they would like to offer physical assessments to their clients while laboring at home, to monitor the health of the mother and baby. ALACE supports labor assistants who perform assessments when they have been appropriately trained and are qualified to perform these skills accurately. However, given the time limitations of the ALACE workshop, graduates are not professionally qualified in these skills after attending the workshop, nor does ALACE certification cover these skills.

ABOUT THE ALACE CHILDBIRTH EDUCATOR CERTIFICATION PROGRAM

ALACE offers the only nationally recognized childbirth educator certification developed by women and midwives. The training grew out of the homebirth movement and was originally developed by midwife Rahima Baldwin Dancy, author of *Special Delivery*.

Most ALACE teachers hold independent classes and offer a seven to ten week series or a weekend intensive, depending on their client's needs. ALACE childbirth educators help expectant parents develop confidence and trust in the birth process by stressing emotional preparation, parent responsibility and informed decision making in addition to labor coping skills.

> The message that birth is not an illness reaffirms the unique foundation of both the childbirth educator and birth assistant training programs . . .

Perhaps the most unique feature of our training is the weight given to mind-body integration and the psychological aspects of pregnancy, birth and parenting. ALACE instructors teach relaxation and coping tools to work with pain and discomfort, rather than techniques for avoiding sensation. Our program has long been recognized for its holistic approach to childbirth education.

ALACE training is a comprehensive distance-learning course that involves extensive reading and completion of learning exercises. Students receive the ALACE training manual, which consists of over 650 pages of background material, resources, teaching outlines and learning modules. As they complete the reading and learning exercises in each module, students send their work to the ALACE director of teacher training, who provides ongoing feedback and guidance. After completing the learning activities, students are required to pass a final exam for provisional certification, which is proctored locally and does not require travel or an exam fee. For full certification, students complete the required reading list and submit evaluations from six clients.

ALACE also offers an Accelerated Childbirth Educator Certification program for experienced teachers. This program is open to students who have achieved the following qualifications: prior certification with an approved program and/or who have at least 125 hours experience teaching childbirth classes. The accelerated program honors students' prior experience and training and exempts them from much of the written work, allowing them to earn certification at a faster rate.

The ALACE program includes a complete curriculum and suggested teaching outlines. However, we do encourage teachers to develop their own style and adapt our curriculum to the needs of their communities and clientele.

WHAT DISTINGUISHES CERTIFICATION WITH ALACE?

ALACE values women and prides itself on having woman-friendly policies and programs. We offer payment plans for all our programs, and our all-inclusive fees have no hidden costs. In addition, we recognize that women have many responsibilities—as mothers, daughters, partners, workers, students and so on, so we have created no time limits for completing certification. Finally, because the trainings themselves are comprehensive, there are no prerequisites for taking either program. A college or nursing degree is not required, nor is it mandatory to have given birth to become an ALACE teacher or labor assistant. Women of all backgrounds have taken and succeeded in our program.

ALACE is proud to provide training programs which respect childbirth as a woman-centered and woman-directed passage. ALACE childbirth educators and labor assistants have affected the births of hundreds of thousands of women and families around the world, and prevented countless unnecessary cesareans and other interventions. The positive changes that are seen in childbirth come about primarily through the efforts and raised voices of women themselves. Becoming a childbirth educator or labor assistant with ALACE is an excellent way to work for institutional change while directly influencing the lives of women and their families.

For more information, contact: ALACE, P.O. Box 382724, Cambridge, MA 02238. 1-888-22-ALACE (1-888-222-5223).

Where Philosophy Transcends Method:
ICEA Teacher Certification Program

by Kim Dungey

Certification alone cannot guarantee quality in an individual educator, nor can the absence of national certification signal incompetence. Competency does not reside in the program the person has completed, but in the abilities and skills she or he possesses. Certification recognizes a certain standard within the profession. Individuals seeking training or certification must examine the goals and philosophy of all program options available to them.

Some educators do not feel a need for formal recognition of certification. Many others find they must be certified in order to establish credibility as a professional in their community.

ICEA Accentuates the Individual's Knowledge

The International Childbirth Education Association (ICEA) Teacher Certification Program (TCP) is a competency-based certification that verifies an individual's knowledge and skills in providing childbirth education. ICEA supports a woman's right to freedom of choice based on knowledge of alternatives in childbirth. Unlike education-based programs or those which require a specific methodology, ICEA welcomes educators of various childbirth methods, as long as they support concepts of family-centered maternity care. This timeless philosophy which encourages consumer oriented education and birth will be valid long after today's childbirth methods have changed and become less popular.

TCP is a self-motivated, self-study program that has certified over 2,600 ICEA certified childbirth educators (ICCE) since the program started in 1982. Individuals need not travel to distant locations in order to complete the program. This international program has been completed by over twenty educators living in countries including South Africa, Malta, Australia and Singapore.

ICEA Certification Requirements (ICCE)

The ICEA TCP involves four elements. A minimum of eighteen ICEA contact hours must be earned. ICEA contact hours are approved for qualifying local childbirth education training and continuing education programs, as well as ICEA-sponsored programs. The candidate must observe a minimum of three labors and births. This enables the candidate to learn from the "complex simplicity" of birth, no matter what her or his previous experience with birth. An evaluated teaching series is completed within ICEA guidelines. An evaluator meeting ICEA's qualifications verifies the candidate's advocacy of ICEA philosophy and competence in teaching. The evaluation can be conducted on-site or via audiotape or videotape. When the three prerequisites are completed, the candidate sits for the certification examination, which is based on the study guides that are provided to every candidate upon enrolling in the TCP.

An ICEA certified childbirth educator from Texas said, "There is a great feeling of accomplishment when you realize that you've answered all those questions (on the exam). I can feel the knowledge in my teaching."

WHY DO EDUCATORS CHOOSE ICEA CERTIFICATION?

The ICEA Teacher Certification Program meets educators' needs. The program has four basic elements, the first three of which can be completed in any order. These prerequisites can be met in a variety of ways and offer great flexibility within the structure. An experienced educator can expand her or his knowledge base and refine teaching skills. A novice educator will find the TCP is more challenging because it was designed as an upper level program. Nonetheless, many beginning educators have been able to combine their basic teacher preparation with the ICEA TCP. Every ICEA certified childbirth educator has demonstrated her knowledge and skill as an educator dedicated to ICEA philosophy; this commitment to knowledgeable choice becomes a sustaining strength for each one of them.

Because ICEA certifies teachers in the philosophy of "freedom of choice based on knowledge of alternatives in childbirth," prospective educators should begin with questions of themselves and their views of the role of the childbirth educator.

WHO IS A CHILDBIRTH EDUCATOR?

A childbirth educator may be female or male, a parent or not. A childbirth educator spends many hours teaching expectant parents about pregnancy and birth. In so doing, she or he facilitates a greater understanding of the transition into parenthood.

Childbirth education combines aspects of many disciplines, including teaching, sociology, psychology, physiology, midwifery, nursing and medicine. None of these backgrounds alone adequately prepares an individual for the profession of childbirth educator. Childbirth educators are identified by their sensitivity, empathy, compassion and knowledge.

HOW IS A CHILDBIRTH EDUCATOR TRAINED?

The unique profession of childbirth educator requires specialized training or preparation. Many childbirth educators train together in local childbirth education groups. Others are apprenticed to an established educator, are self-educated, or use a combination of these methods. Preparation should include observation of classes, guided readings, workshops or conventions, practice teaching, labor and birth observations, evaluations by peers, parents and self-evaluation. This training should be only the beginning of a lifetime of learning as an educator continues to grow and expand her or his knowledge as a childbirth educator.

This article first appeared in Midwifery Today Issue No. 20.

Kim Dungey is the former administrator of the ICEA Teacher Certification Program where she worked for five years.

BIRTH WORKS!

by Cathy Daub & Michelle Freedman Brill

The problem with traditional childbirth education is that it doesn't aim high enough. Simply teaching about birth is not sufficient. To help women love and believe in themselves, to provide women with experiences that increase their self-esteem and self-confidence—these are the primary educational tools that increase a woman's chances of birthing normally. As I designed the Birth Works course in 1981, the dilemma that presented itself was how to pass on these educational tools in a childbirth class setting. How could we help a woman gain more faith and trust in her body's ability to give birth?

To help answer that need, Birth Works developed an experiential structure for learning about birth; that is, learning by doing. For example, instead of showing a baby fitting through a cloth pelvis, women feel their own pelvises during pelvic bodywork. Instead of looking at pictures or posters of how the baby descends into the pelvis, women experience birth during multi-sensory visualization.

The impact of experiential learning is further deepened when it is sustained within an emotional context. In other words, a woman is more likely to remember an experience that went to her heart rather than information aimed solely at her brain. She is also more likely to develop heightened self-confidence as a result. Through a series of unique and innovative experiential exercises, Birth Works participants are guided to access their inner wisdom and as such, learn to have more faith in their bodies. This is in contrast to the didactic or lecture mode of learning.

Birth Works classes address the body, mind and spirit. Class participants and instructors work on developing increased trust, faith and confidence. This requires taking a closer look at their own belief systems and seeing how these beliefs affect their lives and the choices they make. Because Birth Works is a process, not a method, and because we respect the fact that each woman is an individual, we believe there is no one right way to give birth.

We know, however, that what a woman believes about birth has much to do with how she gives birth. Birth Works addresses this truth with a holistic approach. We know the mind and body are so connected that a thought produces a reaction in the body before we are hardly aware of the thought. Thoughts carry energy which in turn produces a reaction in our bodies. (Just imagine yourself sucking on a very sour lemon at this moment and note what is happening in your mouth. Saliva is being produced just from the thought of a lemon.) In classes, men and women are encouraged to become aware of any beliefs they have that may not be conducive to positive birthing. We ask women to have the courage and determination to change some of their thought patterns if necessary and learn how to believe in their bodies. If a woman believes her body can't birth, she may have a difficult birth. If a woman is afraid of becoming a mother, she may have a longer labor. Identifying these beliefs, and allowing men and women to express fears, concerns, and any pain that may be causing tension in their bodies, are ways in which we facilitate normal birthing.

Many women have lost confidence in their ability to give birth normally without being attached to various kinds of equipment. Their trust and faith have shifted from their own bodies to technology and drugs. They expect others to tell them what to do and/or depend on technology to do it for them, not wanting to accept the responsibility themselves. As well, many women are afraid of the unknown. Because in our society birth and death take place primarily in the hospital instead of at home, knowledge and experience of the normal life cycle are being lost. Most women having their first baby have never seen a live birth; they fear what they don't know. With fear comes tension; "holding in" energy is the antithesis of the "letting go" energy required for successfully giving birth. Women have forgotten that the knowledge about how to give birth already exists within. One woman commented that the most surprising thing she had learned in Birth Works was that "[she] had almost lost the ability to be in touch with [her] instincts."

Michel Odent, MD, tells us that birth is unquestionably an instinctive process. He says that "the less a woman

---

BIRTH WORKS TRAINING

- Birth Works has recently become independent of its parent group, the International Cesarean Awareness Network (ICAN), formerly the Cesarean Prevention Movement, and was that organization's official childbirth education program.

- The first Birth Works classes were designed and taught by Cathy Daub, PT, in 1982. Birth Works' teacher certification program is the cumulative effort of the many well-known birth educators and practitioners who wrote modules for the training manual (newly revised in 1991 after the completion of a new three-year pilot program).

- The eighteen-month program is a correspondence course which only requires the attendance at one teacher training weekend, held regionally.

- To enter the Birth Works program one need not have any background in the medical field, for we do not believe birth is a medical event. Although the training period is eighteen months, we recognize that many educators have prior background and extensive knowledge.

- For educators who are currently certified by another organization but who wish to change their affiliation to Birth Works, we have developed a modified program. Send us your previous certification requirements; we will modify our prerequisite list accordingly. A number of people have become certified for Birth Works within a six-month period in this way.

For more information, contact: Cathy Daub, Director, 42 Tallowood Drive, Medford, NJ 08055. Phone (609) 953-9380.

knows about the right way to give birth, the easier it will be for her." Although Birth Works may help women learn how to change their beliefs about birth, we don't attempt to teach a woman how to give birth. For example, many women expect that, if they follow the "correct" breathing pattern in labor, they will feel no pain. When in advanced labor she finds her breathing pattern isn't working, she cries out for painkillers. She is unable to gain access to her natural coping skills because she is not in touch with her own inner resources. In reality, it is her job to let go and breathe into the contractions, relax into the pain so her body can labor. Birth Works teaches each woman to go inside her body, ride the contraction to the top of the wave, feel the power of her body. She then welcomes the strong contractions that are her body's natural technology for birthing a baby.

A woman's inner wisdom and deepest intuition know well how to give birth. Analytical thinking interferes with her ability to gain access to this primal consciousness. It is helpful to identify and rehearse logically what to expect in each stage of labor, but when it comes, a woman must be able to drop deep into her inner reaches and allow her innate knowledge to take over.

In Birth Works classes, new parents and those with previous vaginal and/or cesarean births all share and learn from each other. We encourage parents to take Birth Works classes either prior to pregnancy or within the first trimester. The last trimester is a time for the nesting instinct to settle in; it is not a time for identifying beliefs or interviewing doctors. Birth Works is a ten-week course that covers nutrition, exercise, information on VBAC, risks and benefits of medical procedures, choosing the birth team and birth place, anesthesia and analgesia in birth, the medical training of doctors, variations and complications in birth, informed consent and breastfeeding and postpartum care.

Because Birth Works is holistic, it facilitates a woman's personal growth through childbearing, growth that will continue throughout the remainder of her life. Through confidence and love, safety and nurturance, birth is returned to its natural, joyous place on the human continuum.

A version of this article first appeared in Midwifery Today Issue No. 20.

Cathy Daub, president of the board of directors for Birth Works, is also a physical therapist who works in the public schools helping children with disabilities.

Michelle Freedman Brill holds a master's degree in Public Health and has been teaching Birth Works classes since 1990. She is a member of the Birth Works board of directors, serves on the National Trainee Review Committee and leads Birth Works Teacher Training Workshops.

See the Resource section for contact information on Birth Works.

BRADLEY™ TEACHERS:
SHARING, CARING AND HELPING
IMPROVE OUR QUALITY OF LIFE

by Marjie Hathaway, AAHCC

The Bradley™ Method is a revolution involving parents who have had wonderful unmedicated births themselves and want to share this experience with other parents. Today with such a wide variety of birth experiences available, people are becoming aware of the ways to embrace the labor of birth without endangering the health of the infant.

Bradley™ teachers around the world enjoy the success that comes from teaching something that works. Nearly every couple can apply the Bradley™ principles, and this makes the educational process, as well as the outcome, emotionally rewarding.

Using the techniques taught in Bradley™ classes, over 80 percent of couples have been able to have beautiful unmedicated births. Why? Because the couples that take Bradley™ classes have learned how to give birth. By attending the standard twelve-week series they have the time to really learn and practice how to give birth.

Bradley™ teachers are independent instructors encouraged to charge 10 percent of the going obstetrical rate in their community; this is a small price for the support and skills couples get in return.

BRADLEY™ TRAINING COMPONENTS

Because we are teaching natural childbirth, to qualify for training as a Bradley™ Method instructor, applicants must have experienced a natural birth themselves (preferably having taken a Bradley™ class) and/or have medical obstetrical experience. Exceptions are reviewed on an individual basis.

The training to become a Bradley™ teacher consists of a three-part program. The first part is the academic portion which is done at home before or after the workshop. During this time, trainees read and report on a list of books, observe classes, La Leche League meetings, hospital surveys and become familiar with services available in their own communities.

The second part involves attending a Teacher Training Workshop. These four-day workshops are held in most regions of the country. Many experts in the field of childbirth education are present—either in person or by way of videotape. We work long hours during this workshop giving trainees an amazing amount of information and experience. Each participant receives the Bradley Method™ Teachers Manual which is more than 600 pages and presents information that has been compiled for over thirty years. Included are detailed class outlines as well as topic outlines and many teaching aids which can be used to enhance their Bradley™ classes. The resource information that is included is extensive. Our workshops are an intense four days of concentrated learning so that our attendees will not have to spend too much time away from their families.

The third portion of training is the provisional teaching period of time which concludes with the final exam. At the successful completion of this program, a teacher may become fully affiliated and use the initials AAHCC after their name. Teachers are required to have continuing education each year. The Bradley Method™ program provides national affiliation so that your credentials follow you if you move. The Bradley™ name is a trademark registered with the United States Patent Office. Only currently affiliated teachers may teach The Bradley Method™ or use the term "Bradley™" in conjunction with childbirth education.

The American Association of Husband-Coached Childbirth (AAHCC) not only trains and supports Bradley™ teachers. The Academy makes available to teachers a 130-page Student Workbook, videotapes, teaching aids, newsletter, and extensive research. The Academy maintains a Childbirth Hotline (800)4-A-BIRTH so interested couples can call free of charge to receive a national directory of Bradley Method™ instructors which lists teachers worldwide and gives them information about the Bradley Method.™

WHY AND WHAT OUR TEACHERS TEACH

Teachers train couples so they can birth as a family together. The coach is generally the husband, but not always. (They are historically and practically the best coaches.) In Bradley™ classes, husbands learn how to coach a laboring woman, something quite other than just being an observer. They know what to do to help her avoid unnecessary pain, how to best handle the pain she will experience, and how to recognize and deal with the stages of labor. They are taught to take care of their own needs in labor as well so they can have the strength and enthusiasm necessary for this labor. They participate as part of the team so they can feel involved and included.

Bradley™ teachers are also trained as Labor Support Educators and offer training for assistant coaches as well as for the expectant couple. Assistant coaches can be very helpful to a laboring couple. They are trained to work with the mother when the coach needs a break to eat or use the bathroom but they spend most of their time doing all of the less glamorous jobs so that the coach can focus on the mother's needs in labor. Bradley™-trained assistant coaches learn the importance of working to empower the family. They do not take over the coach's job but do exactly as their title implies, they assist the coach.

Knowing what is natural can save time, money, pain and unnecessary medical interventions such as cesarean section. Bradley™ techniques and Bradley™ instructors give couples the training and confidence they need to plan and adjust to labor, as well as unexpected situations and the avoidance of the domino effect of intervention.

See the Resource section for contact information on the Bradley Method.™

Marjie Hathaway, AAHCC, and her husband, Jay, worked with Dr. Bradley to develop the Bradley Method™ training program and to establish the American Academy of Husband-Coached Childbirth.™ They bring their personal experience of six births themselves plus over thirty-five years of teaching pregnant couples and training Bradley™ teachers. They have attended hundreds of births and produced over forty videos for the education and enrichment of Bradley™ classes.

FROM DOULAS TO MONITRICES:

DIFFERING PHILOSOPHIES OF LABOR SUPPORT

by Jennifer Rosenberg, ICCE, CD(DONA)

Just as there are a variety of midwives and types of midwifery practice, there are many different kinds of labor support providers. At the most basic level, the "original" doulas, from the Klaus and Kennell studies, were laywomen who were simply there for emotional support, with little or no training in the mechanics of birth. Their qualifications were that they had each experienced positive births and were willing to share their confidence in the process. Now the term "birth doula" is used generally to refer to labor support providers who have training in providing physical and emotional support in the birthing process. The Doulas of North America (DONA) standards of practice specifically state that the scope of doula practice does not include giving clinical care. So when I talk about a birth doula, I am referring to a doula who has training in helping women cope with the emotional and physical issues of labor and birth, but does not normally perform clinical skills such as blood pressure checks or vaginal exams. ALACE trains "labor assistants" who do have some training in clinical care, performing some vaginal exams (usually at home before the mother goes to the hospital, or at home before the primary caregiver arrives) and checking heart tones. Monitrices are generally either private duty nurses or midwives who provide labor support while also providing a more intensive level of clinical care without being the primary caregiver. There are other organizations who train labor support providers, and other names for women who provide labor support, including birth or labor coach, birth assistant, midwife's assistant and of course, the generic "labor support person." The distinct characteristic all these professionals share is that they focus primarily on the emotional and physical comfort of their clients, and don't generally have primary clinical responsibility. That is, labor support people generally don't catch the baby.

You might ask, "Why all the different kinds? Why not one standard, one name, one model for labor support?" The answer is both simple and complicated. The simple answer is that different women need different things from their support people.

The complicated answer is that there are advantages and disadvantages to each kind of practice. Realistically, it falls to the individual to determine what level of responsibility she is interested in taking on, what level of skill she thinks she needs to feel "safe" providing labor support, and what her ultimate career goals are.

The reason birth doulas do not provide any clinical care is twofold. The philosophical objection to providing clinical care is that when a labor support person "crosses the line" and checks heart tones, blood pressure or cervical dilation, she takes on a different role to the woman and a different level of responsibility for the birth. By not providing clinical care, we (I am certified by DONA) leave the medical and clinical responsibility with the client and her care provider, and are better able to focus on the emotional needs of the client. This is a two-edged sword. It is freeing not to take responsibility for the life of the baby and the mother, and allows us to stay with the woman, talking to her, explaining to her, if problems do arise. On the other hand, my clients go to the hospital a couple hours sooner than they might if I were doing vaginal checks. It is a two-edged sword professionally as well. On the one hand, care-givers are less threatened by my presence when they learn that I'm leaving the clini-cal duties to them. On the other hand, my opinion weighs less with them, I believe, than if I had the weight of several years of formal training behind me.

There are equally compelling arguments for labor support providers to provide basic clinical care, by which I mean cervical exams, fetal heart tones and blood pres-sure. The first argument is that having those skills means it is safer for the mom to labor longer at home. This is absolutely true. In my doula practice, I do go to my clients' homes to labor with them, but generally go very early in labor when they would not be in a hospital anyway. Most of my clients get to the hospital at three cen-timeters dilation, and I've usually been with them for a few hours before they go in. I'm torn about this. It is what my clients want, but as a believer in natural birth, I wish they didn't really want to go in at all. I would like to see them stay home longer. Having the exam skills would make it possible for me to help them do that, but I would also take on a much greater level of responsibility for their care, and a greater liability. Since it is not my goal to be a midwife and I'm not really interested in per-forming clinical skills, I provide them with emotional and physical support and my clients retain the responsibility for the decision making. I don't tell them, "It's time to go." Instead, I watch, look, listen and give them feedback on what I'm seeing. They make the call.

It is important to note here that although DONA's training and standards of prac-tice do not include clinical skills, DONA does not "forbid" its doulas to use skills they have from other training. Thus a DONA certified doula who is also a certified nurs-ing assistant (CNA) may, if her client requests it and it is within her training, take the client's blood pressure. A DONA certified doula who is also a chartered herbal-ist, "wearing the hat" of the herbalist, may suggest specific herbal remedies to her client. And a DONA certified doula who is trained as a midwife's apprentice, may, if the circumstances justify it and the client requests it, perform a vaginal exam.

It is important, in my opinion, for the doula to be clear with her client which training she is using when she goes beyond the normal scope of doula care. When I offer breastfeeding advice, I do so from my experience as a mom, my training as a childbirth educator, and extensive reading and experience helping other women. My clients know that I am not a lactation consultant. Similarly, a doula who is also a midwifery student may find that she occasionally will measure or palpate her client's belly or do a cervical exam because she is a student, not because she is a doula. I've had doctors or nurses offer to let me do clinical care, and politely refused. Then I've suggested that the midwifery student accompanying me take the opportunity to learn, because while the clinical care is not within my scope, it is within hers.

For my own daughter's birth, having a full-fledged midwife as my monitrice was a godsend. Having her come check my cervix at home kept me from going to the hospital on three or four separate occasions during a month-long prodromal labor.

Having her there at the hospital helped my support people weave a protective shield around me. I was a terrified, high risk, first-time young mom, and she really helped ground me. I felt very safe knowing she had oxygen in the car and could come out to my house on a moment's notice. I knew that if I didn't go to the hospital, we'd be quite safe. (At that point, I still thought of myself as high-risk and didn't consider myself a candidate for planned homebirth.) All the same, she was focused both on my clinical care and my emotional care, and in the chaos of the hospital setting some of the things a doula might have been able to do did not get done. My needs were met fairly well, but my partner's needs were not. I believe that if my midwife/monitrice had been less focused on my clinical care, it would have been easier for her to address some of the emotional needs of both my partner and me.

When problems arise, and even when everything is normal but intense, as in transition, I'm there for the mom and I'm there for the dad, explaining, reassuring, helping them understand the process and the procedures. It seems to me that when the line of clinical care gets blurred, it is very easy for the labor support person to lose that focus even if they don't have primary responsibility. Thus, in my own practice, while I know how to take blood pressure, measure a belly and palpate for position, I rarely do so. More often I'll teach my client or her husband how. I just don't want to cross the line between being "with" her and doing things "to" her.

It is clear, both from studies and from the experiences of many doulas and support providers, that any support is better than none. I personally believe that there are places and needs for all kinds of labor support providers, from loving mothers holding their daughters' hands, to doulas, to monitrices, and everything in between.

The following excerpt is from an article printed in the first edition of this book, *Getting an Education*. The article was replaced primarily by the article on ALACE for this edition. **I include the following because it clearly explains the rationale behind teaching birth assistants clinical skills and thus provides a good counterpoint to my own perspective.**

This article was written especially for this book.

Jennifer Rosenberg is an ICEA certified childbirth educator and a DONA certified doula. She is also a single mom and works at Midwifery Today.

Counterpoint: An excerpt from "HOMEBIRTH AS THE STANDARD OF CARE"

by Rahima Baldwin Dancy

When I spoke at the First International Conference on Home Birth in London in 1986, I was struck by the conferees' bold formulation that birth at home is not "alternative birth," but rather the standard by which all maternity care ought to be measured. Western obstetrics, in reality, is a hundred-year aberration in the history of giving birth on the planet.

The message that birth is not an illness reaffirms the unique foundation of both the childbirth educator and birth assistant training programs formerly offered by Informed Homebirth/Informed Birth and Parenting and now directed by ALACE, the Association of Labor Assistants and Childbirth Educators. Developed by practicing midwives, both programs take homebirth and the midwifery model as standards of reference. Offering what has been learned from the "laboratory of the normal" (physiological birth at home), our programs also make this knowledge available to couples birthing in a hospital or birth center setting. Childbirth educators and birth assistants trained with Informed Homebirth are professionals who know how to interface with the medical community. But they also maintain that giving birth is the healthy expression of the way we all come into the world, through a woman's body.

BIRTH ASSISTANT EDUCATION

Our Birth Assistant Training (offered nationally since 1983) was developed by midwife Karen Parker from the training she originally designed for her own birth assistants. It differs from other programs in this regard: Students learn skills which may later allow them to become an assistant (apprentice) to a midwife or other primary caregiver, as well as the skills necessary to accompany a woman or couple to the hospital as a labor assistant or doula. Of the over 2,000 women who have trained with our program, many find it a valuable step toward becoming an apprentice with a midwife; numbers of others are equally satisfied with the developing role of the birth assistant as a paid professional in her own right.

If women are asking birth assistants to stay home with them as long as possible before going to the hospital, basic skills such as monitoring fetal heart tones and checking dilation increase the safety of both mothers and babies. (The fact that women want to avoid their primary caregivers until the last minute is obviously less than optimal, and certainly a strong indictment of the current medical system.) But as this trend develops, we feel most comfortable teaching birth assistants the basic skills of labor monitoring. A distressed infant or a mad dash to the hospital with delivery en route is to the advantage of no one, least of all to the newborn and her mother. Mastery of monitoring skills in application with midwifery principles can smooth the "transition" between home-attended early labor and the hospital.

Our training consists of two and one-half days of training intensives. Certification follows the completion of a reading list and an evaluation from couples. Basic midwifery skills are taught to enable the birth assistant to help the primary attendant with record keeping, sterile technique, assessing vital signs and monitoring the fetal heart rate. Care and assembly of equipment is discussed, as well as methods to assist the midwife in critical care situations.

Rahima Baldwin Dancy is the founder of Informed Homebirth/Informed Birth and Parenting (now ALACE) and the author of Special Delivery, Pregnant Feelings *and* You are Your Child's First Teacher.

BIRTH COMPANIONS:

THE KEY TO A POSITIVE HOSPITAL BIRTH EXPERIENCE

by Lily Fountain Werbos

There are numerous ways in which the childbirth educator can assist expectant families aside from teaching consumer-oriented childbirth classes. One such option is to become a birth companion to couples birthing in the hospital.

A birth companion, who offers her services in addition to those of a labor coach, is experienced in birth and provides support and information to a woman during pregnancy, labor and birth and the early postpartum period. She is part of a contemporary movement focused on bringing the ancient tradition of woman-to-woman support to the birth process.

The advantages of using a birth companion are considerable. The birth companion provides continuity of care, knowledge about labor, coping skills, physiology, natural remedies and natural baby care, and is experienced in birth as both a woman and professional. The birth companion can also relief coach during a long labor. She acts as a personal advocate for the birthing mother in cases where birth plans must be changed or are challenged. Research has documented shorter labors with fewer complications, healthier babies, more successful breastfeeding and mothers that interact more favorably with their newborns if the woman has been "mothered" during pregnancy and especially during birth.

The birth companion develops her profession by learning and utilizing many midwifery skills. She has the opportunity to nurture positive and ongoing work relationships with birth practitioners in her area and learn firsthand the ins and outs of the facilities they use. The role she has chosen can serve as a significant first step on the path to midwifery, and her familiarity with hospital procedure can qualify her to serve as an especially effective midwife to the majority of American women who are still choosing to birth their babies in the hospital.

Note that a birth companion differs from a birth assistant. The birth companion provides extra support for the family who plans a hospital birth, whereas the birth assistant's primary focus is the family giving birth at home.

Specific skills enable the birth companion to be an effective support person:

- She is knowledgeable about normal labor patterns.
- She is knowledgeable about labor coping skills, positioning, etc.
- She has good counseling skills.
- She has the ability to develop rapport with different kinds of people.
- Her familiarity with area hospitals is helpful and improves with experience.
- When measuring vital signs she has the ability to monitor temperature, pulse, respiration, blood pressure and fetal heart rate and she knows the normal ranges.

(This is not essential, but very important to clients such as VBACers who want to stay home until active labor.)

- During pelvic exams she knows how to check for dilation, effacement, station, character and position of the cervix, fetal position and membranes status.
- She has the ability to use effective communication skills and professional terminology in dealing with hospital staff.
- She understands sterile technique, essential for vaginal checks and helpful when dealing with the doctor and nurses in the hospital.
- She knows how to use perineal massage and support using hot compresses and oil.
- She is informed about breastfeeding skills.
- She understands normal postpartum changes in mother and baby.

The aspiring birth companion learns her skills in a variety of ways. Being a childbirth educator is a good first step, and provides clients easily and naturally. Local clinics often serve single or non-English speaking mothers who will also welcome her services. Much of the technical information she will need to learn is covered in professional midwifery texts, obstetric nursing texts, nursing fundamentals textbooks, and hands-on experience comes from not being afraid to put the information to use. The aspiring companion can take her partner's blood pressure or check her best friend's dilation during labor. Her technique can be checked by a midwife, nurse, another birth companion or birth assistant. She can gain skills by volunteering at a prenatal clinic. She might try teaching her students how to palpate and take fetal heart rates as she practices on them. Obviously, going to births is a must. Working out a cooperative arrangement with one or more other birth companions is extremely helpful. In this arrangement babysitting and backup duties can be shared and a support/study group can be organized.

> The role of birth companion provides the woman who loves the birthing experience with many opportunities to expand her skills and knowledge. She also offers woman-to-woman support often missing in our society.

Formal training programs are provided by ALACE (Association for Labor Assistants and Childbirth Educators), Ancient Arts Midwifery Institute/Apprentice Academics, Birth Support Providers International (BSPI), Doulas of North America (DONA), Birth Works, and by the Utah School of Midwifery. The National Association of Labor Assistants (NALA) maintains a national directory of labor assistants.

Aside from the immediate skills that the birth companion learns and puts into practice, she must also consider the business aspects of her occupation. Advertising is essential, and an attractive and informative brochure is an excellent means to inform the public about her service. The brochure can be sent to libraries, hospitals, doctors, midwives, clinics, Red Cross chapters, and other childbirth educators as well as to childbirth resources. Good public relations involves giving free public lectures at local libraries and speaking at childbirth classes and conferences.

Good business practices include keeping a record of expenses and income. The probable range of fees is between fifty dollars and five hundred dollars depending on services provided, level of experience and the area's standard of living.

Various equipment and supplies will be needed. An answering machine and a pager will be helpful. A birth bag can contain the following items: fetoscopes, blood pressure cuff and stethoscope, client's file and forms, sterile gloves and K-Y jelly packets, emergency OB kit (available from medical suppliers such as Moore), natural remedies if you are knowledgeable in their use, massage oil (lavender is my favorite) and kidney-shaped emesis basin to put it in, improvised portable Crockpot, pint jar, water-boiling element, mug-warming plate, washcloths, gauze sponges, unbreakable 5" x 8" mirror, nutritious snacks, and personal items such as Chapstick, contact lens case and sanitary pads. I include colorful elf caps as gifts for each baby.

The birth companion gets to know the couple prenatally and teaches them about aspects of prenatal care such as palpation, fetal heart rate and fundal height. Together they discuss the birth plan and note whether the physician's and hospital's attitudes and procedures match the mother's desires and expectations. The companion makes sure the couple's childbirth education has been adequate and reviews areas where there may be questions. She notes whether the mother is getting along well with the father, if finances are working out and if there are any other pressures on the family. She facilitates discussion and refers to professionals as necessary.

A birth companion continues to offer her skills and knowledge as well as support as the due date approaches (and sometimes passes). Once labor has started, she and the couple decide when they will go to the hospital. If the companion can monitor vital signs, the couple may decide to remain in the comfort of their own home until active labor begins.

If the birth companion dresses professionally, wears a nametag and learns the names of her client's nurses, she can more easily develop a friendly rapport with the hospital staff. Ideally, her presence will encourage the staff to be more conscious about how they treat her client. A verbal explanation of procedures enhances this tendency. (For example, "Mary, Dr. Miller is preparing a tray of instruments in case you're not stretching well—you are planning to birth without an episiotomy, correct?")

During second stage the birth companion can be the extra arms that get the mother into non-traditional positions if progress is slow, and help guard the perineum. I once helped resolve a shoulder arrest by hauling the mother up into a squat. Perineal massage and support may or may not be possible or necessary. Some physicians allow it and others don't, and may or may not object to it.

Getting the baby to breast immediately after birth is important and the companion's encouragement and assistance can help ensure that it happens. The companion can also stay with the mother until the baby has nursed and they are settled in her room.

At the postpartum visit, the birth companion hones her postnatal midwifery skills and provides continuing support, especially if the mother came home in less than three days. I use the mnemonic phrase, For Every Lady Be Vigilant (Check her Fundus, Episiotomy site or perineum, Lochia, Breasts and breastfeeding, and Vital signs). She makes sure household maintenance is set up and everyone is coping adequately. Her support might be the only contact the couple has in those early, intense weeks.

The role of birth companion provides the woman who loves the birthing experience with many opportunities to expand her skills and knowledge. She also offers woman-to-woman support often missing in our society. The following excerpt from my brochure sums up my approach to my work as a birth companion:

"I feel most women can derive great personal satisfaction and self-esteem from a positive birth experience. An easy or a difficult birth, and parenthood, provide us with opportunities for much personal growth. I've found that women who prepare physically, emotionally and intellectually during pregnancy, and who have good support during labor, can usually give birth safely without a lot of medical intervention. My years as a childbirth educator convinced me that nearly every woman benefits from having an experienced woman stay with her and her husband during labor and birth. Mother, sisters or friends can fulfill this role too, but are often unavailable or inexperienced as birth companions. I tremendously enjoy helping women and their families during this time of natural but intense physiological and psychological transformation."

To all those readers who are aspiring or studying to be a birth companion: May you enjoy sharing your love and talents!

This article first appeared in Midwifery Today Issue No. 5.

Lily Fountain Werbos lived in College Park, Maryland, when she wrote this article, and was a birth companion, birth assistant, nursing student, mother and midwife-to-be.

DOULAS DELIVER SUPPORT

AN ANCIENT TRADITION OF WOMEN HELPING WOMEN IN CHILDBIRTH FINDS NEW RELEVANCE

by Annie Kennedy & Penny Simkin, PT

High maternity care costs, high cesarean rates, a shortage of nurses and midwives—all are serious problems for today's expectant parents. There is a solution, and it's not a new technology and not a new medication. It's the oldest idea in childbirth today—the labor support person, or doula. This person has become the object of much media attention, due to the publication of a study, "Continuous Emotional Support During Labor in a U.S. Hospital," published in the *Journal of the American Medical Association* by doctors John Kennell and Marshall Klaus. Their study, which took place in a large and medically advanced hospital in Houston, found numerous benefits for both mother and baby from continuous emotional support of the mother throughout labor by a trained and caring individual, called a doula (a Greek word meaning caregiver for women in childbirth).

They compared women who labored alone with women who were assigned a doula. Those who had a doula had shorter labors (25 percent shorter), needed less pain medication (narcotics and epidural anesthesia), and had fewer forceps and cesarean deliveries. In addition, there were fewer newborn complications, and maternal-infant bonding was measurably enhanced in the doula group.

Kennell and Klaus' study confirmed what we had already learned from several previous studies in Guatemala, Dublin, Toronto and Australia. All these studies, which included couples who had taken childbirth classes, couples who had not taken classes, and women who labored without a loved one present, found similar benefits—equal or better obstetric outcomes for mother and baby in the supported groups, fewer labor complications, less need for pain medications, and greater satisfaction on the mother's part.

Woman-to-woman support in labor is hardly a new idea. Throughout recorded history, mothers, sisters, friends and other women have always helped each other through birth and afterward. In paintings, sculptures and artifacts from traditional cultures birth is almost always portrayed with a trio of women: the laboring woman, always large and in the center; a midwife, smaller and kneeling in front of the woman; and a helper supporting the woman from behind. It was the same from pre-colonial times until the 1930s in the United States. A woman's pregnancy, labor and postpartum were a time for social connection, emotional support, advice and help from other knowledgeable caring women.

When birth moved into the hospital in the 1930s and 1940s, there was no longer any emotional support available to laboring women. The father was left out and nurses had little time for this role along with their clinical responsibilities. By the 1970s the woman's husband was allowed in the hospital maternity suite to make up for this lack. Today women can invite whomever they wish to accompany them in labor, but many partners feel uneasy with their heavy responsibility of being the woman's main source of emotional support and provider of physical comfort. It is a difficult role to play, especially in the highly technological environment of the hospital.

Although most nurses are fully capable of giving excellent emotional care, they are really not free to do it because of other job requirements and heavy clinical responsibilities (for example, conducting observations of mother and baby, looking after more than one patient, responsibility to keep equipment functioning properly, and an inability to provide continuity of care through shift changes). Emotional care has had to take a back seat to these other duties. And as obstetric care continues to become more complex and confusing, fathers as well as laboring women want and need help and emotional support. So parents once again are turning for help to women with greater experience and perspective.

A recent study by Penny Simkin of women's long-term memories of their birth experiences found that even twenty years later, women still remember their own feelings and actions and the words of their partners, nurse and doctors. Their memories are poignant, vivid and accurate. Women who had satisfying birth experiences still remember them with joy. Those with disappointing birth experiences still express anger or remorse. Their strongest feelings, positive and negative, focus on the way they were treated by caregivers.

Today's labor support providers recognize the lasting psychological impact of the birth experience and work very hard to help make every birth a positive memory. Trained and experienced, they provide a continuous caring source of knowledge, comfort and encouragement both for the laboring woman and her partner. As one woman said, "Her voice was kind and gentle, yet strong. I needed that because I wasn't sure how long I could go on."

The fee for labor support services, including one or more prenatal meetings with the client, attendance at her labor and birth, and at least one postpartum meeting ranges from one hundred to four hundred dollars in the Seattle area. Sliding fee scales are also available for those clients who cannot pay the full fee. In addition, a few health departments, hospitals and group practices pay for labor support services for their clients. Women who wish to become doulas or learn more about labor support services, or who want a referral to a doula should contact:

Doulas of North America, 1100 23rd Avenue East, Seattle, WA 98112 (206) 325-1419

This article was written especially for this book.

Annie Kennedy is past president of Doulas of North America (DONA), a former president of the Pacific Association for Labor Support, a doula, and extension education director at the Seattle Midwifery School.

Penny Simkin is a childbirth educator, a doula and doula trainer, and author of numerous books and publications in the field of childbirth. She is the founder of the Pacific Association for Labor Support (PALS) and Doulas of North America.

EARNING MONEY DURING YOUR EDUCATION

by Jennifer Rosenberg, ICCE, CD(DONA)

Nearly every student doula, midwife and childbirth educator will be faced with some sort of money issue during her training. Some women have full-time jobs and pursue education in midwifery or related fields on the side; others are full-time students or perhaps single moms who work on the side. Because midwifery, childbirth education and doula work can be fairly expensive—between books, equipment, teaching aids, videos, gas costs and childbirth education—it's important to start earning while learning to help defray costs.

One of the best ways I've found to make money while helping moms is as a postpartum doula or mother's helper. I charge on a sliding scale from eight to twelve dollars per hour. I've learned to clean very efficiently and prioritize tasks to get the maximum benefit from limited time. I've learned to listen while I clean, and so often end up doing postpartum counseling and breastfeeding support—helping moms gain an understanding of the chaos which often accompanies postpartum. I saw such a benefit for the moms I was working with that as soon as I returned to the "regular" workplace myself, I hired a student midwife to clean for me so I wouldn't have to be a single mom, working thirty hours per week, parenting, cooking, laundering AND cleaning. Now I forget the cleaning, sometimes get help with the laundry, and my house is spotless once a week. This help brings sanity and stability into my life, and since my doulas can clean my two bedroom townhouse from top to bottom in two to three hours, it only costs me twenty-four dollars per week or less for this marvelous service. Because I'm a doula and childbirth educator myself, my doulas get clients from me, pick my brain about birth, and are welcome to peruse my library when they're done working.

Because I'm working at Midwifery Today and only occasionally take doula clients, I do this work on a volunteer basis for my neighbors and friends. I help one friend, who is on bedrest and six months pregnant, do her dishes and chat with her about what's going on. Another neighbor just had her baby, and I visit every couple days to see how breastfeeding is going and give her some of the freebies I get as a childbirth educator. She doesn't need help with her house, but she does need reassurance that her daughter is gaining weight well even though she can't tell how much she's drinking. The volunteer work I do often leads to referrals and paying clients or brings me valuable experience to expand my abilities to work with birthing women.

There are many postpartum doula training programs and organizations, but one of the simplest ways of learning how to help people at home is to become a certified nursing assistant (CNA) and work for a home health agency on a part-time basis. Most agencies pay CNAs seven to eight dollars per hour in my area, and many agencies are developing programs of home healthcare for pregnant women and babies with ongoing medical problems. Most CNA programs are inexpensive and can be completed quickly; there is a high demand for nursing assistants. Any background in maternal health as a student midwife, doula or childbirth educator will help you find work, though experienced postpartum doulas are especially successful.

I found the CNA training very informative; it helped me understand better the routines and driving forces behind hospital policies and procedures. I can better communicate with staff and help my clients work with their caregivers to "bend" the policies that are less than client-friendly. Knowing medical terminology is also helpful to me because it enables me to read charts easily and help interpret for my clients. It also gives me an advantage when a client asks me "Is this normal?" because if I see something that needs reporting to a doctor, I can tell them the right terms to use with that caregiver. For example, a friend's baby was breathing rapidly and her chest was seesawing as she breathed. I was able to tell the mom, "Call your doctor and let him know that the baby is tachypnic and that I'm seeing some retractions." I explained what the words meant to the mom, and the doctor knew exactly what was going on. At the same time, when she asked if her baby was getting enough to eat, I looked at the baby, saw there were no signs of dehydration, asked about dirty diapers and was able to reassure her that her baby didn't need a supplement. A day later a weight check confirmed the baby was gaining almost two ounces per day.

> This help brings sanity and stability into my life. . . .

Having been on both the giving and receiving ends of home help, I can say that it's a positive and educational way to earn extra money and experience. This support also transitions well into doula work, childbirth education, midwifery and lactation consulting. It's something you never really have to stop doing, and I try to make sure that all my doula clients know the service is available, whether through me or through my doula.

This article was written especially for this book.

Jennifer Rosenberg is an ICEA certified childbirth educator and a DONA certified doula. She is also a single mom, and works at Midwifery Today.

MILK ANGELS

by Jennifer Rosenberg, ICCE, CD(DONA)

Via my computer, I speak with many women around the world who plan to breastfeed, try to breastfeed, and then struggle with breastfeeding until they wean to formula. The most common barrier to successful nursing for these women seems to be a lack of support at critical times.

We've known for years that the strongest predictor of nursing success is good advice and support for breastfeeding moms. Today we have more resources, more knowledge, and more support for breastfeeding than we've had for years, such as lactation consultants and La Leche League.

Why isn't this enough?

I believe the problem is simple: Babies' needs can't be scheduled.

Many moms tell me "I got great help in the hospital, but once I got home, everything fell apart"; or "I had my baby on the weekend, and the hospital's lactation consultant only works on weekdays"; or "The lactation consultant can see me tomorrow at two in the afternoon, but my baby is hungry now and I can't get her latched on!"

As a doula, I'm comfortable with the concept of being on call. If a client goes into labor, I can't tell her, "I'm sorry, I have room for you in my schedule tomorrow morning at ten." I don't expect her to put up with her contractions knowing help will be there tomorrow. Tomorrow may be too late.

We need a similar approach when it comes to the first weeks of breastfeeding. I tell my nursing mothers, "I want you to call if nursing hurts, I want you to call if you're getting frustrated, and I want you to call if you're even thinking about giving your baby a bottle of formula." More often than not, I call them when their baby is a few days old and ask them how nursing is going. If they indicate any problems at all, I go to them—not the following day, not three hours later, but within the hour. I rarely spend more than a half hour with them at their houses. When I sit with them and watch them struggle to nurse, I usually only need to help make a small adjustment, pull a lip here, place a hand there, calm the baby down, calm the mom down. Small things. The baby will latch and the mom will see it can be done. This might happen at eleven in the morning, but just as often it happens at ten at night. If it happens during the day, I call a few hours later and ask how it is going. If it happens at night, I call the next morning. I always get one of two answers: either everything is fine (in which case I will call back the next day just to make sure), or there is still a problem. Sometimes I refer my clients to lactation consultants, other times I simply get back in my car and go sit with them.

One client had a baby who would only latch on well when I was there. So I told the mom if she had to call me eighteen times in the next twenty-four hours in order to get it to work, that would be fine with me. I took the pressure off her—gave her permission to ask for help. We discussed strategies, options, talked about her alternatives. She called two or three times. I called her a couple of times to check in with her; two days later, her answer to "How is nursing going?" was "Just fine! No problems!" She's still nursing her daughter, several months later.

We have an extraordinary pool of talent and resources to draw on right now. We have doulas, La Leche League, lactation consultants, midwives, childbirth educators, nurses and postpartum doulas. We have telephones, pagers, email and the Internet. We also have a growing foundation of scientific and practical knowledge about breastfeeding.

Every woman who wants to nurse her baby should have all the support she needs to do so successfully. But these resources are not being utilized, and in many areas, the resources are not available.

My dream is that a mother learning to nurse her baby will be able to pick up her phone, call someone knowledgeable, talk about what is going on with her and her baby, and have a "milk angel" sitting on her couch to help her through any crisis within forty-five minutes. It would be a form of triage.

I am in favor of an on-call crisis breastfeeding support service which would be offered by doulas, experienced moms and La Leche League leaders. For the majority of

> **A MODEL FOR IDEAL BREASTFEEDING SUPPORT:**
>
> 1. From the beginning, moms need good help getting the baby latched on.
> 2. When the milk comes in, it is important that someone touch base with moms to make sure they are doing well emotionally and that nursing is going well.
> 3. If nursing is not going well on the second or third day (when someone checks in with the mom via phone), a milk angel will be sent to observe the mom breastfeed and provide basic assistance.
> 4. Breastfeeding help via phone should be available twenty-four hours per day. If phone help is not enough, a milk angel should be sent to help the mom in her home.
> 5. Lactation consultants will be available for more intensive help for more complicated cases.
> 6. Breastfeeding support groups, such as La Leche League and peer support programs should be available for all women who want them.

women, a half hour or hour of assistance will be all that is necessary—as long as it is provided when it is needed. When that crisis visit does not solve the problem, a visit with a lactation consultant would be scheduled for more intensive help.

Think about it. Instead of moms giving babies bottles out of frustration and panic because their screaming baby can't wait until tomorrow morning at ten o'clock to get help latching on, moms would know help is forty-five minutes, not fifteen hours away. The milk angel can help them find alternatives to bottles so the baby does not have nipple confusion to contend with as well.

I am not a lactation consultant. When I do breastfeeding support, I do basic things, like untuck the bottom lip, correct the position of the hand on the breast, get the baby to latch on quickly to my finger without chewing before the mom puts the baby to her tender nipple.

Sometimes when I first walk in, if the mom and baby are both frantic and there is milk expressed already, I will show the mom how to use a spoon or small cup to drip the milk into the baby's mouth. This calms the baby down and soothes the mother's fear that her baby isn't getting anything to eat.

I don't set moms up with breast pumps or nipple shields or supplemental nutrition systems (SNS). I don't do intensive suck training or teach them how to finger feed. I always refer moms with inverted nipples and babies with weak sucks.

Perhaps the most important thing I do is respond quickly and go to the clients, rather than make clients come to me or schedule an appointment. I know that if I go right away, I'll only have to take a half hour or an hour of my time to help them. If I wait, we may have a much longer row to hoe.

If I didn't go to my client at 10:30 at night—what would she do? Tough it out? Send her husband to the store to buy formula and bottles? But then the mom may have to use a breastpump to get her supply back up. She may be engorged. She may get a breast infection. She may not go to the lactation consultant at all, but simply wean to formula and bottles because her baby stopped screaming and drank four ounces and slept through the night. Maybe she nurses through the pain of a bad latch for months. If she has suffered through any of these possible scenarios, she remembers those first months as a time of pain, a time of failure and a time of crisis. I'd rather she is able to enjoy nursing, feel the success of a baby who doubles her birthweight in her first two to three months, feel the pleasure of nursing when it doesn't hurt, and experience the wonder of a baby falling asleep on her breast, completely content.

MONEY

Ideally, a program such as "Milk Angels" would be funded by grants, insurance companies, doctors and hospitals. It should be part of standard care. Another option would be to have clients of the program pay on a sliding scale, ranging from five to thirty dollars per visit. Realistically, given the skill level and time involved in an average visit, fifteen to twenty dollars would be a reasonable reimbursement for a milk angel for a single thirty to sixty minute home visit with phone follow-up. I base this on the average rate that childbirth educators and doulas make per hour (ten to twenty dollars), and considering that each visit may require child care, driving time and the on-call nature of the work. As a doula, I do many of these visits for free because I feel it is so important for women to get the help they need. Many of my clients tip me substantially which makes up for those who cannot afford to pay me extra for milk angel visits.

Given the fact that lactation consultants often charge between forty-five and sixty dollars per visit, this seems very reasonable and a good way to help families feel that if they do end up hiring a lactation consultant, that it is really necessary to have someone with that level of training to help.

This article first appeared in The Birthkit, Issue No. 17.

Jennifer Rosenberg is an ICEA certified childbirth educator and a DONA certified doula. She is also a single mom and works at Midwifery Today.

Chapter

6

Midwifery into the Future

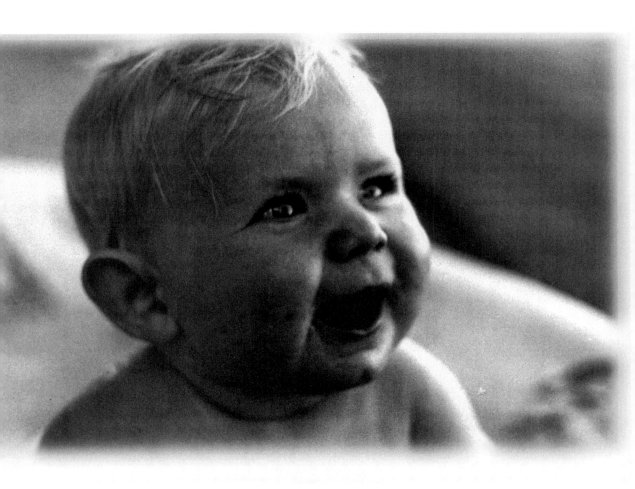

NATURE OF THE INTERNET

AND THE FUTURE OF MIDWIFERY

by Midge Jolly, LM

"The real voyage of discovery consists not in seeking new landscapes, but in having new eyes." —*Jonathan Swift*

My great-great-grandmother, Clara Dove, was a midwife and herbalist in the Appalachian Mountains of West Virginia in the 1920s. Though she was a forward-looking woman for her time, she would not recognize midwifery today. Considering the way our field is changing, I am not sure I will recognize the midwifery of tomorrow if I don't keep my eyes open and focused not only on my sister midwives, but also online—the world of the Internet. I resisted computers until midwifery school forced me to have a relationship with them. It didn't take long, however, before I began to share a worldview (with Jonathan Swift) that becomes more pertinent every day. With the Internet, my eyes have been forced open to an entirely new way of viewing the future of midwifery as an independent, viable art and profession. It is a fresh new vision, pregnant with possibility that I want to share with my fellow midwives.

Without a lot of fanfare or media attention, the midwifery model of care is gaining momentum and promoting change via the Internet through the cooperative efforts of midwives and advocates for the midwifery model. While there are serious midwifery-related witch hunt fires cropping up all over the country, positive attention to midwifery on the Internet is alive and well. The witch hunt today seems to be a response to the growing positive attention and empowerment of those seeking out the midwifery model, and by those increasing advocacy for ourselves and our place in the women's health community. It is also possible that the current escalation of the midwifery witch hunt mentality may be related, in part, to our increasing presence on the World Wide Web.

The informal, almost friendly, nature of Internet communication has allowed doors that have long been closed to be flung open and the information contained therein to come tumbling out. Most folks on the Internet have never seen one another and only share their experiences via the electronic medium of cyberspace—email, electronic bulletin boards and Web pages. Most of these women and men, professional and consumer alike, are unaware of the impact of their presence, even without their participation, in this medium. To me this is a fantastic thought: hands on, face to face midwifery is growing in its ability to promote change, and is facilitated by a medium that appears to be anathema to the midwifery model.

The benefits of rapid information exchange far outweigh any risk that I can contemplate (not discounting confidentiality issues). As this medium expands so does the number of people exposed to the midwifery model of care. Women are exposed to a greater variety of possible choices in healthcare than ever before, and midwifery information on the Internet is in the forefront of this information explosion.

One of the most integral components of the midwifery model is the amount of time we spend building relationships with clients. The midwife's intimate bond with women has long been at the core of this relationship, requiring time to develop. Time. Midwives spend so much time being with women there has often been little time for advocacy and politics outside of our immediate spheres, unless there is a threat to our immediate survival. On the Internet it is possible to spend time with women and talk with other midwives, students, midwifery advocates, MDs, world renowned birth activists and consumers without leaving home or office, gaining much needed clinical information, support and inspiration while saving time. On a daily basis, many of us are making contact with one another via the Internet. There are web pages, mailing lists, bulletin board forums, newsgroups and email loops dedicated to midwifery, pregnancy, parenting and birth. The variety of discussions found on the Internet is mind boggling. There exists everything from professionals on clinical issues, traditional and allopathic therapies, to professionals and consumers on the merits of home or hospital as a birthing site, international homebirth support email loops, midwifery mailing lists that welcome OBs to their forum, and vice versa. Midwives are being seen and heard and are making change in a way imagined but never realized before the Internet. Women on message boards everywhere are avidly seeking information on alternatives to the medical model of healthcare and birth.

. . . the Internet gives us the opportunity and ability to address assaults to the profession in a timely and professional manner with more support than ever.

Grassroots political action is also taking great leaps forward on the Internet. We can now be kept up to date about local, national and international midwifery activity via grassroots updates from MANA/NARM/MEAC, the OBCNEWS, <sci.med.midwifery> newsgroup, Citizens for Midwifery (CfM) and discussion lists for midwives, to name just a few of the many sources of information available. We are also able to garner support for time sensitive issues without the delay of traditional "snail" mail, phones and faxes. When, for example, it was announced on the Internet through OBCNEWS that Ste. Thérèse birth center in France would close in three days without additional support, the online community rallied to their aid. The rapid nature of communication on the Internet gives us the opportunity and ability to address assaults to the profession in a timely and professional manner with more support than ever. Recently a public poll held in support of midwifery in Illinois with only a several hour window of time to reply was greatly enhanced by posting it on various midwifery-friendly sites. With groups popping up such as the America Online home and hospital discussion group, midwives are finding support in surprising places.

The diverse midwifery populations I have encountered on the Internet have helped me gain a different perspective on old issues that bear watching as the national midwifery struggles continue. Whatever our position, working to promote midwifery and taking great care to maintain autonomy and individuality is essential. Keeping abreast of the current tug-of-war in our own back yards is difficult but necessary to our continued survival. As we keep adding our voices to the shared pool of information, midwifery will be better able to survive. As our voices join together and become stronger, midwifery will be more likely to flourish.

Thankfully, not only the struggles are out there to be watched on the Internet. My new eyes have allowed me to see many things in the last year that offer hope for the future of natural birth. I see midwives sharing information and learning a new respect for one another in spite of a personal alphabet soup of issues. I see the potential for midwifery advocacy via the Internet to increase exponentially as we begin to "meet" and interact more with one another. Old habits can be difficult to change and midwives in the United States have too long existed in a survival mode. Internet communication is allowing us to see how midwifery operates in other parts of the world. If we use the Internet to its full advantage, I believe midwifery might actually find the energy to advocate for itself rather than spend so much energy doing damage control.

The varieties of personal Web sites promoting midwifery, homebirth and advocacy issues are becoming too numerous to count. Since most servers offer quick and easy help to set up a Web site, I encourage all of us to develop our own Web pages, join midwifery mailing lists, grassroot updates, state and national midwifery advocacy organizations, and respond to requests for information and or action. Midwifery advocacy can be as simple as signing a guest book and telling folks you are a midwife. If you are experienced on the Internet, offer your help to a novice. If you are a novice, the help is there; all you need is a little time to find the help that fits your needs. I have great hope we can all use new eyes to see ways to promote the midwifery model of care as a safe and sane choice in a quickly changing world. Growing connected with one another is the key to our survival and growth.

Please see the Resource section for a list of Web sites.
This article first appeared in Midwifery Today Issue No. 45.

Midge Jolly is a Florida licensed midwife and graduate of the Miami-Dade associates in midwifery program. She has been active in midwifery advocacy and homebirth since the early 1980s and offers home-based midwifery care in the Florida Keys. If you wish to share information about sites, lists, or want to know more about midwifery mailing lists, building your own Web sites or ways to promote midwifery using the Internet, email Midge at <midgewife@aol.com>. Visit her Web site at <http://members.aol.com/Midgewife/midwifesdream.html>.

MIDWIFERY TRAINING IN ENGLAND

by Irene Walton

Editor's Note: We have discussed many paths to becoming a midwife in this volume. Another viable choice is to get your schooling in the UK, especially if you can find a school that is philosophically akin to your own. Consider this article in that possible context.

Prior to 1902 midwifery training in England was not regulated. In 1864 the Ladies Obstetrical College was founded in London which provided educated women with facilities for learning theory and practice of midwifery, and the accessory branches of medical science. The training consisted of attendance at lectures during the winter, and attendance at a lying-in hospital or maternity charity hospital during the summer, with personal attendance at twenty-five births. In 1869, following an investigation and report on the causes of infant mortality by the London Obstetrical Society, a recommendation was made that an examining board be established so that midwives could be tested and granted a diploma. This was not acted upon by the government and so the London Obstetrical Society went ahead and created their own board which commenced its own (voluntary) examinations in 1872.

In 1902, following years of lobbying, the first Midwives Act (H.M.S.O. 1902) was passed by Parliament; it aimed to secure better training for midwives and to regulate their practice. Its main objectives were: to have the title "midwife" protected in law, the profession restricted to those who were qualified, to set up a Central Midwives Board (CMB) which would maintain and publish a roll of midwives and publish accounts, to develop a system of statutory supervision of midwives and to produce a handbook of rules for midwives.

There have been a succession of acts since that time which have closed the perceived loopholes. Initially as described, midwifery was governed by its own regulating body, the CMB but, following the 1979 Nurses, Midwives and Health Visitors Acts (HMSO 1979), it came under the United Kingdom Central Council for Nursing, Midwifery and Health Visiting (UKCC) which keeps the register. I do not propose to go into the history or for that matter the politics of regulation here, but will be content with describing how one becomes a midwife today and what is the scope of practice.

Until recently there were two ways of becoming a midwife which were either a short programme following registration as a nurse, or more rarely by direct-entry. The shortened programme for nurses was twelve months long until 1982 when it was lengthened to eighteen months (78 weeks), and the direct-entry programme was two years and then lengthened to three years (156) weeks. These programmes were delivered in small schools of midwifery on site in a maternity hospital, and were funded and resourced by the National Health Service. The training was an apprentice type training where the student worked in the clinical area and was released to attend a weekly study day or week-long study blocks. The formal clinical and theoretical teaching was delivered by a midwife teacher holding the midwife teacher's diploma

(MTD). The teacher was usually responsible for all the teaching of a set of students—usually from two to ten—and the informal teaching was performed by clinical midwives. The award granted was by the English National Board for Nursing, Midwifery and Health, and conferred eligibility to seek entry to the Register held by the UKCC. Although both programmes were substantive in their content and rigorous in their assessment of competence, they were deemed to equate at the point of exit with the first year of a degree in a university, i.e., certificate level.

In the early 1990s the government facilitated a move of the schools to the higher education sector, and now most midwifery schools throughout England are sited in either a university or a college of higher education accredited by a university. The students are now university students undergoing a programme of education which leads to a joint award by the English National Board. The Board requires the student be fit to practice and achieve the learning outcomes as outlined in the Midwives Rules (UKCC 1993).

In addition each university expects the programme to meet its own exacting quality and standards requirements for the award. The academic level of the award can be at either diploma (level two) or honours degree (level three). The programme is planned and validated at a particular level and inextricably linked to the ENB requirements for eligibility to register as a midwife. What this means in practice is that a student entering a programme which has a degree level exit award must achieve level three to be eligible to practice as a midwife. So a student who enters a degree programme and fails to meet the requirements to graduate cannot have a "fall back" award at diploma level with the word midwifery in the title. Such a student could exit at diploma level with an award entitled, for instance, diploma in higher education healthcare studies. This would give academic recognition for study but would not allow any confusion regarding the person's eligibility to practice midwifery. The same situation stands for a student entering at diploma level. The fall back award in this case would be certificate in healthcare studies. Because both programmes conform to the legal requirements for midwifery education, a student in either programme will exit as a knowledgeable, clinically competent practitioner.

The aim of the profession is that all graduates be degreed; to this end, many institutions have part-time programmes which enable qualified midwives to "top up" to degree level. However, in the interim, the Institutions are still offering diploma level programmes because these are often funded through contracts with the National Health Service which provide students with a bursary, uniform and other limited expenses. These can be very attractive to students who otherwise would be funded by a lower rate grant system.

One of the changes that such a move into higher education has entailed is the physical move off site into university buildings. This combined with the amalgamation of the small midwifery training schools into large multi-disciplinary schools of health or nursing and midwifery did have the effect of loosening the previously strong links between clinical practice and education. There was also a great emphasis on the academic aspects of the programme in an endeavour to be credible. In the early 1990s some of the institutions were offering programmes some practitioners felt were too academic as distinct from being clinically focused. Most educators would have disagreed with this by pointing out that the curriculum was delivered fifty percent as theory and fifty percent as clinical practice. In most institutions the academic credit was awarded for the theory and competence was assessed in clinical practice but not credited toward the academic award. The nature of modular structures made designing a curriculum which gave continuity in the clinical areas quite difficult.

At John Moores University we think we have combined the best of the old and new academic forms of teaching midwifery. We offer two programmes leading to registration as midwife. Both are three years in length, and one leads to diploma level and the other to degree level. There is a slightly lower entry requirement for the diploma level, but both programmes are structurally very similar. The University acknowledges that learning takes place in practices and so what students demonstrate is accredited as fifty percent of the programme. For one whole year the student practices full-time and has the opportunity to give care for a few women, from booking to the end of the postnatal period. Emphasis is on woman-centred care so it is acknowledged that some women may have a complicated labour or delivery and that the midwife's role is to offer choice, continuity and control. During the clinical placements, a midwifery lecturer facilitates on a one-to-one basis with the student. Student's competence is assessed by the clinical midwives acting in an assessor role.

The programme's philosophy encourages the woman to exercise informed choice, autonomy of decision making and continuity of care within her maternity experience. Subjects within the modules are not taught in isolation but are consistently related to the woman's psychological, social or physical needs. Each module is structured carefully to obtain a balance between the different teaching strategies to promote student empowerment. The combination of teaching and clinical strategies encourages the student to becoming an autonomous practitioner whose practice within the clinical setting is woman-centred.

A key hope of a graduate midwife or diplomate is that she will be a change agent. Yet, as pointed out by an ENB study, "Developing confidence is daunting enough without also having to develop the confidence to change the system itself." To enable this development, students need to develop academic and professional confidence, ability and prowess. They need the ability to critically analyse, reflect and meaningfully synthesize information and contemporary practice. They must be able to articulate their thoughts and feelings and have insight into the needs of women. They must be clinically credible, know how the service is planned and delivered, and most importantly, they must have the courage to be challenging, to stand up for and be the advocates of women in their care. Midwives in England are committed to making the experience of birth as fulfilling as possible for all women regardless of their social background or type of pregnancy and birth.

References:

H.M.S.O. (1902). Midwives Act 1902. London. H.M.S.O.

H.M.S.O. (1979). The Nurse, Midwives and Health Visitors Act 1979. London. H.M.S.O.

English National Board. (1996). An evaluation of pre-registration undergraduate degrees in nursing and midwifery programmes. London. ENB.

United Kingdom Central Council Requirements Midwives Rules:

Is provided at an approved educational institution.

Will enable the student midwife to accept responsibility for her personal professional development and to apply her knowledge and skill in meeting the needs of individuals and of groups throughout the antenatal, intranatal and postnatal periods and shall include enabling the student to achieve the following outcomes: (Rule 33)

(i)   The appreciation of the influence of social, political and cultural factors in relation to healthcare and advising on the promotion of health.

(ii)   The recognition of common factors which contribute to, and those which adversely affect, the physical, emotional and social well-being of the mother and baby, and the taking of appropriate action.

(iii)   The ability to assess, plan, implement and evaluate care within the sphere of practice of a midwife to meet the physical, emotional, social, spiritual and educational needs of the mother and baby and the family.

(iv)   The ability to take action on her own responsibility, including the initiation of the action of other disciplines, and to seek assistance when required.

(v)   The ability to interpret and undertake care prescribed by a registered medical practitioner.

(vi)   The use of appropriate and effective communication skills with mothers and their families, with colleagues and with those in other disciplines.

(vii)   The use of relevant literature and research to inform the practice of midwifery.

(viii) The ability to function effectively in a multi-professional team, with an understanding of the role of all members of the team.

(ix)   An understanding of the requirements of legislation relevant to the practice of midwifery.

(x)   An understanding of the ethical issues relating to midwifery practice and the responsibilities which these impose on the midwife's professional practice.

(xi)   The assignment of the midwife of appropriate duties to other and the the supervision and the monitoring of such assigned duties.

EEC Directives

European Community Directives 80/155/EEC and article 27 of the EC Directive 89/594/EEC state:

The training is to be dispensed under appropriate supervision:

1.   Advising of pregnant women, involving at least 100 prenatal examinations.

2.   Supervision and care of at least 40 women in labour.

3.   The student should personally carry out at least 40 deliveries; (when this number cannot be reached owing to the lack of available women in labour, it may be reduced to a minimum of 30, provided that the student participates actively in 20 further deliveries).

4. Active participation with breech deliveries. Where this is not possible because of lack of breech deliveries, practice may be in a simulated situation.

5. Performance of episiotomy and initiation into suturing. Initiation shall include theoretical instruction and clinical practice. The practice of suturing includes suturing of the wound following an episiotomy and a simple perineal laceration. This may be in a simulated situation if absolutely necessary.

6. Supervision and care of forty women at risk in pregnancy, or labour or postnatal period.

7. Supervision and care (including examinations) of at least a hundred postnatal women and healthy newborn infants.

8. Observation and care of the newborn requiring special care including those born preterm, post-term, underweight or ill.

9. Care of women with pathological conditions in the fields of gynaecology and obstetrics.

10. Initiation into care in the field of medicine and surgery. Initiation shall include theoretical instruction and clinical practice.

UKCC REQUIREMENTS

It will also meet the UKCC requirements (UKCC 12/1991) which states that:

UKCC 5.4 Education Programmes should aim to:

1. prepare the student midwife for her specific role (as described in article 4 of Directive 80/155/EEC);

2. enable the student midwife to be competent to fulfill her role as an accountable practitioner at the point of registration;

3. promote client-centred understanding and development of caring skills;

4. place emphasis on the student as a focus for educational strategies;

5. integrate theory and practice;

6. encourage self-directed learning;

7. promote the development of analytical thinking and creativity;

8. enhance personal and professional growth and development of the student;

9. promote the concept of holistic care;

10. promote understanding of research-based practice; and

11. motivate the midwife toward continuing education.

This article was written especially for this book.

Irene Walton is the principal lecturer in midwifery at the John Moores University in Liverpool, England.

HOW MIDWIFERY TODAY CAN HELP YOU BECOME A MIDWIFE

1. Attend Midwifery Today conferences.

Most Midwifery Today conferences include a beginning midwifery all-day pre-conference session. Attend this workshop for a good overview of the profession, one that will help you decide if midwifery is truly your calling. Then, choose from classes on a wide variety of topics including prenatal care, the various stages of labor, delivery complications, newborn assessment, basic and advanced suturing, waterbirth, herbs for pregnancy, sexual abuse and much more.

You'll also:

- Receive support and advice from senior midwives,
- Learn from some of the best teachers in the country,
- Meet a wide variety of birth practitioners: doctors, nurses, doulas, childbirth practitioners, birth activists and midwives of all kinds, and
- Begin to create your own identity as a birth practitioner as you learn about different styles of practice that can be combined into one that is uniquely yours.

Visit our Web site at http://midwiferytoday.com and follow the links for information about current conferences. Or call, write or email us and ask for the current conference programs.

2. Read *Midwifery Today* magazine.

Read this quarterly, 74-page journal to keep informed and inspired about birth and midwifery. It's a wonderful way to keep in touch with your sister midwives all around the world.

- Learn from news, reviews, birth stories and informative articles.
- Enjoy poetry and beautiful black-and-white birth art.
- Benefit from an in-depth look at a particular topic, as each issue explores a theme.
- Learn birth information and techniques from other cultures in the International Midwife section.
- Discover new ideas to improve your practice in the Tricks of the Trade column.

3. Subscribe today.

Regular price is $50 for one year in the United States, $60 in Canada/Mexico, and $75 in all other countries. Two-year prices are $95, $113 and $143. Take advantage of the Aspiring Midwives New Subscribers Special:

Mention code <u>857</u> with your order and save $5 on a one-year or $8 on a two-year subscription. This offer is good only with new subscriptions.

4. Back issues are also available—be sure to ask for the list.

Many aspiring midwives order the entire set. You will have an entire midwifery education at your disposal. Within these pages you will learn midwifery and birth from hundreds of teachers, and learn about all the vital issues related to your new profession. Perusing the past years of midwifery research and education is an excellent way to build a strong midwifery foundation. Mention code <u>857</u> and receive 10 percent off the entire set.

5. Listen to the educational audiotapes from our conferences.

Take advantage of this repository of wisdom from over seven years of Midwifery Today conferences! With over 600 tapes on hundreds of topics, you'll find information to help you at all stages of your career.

Ask for the Beginning Midwives Audiotape Special, and we'll send you a flyer of tapes especially chosen to guide the aspiring and beginning midwife.

6. Learn from a selection of midwifery books published by Midwifery Today.

You'll gain from having the experiences and opinions of several different authors in one volume—distilled insights that you'll turn to again and again. We also carry a small selection of books by other publishers, including Anne Frye's *Understanding Diagnostic Tests; Healing Passage, A Suturing Manual* and *Holistic Midwifery: Vol 1: Care During Pregnancy.*

7. Get the companion volume to *Paths to Becoming a Midwife* —
**   *Life of a Midwife: A Celebration of Midwifery.***

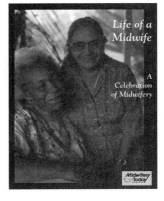

Designed to let you experience what it is like to be a midwife.

8. For more information, ask for the Books Flyer.

To contact us, call, write or email: Midwifery Today, P.O. Box 2672-350, Eugene, OR 97402, 541-344-7438, 800-743-0974 (USA only), fax 541-344-1422, email: Midwifery@aol.com

Be sure to mention code <u>857</u> and receive 10 percent off the entire set of back issues or $3 off *Life of a Midwife.*

AFTERWORD:
MAKING SENSE OF IT ALL

by Jennifer Rosenberg, ICCE, CD(DONA)

The process of becoming a midwife is not unlike the birth process.

Consider the pregnant woman. She is faced with an array of choices, a daunting spectrum of options. None is perfect. None will make everyone in her life happy. There is no consensus from the powers that be as to which option is best for her. She may choose between having a doctor and having a midwife. She may choose between having her baby at home or in the hospital. She can take birth classes or not. She can take classes sponsored by a doctor or hospital that last only a few weeks, or she may take an in-depth course that lasts a couple of months. She can hire a doula or have a friend with her. She may go through the pregnancy nestled in the arms of her partner and community, or she may face the road alone. She can choose to focus on nutrition, fitness and staying healthy. Or she may simply coast along, letting her care provider respond to whatever comes up. She may have to choose between a highly medicalized birth or the risks of doing nothing if a risk factor or potential complication shows up. She must choose between working through the process of her labor and numbing the pains away with an epidural or narcotics. She will choose to either take responsibility for her health and education, or do nothing and simply take what comes. No matter what she decides to do, someone will think she's either crazy or selling out. Someone will tell her she's risking everything to follow the course she's chosen, no matter what that course is.

Somehow each and every pregnant mother manages to find a way through this forest of choices and condemnation. Every day women choose to have an epidural or to breathe through one more contraction. Every day women choose to hire a midwife rather than go to the doctor a neighbor or sister used. Every day women choose to ask questions and every day women evaluate and decide which answers work for them and which do not.

Likewise with midwifery. There are no easy answers—no consensus, no one course to be followed. Some issues will never be fully resolved one way or the other. There is no one ideal path to follow, no clear single goal to be achieved. This book has already shown that in many ways. We have attempted to present the full spectrum of midwifery education and midwifery as a profession, warts and all. Someday, perhaps there will be more harmony between the various organizations and kinds of midwives. At this point, however, it is difficult, even impossible to point to one group or one philosophy and say, "This is the ideal truth; this is how we all should be."

What is true is this: you, the aspiring midwife, are the only one who has the authority and the self-knowledge to choose which path is right for you. No matter which path you choose, someone will tell you that you're either crazy or you sold out. But that's okay. That person is not the one who has to walk your path. As you have seen, each path has its glories and its pitfalls. But one path will likely fit you better than any other. The advantage of so many choices, both in birth and in midwifery, is that each of us has a chance to find the choice that fits us best.

Remember, the reason there are so many different midwives and so many different ways of becoming a midwife is that there are four million women giving birth each year, and each of them is unique. There are so many different kinds of midwives and doulas and childbirth educators because there are so many different communities and families and women.

The best thing you can do is keep your sense of humor and your sense of self. Even if the path you choose at first does not turn out to be the path you ultimately take, if you learn from everything you do, none of it will be wasted. When you get away from all the politics and philosophical disagreements, the fundamental truth is still there. Midwife means "with woman."

> You, the aspiring midwife, are the only one who has the authority and the self-knowledge to choose which path is right for you.

Jennifer Rosenberg is an ICEA certified childbirth educator and a DONA certified doula. She is also a single mom and works at Midwifery Today.

NOTES:

Resources

Directory of Schools & Programs

ACNM & MANA:

Core Competencies • Code of Ethics/Values

Standards of Practice

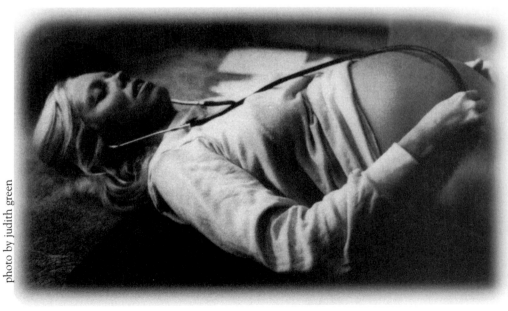

photo by judith green

Midwifery Education Accreditation Council
(MEAC)

by Mary Ann Baul, CPM

Midwifery Education Accreditation Council (MEAC) supports quality and innovation in direct-entry midwifery education. What does this mean to students looking into midwifery education?

Direct-entry midwifery is based on the European model of professional midwifery practice which does not require becoming a nurse as a prerequisite, although nursing skills are taught as part of a comprehensive midwifery education. Programs of study encompass both clinical and theoretical learning experiences.

MEAC accredited schools have met educational standards based on the nationally recognized core competencies of midwifery practice set by the Midwives' Alliance of North America (MANA). However, that does not mean all schools are alike. MEAC accredits midwifery programs that come in many colors, from apprenticeships to private schools, from at-a-distance programs to programs within other institutions. Some programs offer degrees or certificates in midwifery. All programs meet requirements to prepare the student to qualify for the North American Registry of Midwives national examination to become a certified professional midwife (CPM).

MEAC's standards were developed by a coalition of expert direct-entry midwifery educators. Our mission is to promote quality education in midwifery through accreditation. Our goal is to be a "federally recognized accrediting agency" by the Department of Education (DOE), and we plan to apply to the DOE next year.

Once MEAC is a federally recognized accrediting agency, MEAC schools will be able to apply to become providers of Title IV funding (student loans under the Higher Education Act).

MEAC accredited programs have opened their doors to a thorough inspection by an outside examining committee of peer educators. Each school shares a comprehensive self-evaluation of its mission, curriculum, student policies and services, facilities, faculty policies, financial management and record of graduates' success. Accreditation provides an assurance of institutional and educational quality for employers, educators, governmental officials, and the public, because the school or program adheres to established criteria, policies and standards.

Programs which are pre-accredited meet all of MEAC's standards except they do not have any graduates from their midwifery program yet. They should be accredited within a three year period. All schools must reapply for accreditation every three to five years. MEAC provides a directory of accredited schools to anyone who requests it.

Some students ask whether their credits will transfer if they attend a MEAC-accredited school. This depends solely on the discretion of the receiving institution. We recommend that students speak to a receiving institution ahead of time to determine which credits the institution accepts.

Other students ask if MEAC accreditation guarantees that the educational program will be comprehensive enough to qualify the student to become licensed or certified in her state. Each state has its own laws regarding certification and licensing, although some states accept the certified professional midwife credentials. It is the student's responsibility to become familiar with her state's requirements.

As a separate service, MEAC also approves programs and workshops providing continuing education units for professional midwives to maintain and upgrade their standards for practice. MEAC is a member of the International Association of Continuing Education and Training.

The following is a list of programs and schools accredited by MEAC.

Maternidad La Luz: The Birth Place, 1308 Magoffin Ave., El Paso, TX, 79901 (915) 532-5895 Fax: (915) 532-7127 Deborah Kaley, Director. (Accreditation period: 11/95-11/98)

Seattle Midwifery School, 2524 16th Ave. S., Rm. 300, Seattle, WA 98144-5104 1-800-747-9433, (206) 322-8834, Fax: (206) 322-2840 JoAnne Myers-Ciecko, Director. (Accreditation period: 8/96-8/99)

• Utah School of Midwifery, 190 S. Canyon Ave., Springville, UT 84663 (801) 489-1238 Dianne Bjarnson, Director (Accreditation period: 8/96-8/99)

Programs Pre-Accredited by Midwifery Education Accreditation Council

(They did not have graduates from their generic track of midwifery education during the accreditation process.)

Birthingway Midwifery School, 5731 N. Williams, Portland, OR 97217 (503) 283-4996 Holly Scholles, Director (Pre-accreditation period: 8/96-8/99)

• Midwifery Institute of California, 3739 Balboa #179, San Francisco, CA 94121 (415) 248-1671 Shannon Anton & Elizabeth Davis, Directors (Pre-accreditation period: 8/96-8/99)

• Oregon School of Midwifery, 342 E. 12th Ave. Eugene, OR 97401 (541) 338-9778 Daphne Singingtree, Director (Pre-accreditation period: 5/96-5/99)

Sage Femme Midwifery School, P.O. Box 2014, Clackamas, OR 97015 (503) 786-1460 Patricia Craig-Downing, Director

Portland Campus: 2702 SE Lakewood Dr., Milwaukie, OR

Santa Cruz Campus: Pacific Cultural Center, 1307 Seabright, Santa Cruz, CA Cindy Bacon, Regional Director (Pre-accreditation period: 8/97-8/2000)

• Have distance education program

Contact programs for their accreditation status.

This article was written especially for this book.

Mary Ann Baul, LM, RN, CPM, has been president of Midwifery Education Accreditation Council (MEAC) since 1996. In that time, MEAC has accredited or pre-accredited eight direct-entry midwifery programs, and has approved over thirty continuing education programs for professional midwives.

Mary Ann regularly speaks to midwifery educators, state agencies and aspiring midwives regarding midwifery education and accreditation. She has served as a site visitor and reviewer for midwifery education programs undergoing accreditation. She works closely with her board of directors, who represent diverse midwifery education programs in the United States as well as consumers and members of the public. She is past president of the Arizona Association of Midwives, she has been a licensed midwife for over fifteen years, and is co-owner of Womancare, a homebirth practice in Flagstaff, Arizona.

Midwifery Education in the United Kingdom

by Sara Wickham

Midwifery education in the United Kingdom is now taught through universities and colleges of higher education. In the UK, over 99 percent of women have midwives to care for them throughout pregnancy, labour and the postpartum period, and midwives work in hospitals, community practice and women's homes. Most midwives work for the National Health Service, although a few midwives also work independently and care for women birthing at home, in birth centres or in hospitals.

Most midwifery courses are now pre-registration or direct-entry. They last between three and four years, and also offer a diploma or a degree to successful students. Theoretical classes are usually held in the university, and practice placements are offered in both hospital and community settings, where midwifery students are attached to experienced mentors. There are also a few eighteen-month courses for students who are already registered nurses.

Upon qualification, midwives can work in any setting, although most practise in a hospital initially. There are a large number of specialist and advanced courses for qualified midwives, and some midwives choose to work within a specialist area, such as research and development, midwifery education or a special care baby unit. Currently, there is a great demand for midwives in the UK, and there are jobs available in most areas. It may be possible to convert a foreign midwifery qualification, but full and up-to-date details should be sought from the relevant professional organisation. Foreign students who require a work permit or visa will usually need to cover the cost of course fees themselves, although further details of costs can be obtained from individual institutions.

The United Kingdom Central Council for Nurses, Midwives and Health Visitors (UKCC) holds the professional register for midwives. There are separate National Boards for each country who have an up-to-date listing of schools of midwifery. The addresses for these organisations are:

United Kingdom Central Council for Nurses, Midwives and Health Visitors
23 Portland Place, London, W1N 4JT England

English National Board Careers Department
P.O. Box 2EN, London, W1A 2EN England, Tel; (0171) 391 6200 or (0171) 391 6205

Welsh National Board
2nd Floor Golate House, 101 St Mary Street, Cardiff, CF1 1DX Wales, Tel: (01222) 261400

Scottish National Board
22 Queen Street, Edinburgh, EH2 1JX Scotland, Tel: (0131) 226 7371

National Board – Northern Ireland
Centre House, 79 Chichester Street, Belfast, BT1 4JE, Northern Ireland, Tel: (01232) 238152

Sara Wickham, RM, BA, is a British direct-entry midwife who has also practiced in the US. She is studying for a master's program and is researching the issue of routine Rhogam administration.

RESOURCE LIST:
ORGANIZATIONS THAT PROMOTE MIDWIFERY

ACNM, The American College of Nurse-Midwives
Organization committed to promoting nurse-midwives in the United States
818 Connecticut Avenue NW, Suite 900, Washington, D.C. 20006
(202) 728-9860 • http://www.acnm.org or http://www.midwife.org

Birth Gazette
42-MT The Farm
Summertown, TN 38483
(931) 964-3798

MANA, The Midwives Alliance of North America
P.O. Box 175, Newton, KS 67114
(888) 923-6262 • ManaMW@aol.com • http://www.mana.org/

MEAC
220 W. Birch, Flagstaff, AZ 86001
(520) 214-0997

DONA, Doulas of North America
Doula support and education organization
1100 23rd Avenue East, Seattle, WA 98112
(206) 325-1419 • http://www.dona.com

ICEA, International Childbirth Education Association
P.O. Box 20048, Minneapolis, MN 55420
(612) 854-8660 • http://www.icea.org • Orders only: (800) 624-4934

La Leche League
Breastfeeding support organization, promoting breastfeeding internationally
1400 N. Meacham Road
Schaumburg, IL 60173-4840
(800) La-Leche • (847) 519-7730 • http://www.lalecheleague.org/

Lamaze International
Lamaze childbirth preparation organization
1200 19th Street NW, Suite 300
Washington, D.C. 20036
(800) 368-4404 • (202) 857-1128 • http://www.lamaze-childbirth.com

NARM, North American Registry of Midwives
P.O. Box 15, Linn, West Virginia 26384
(888) 84-Birth • (888) 842-4784

Midwifery Today, Inc.
P.O. Box 2672
Eugene, OR 97402
(800) 743-0974 • http://www.midwiferytoday.com

The Online Birth Center
http://www.efn.org/~djz/birth/birthindex.html

NARM REQUEST FORM

For more information from the North American Registry of Midwives (NARM):

Call toll-free 1-(888)84-BIRTH (842-4784) for general information and brochures on how to become a certified professional midwife (CPM). For CPM applications, make all checks and money orders payable to NARM, and send to our new address:

NARM Applications
P.O. Box 6449
Bend, OR 97708-6449

Request form for NARM Certification Application Packet and Candidate Information Bulletin

(Please photocopy this page & print in black ink)

Name: _____ Date: _____

Address: _____

_____

City: _____ State/Province: _____

Country: _____ Postal code: _____

Home phone: _____ Work phone: _____

Pager: _____ Fax: _____

ATTACHED IS MY NON-REFUNDABLE:

__Certified check __ Money order (made out to North American Registry of Midwives (NARM) in U.S. funds.

IN PAYMENT FOR:

__Application Packet (includes application and Candidate Information Bulletin (CIB)) $50

__Candidate Information Bulletin (only) $10 (Note: The CIB contains general information and policies regarding the CPM process and study guides for the required exams.)

Direct-Entry Midwifery Programs

This list is not comprehensive and reflects only our current database. If you know of schools not listed here, please let us know. We have included a form on page 331 for schools and programs to send us so that we can keep our directory current. Call for updates.

Ancient Arts Midwifery Institute

P.O. Box 788, Claremore, OK 74018-0788 918-342-2926, 818-902-0449
fax: 918-342-2956, http://members.aol.com/anctartmi/index.html

Our goal is more midwives. Our emphasis: the preservation of apprentice trained midwives; honoring midwifery as the ancient art of touching the future! We offer superior education at a reasonable fee so that we can help more women reach their goals. We began as Apprentice Academics in 1981, setting the standard for academic midwifery education with the original midwifery homestudy course. Introductory program, advanced options, childbirth educator certification, online study group and assistance, documented apprenticeship and annual proficiency exams.

Arkansas Midwives School & Services

4528 E. Huntsville Rd., Fayetteville, AR 72701, P.O. Box 4426, Fayetteville, AR 72702-4426 501-571-2229, Midwives@dicksonstreet.com

Our mission is to train professional midwives to provide safe, affordable and personal care to women; to offer family-centered maternity care, and to promote cooperation and communication among all those providing maternity services. Some scholarships available.

Association of Texas Midwives

Ste.1A-202, 603 W. 13th St., Ste 1A, Austin, TX 78701-1796 512-928-2311, atmed@juno.com

Self-paced, home-study format makes the course extremely flexible; students can become certified with Assoc. of Texas Midwives Professional Certification and Preceptor Certification. Course has just been revised for the third time with required reading lists and program structure designed for at-a-distance learners, with observation and apprenticeship incorporated into its academics. Students may find own qualified preceptors, as long as they use ones that are ATM-certified. This is one of the mandatory education courses required for Texas documentation (incorporates 1991 draft of core competencies of MANA). Program is designed for beginning students or midwives with no formal training to complete within three years, is based on independent reading and research; courses and workshops are available. Experienced midwives can challenge course by testing.

Austin Area Birthing Center, Inc.

8500 N. Mopac Suite 502, Austin, TX 78759-8347 512-346-3224, fax: 512-345-6637

The Austin Area Birth Center is a beautiful facility dedicated to providing moms and families with a healthy birth in a nurturing environment. Apprentices get lots of firsthand experience, live on-site, and get ample training and supervision one-on-one with an experienced midwife. Call for an application packet. Primarily intended for students who have completed didactic and academic training and taken part in a number of births. This is an opportunity for the student midwife to "primary" at births and gain the experience needed for independent practice.

Birth Rite Education Center

P.O. Box 276, Madisonville, LA 70447-0276   504-845-4247, fax: 504-845-1760

We are dedicated to improving maternal and child healthcare by providing quality midwifery education. While training kind, loving midwives, we also teach competency in the skills and procedures of birthing, complementing the science of obstetrics with the natural art of midwifery. By respecting birth as a fundamentally spiritual event, we recognize that a joyous, peaceful birth leads toward world peace. Preceptor sites available locally, nationally and internationally. New site recently secured in Honduras. No correspondence course. Pre-accredited thru MEAC.

Birthingway Midwifery School

4620 N. Maryland, Portland, OR 97217   503-282-5729

The purpose of the school is to train practitioners in a traditional midwifery model of care, using their intellect, senses, intuition and judgment to integrate new medical approaches with age-old wise woman practices. Birthingway's program provides a balance of textbook and empirical knowledge, along with clinical skills emphasizing low-tech methods, in an environment of respect for the physical, psychological and spiritual dimensions of childbirth. Write or call for a free catalog. Washington state accreditation pending.

Birthwise Midwifery School

66 S. High St., Bridgton, ME 04009-1110   207-647-5968
http://www.birthwisemidwifery.org

Birthwise is committed to training certified professional midwives (CPMs) in an intimate, relaxed environment. Faculty members are varied in their training and background to represent the wide spectrum of midwifery. Students learn actively through discussion, case studies, research, role play and hands-on practice. Contact us for our changing accreditation status.

Casa de Nacimiento

1511 E. Missouri Ave., El Paso, TX 79902-5615   915-533-4932

An intern program that offers intensive study in prenatal care, risk assessment, labor and delivery experience, newborn assessment and postpartum care. Interns accepted learn to do Paps/GCs, PKUs, venipuncture and nutrition counseling, see about 100 women for prenatal care weekly, with 30–50 babies delivered per month. Two interns are accepted every six weeks, four at any one time, with the interns living on the premises as part of one family. Individualized programs, shorter programs for those with much experience, longer ones for those with little experience, split programs with time in between to help interns fulfill family requirements, and programs tailored to those trying to meet new legal requirements.

Delphi Center for Midwifery Studies

2514 Kennedy Blvd. W. Tampa, FL 33609   813-873-7135, fax: 813-873-0274,
Delphicntr@aol.com

The Delphi Center's mission is to promote excellence in midwifery and maternal healthcare delivery through community and professional education, vocational training and direct maternity care services. School offers training for CBE, doulas, LA, MA and DEM. Midwife assistant program.

Family Birth Services Midwifery Course

814 Dalworth, Grand Prairie, TX 75050 972-263-0299, fax: 972-642-4177

The Farm

Ina May Gaskin, 156 Drake Ln., Summertown, TN 38483-5011 931-964-3798

Florida School of Traditional Midwifery

P.O. Box 5505, 4220 NW. 20th St., Gainesville, FL 32627-1818 352-338-0766, fax: 352-338-2013, fstm@juno.com, http//flmidwife.gainesville.fl.us/fstm/index.html

Our program blends a strong academic curriculum with the invaluable direct learning experiences that can only be provided by working with seasoned midwives. This sharing of the art of midwifery is one of the most vital components of a student's education. One year midwife assistant program.

Hands-On Midwifery Workshops

8274 S. Bright Rd., French Camp, CA 95231 209-982-5640, fax: 209-983-0137

Provides hands-on training in midwifery skills, allowing students one week of intensive training, networking, building confidence and having lots of fun while being totally immersed in midwifery. Food and lodging in our newly remodeled three bedroom mobile home (just for students) included.

Heart & Hands Midwifery Intensives

555 Pistachio Pl., Windsor, CA 95492-8166 800-594-3644

Intensive format designed to meet students' level of understanding. Coursework embraces a comprehensive study of midwifery technique and philosophy, includes hands-on training in blood pressure and fundal height assessment, fetal palpation and heart auscultation, pelvic and breast exams, nutritional analysis, intramuscular injections, and suturing. Blends academic with clinical, while teaching students to value and assess the role of the emotional and intuitive in midwifery care. Also available in at-a-distance format. Credit granted by Midwifery Institute of California. Good for aspiring midwives still exploring educational options.

The Holistic Midwifery Institute

128 N. 7th St., Ann Arbor, MI 48103-3317 734-663-1523, fax: 734-668-0016, GBrennan@umich.edu; Contacts: Patty Brennan, Patty Kramer

The Holistic Midwifery Institute offers a classroom-based learning experience for the purpose of training midwives in the full scope of homebirth midwifery practice. The institute specializes and provides training in the use of holistic modalities such as homeopathy, herbology, principles of nutritional support, cranial/sacral techniques, essential oils, aromatherapy, flower essences and yoga. Midwives are understood to be "partners in care" with the women and families they serve and a philosophy of informed consent is emphasized. All classes are taught by Patty Brennan and Pat Kramer, RN, two experienced midwives with homebirth practices of over 15 and 20 years respectively. Programs available include "The Art Of Midwifery" intensives, midwifery basics, clinical midwifery skills, infertility and miscarriages, introduction to holistic modalities, childbirth preparation series, vaccine choices, homeopathic alternatives and parental rights, herbal and homeopathic remedies for children.

Holistic Midwifery Training: Elizabeth Mazanec

P.O. Box 137, Acworth, NH 03601-0137

Hygieia College & Home Study Course

Jeannine Parvati Baker, P.O. Box 398, Monroe, UT 84754-0398 801-527-3738

Every mother is a midwife: Reclaim birth from the cult of the expert back to the lap of the family. Earth-based midwifery presented as evaluative dialog between founder Jeannine Parvati Baker and each Hygieia student. Healing the earth by healing birth. An international mystery school "in the manner of a midwife." Application/interview $108.

Informed Homebirth, Informed Birth & Parenting

P.O. Box 1733, Fair Oaks, CA 95628 916-961-6923, IHIBP@aol.com

Institute of Maternal & Child Health

6115 Woodrow Bean, Transmountain Rd., El Paso, TX 79924-5056
915-757-3700 fax: 915-751-6754, vcsneep1@aol.com, www.mercyinaction.org

This is a Christian mission training through The Vineyard Church to prepare missionary midwives for charitable service to the poor. Training follows guidelines for World Health Organization/International Confederation of Midwives standards of midwifery skills/training.

International School of Midwifery

711 S. Rue Notre Dame, Miami Beach, FL 33141 305-866-1095

Clinical site in Jamaica.

IXMUCANE

4A Avenida Norte #32 Antigua, Guatemala, Mailing address: Attn: Jennifer Houston, 7907 NW. 53rd St. Suite 409, Miami, FL 33166,
http://members@aol.com/womanway

Providing nurturing, respectful and affordable training, supplementing previous schooling in a Central American site that practices traditional midwifery arts. Providing a model of midwifery that is independent, yet affiliated with local hospitals and works cooperatively with physicians, blending the art of midwifery with medical resources as appropriate. Provides training that is not only compassionate and respectful to the women we serve but to learn how to care for ourselves as midwives also. $100/week room and board includes four hrs/day of Spanish. $25/wk for the training.

Maternidad La Luz: The Birth Place

1308 Magoffin Ave., El Paso, TX 79901-1626 915-532-5895 fax: 915-532-7127

Philosophy of Maternidad La Luz is based on respect for pregnancy and childbearing women as healthy and normal; that women have a right to birth in a safe, nurturing place assisted by the attendants of their choice. Maternidad La Luz (MLL) provides academic and clinical experience to those with the calling to the art and practice of midwifery, midwives who will answer the need in our society of supporting women and their families through the natural, healthy process of pregnancy and birth. Students work rotating clinic schedule, academic classes held three times a week for three hours, include case discussion. Community birth center serves 400+ women a year, mostly Spanish-speaking. Students diverse, from all over the world. Study is very intense: major topics in class and opportunity to train by interning for over 100 clinical hours. Students supervised by diverse staff of experienced midwives, with opportunity to learn from several teachers. Advanced classes, short terms also available.

Miami-Dade Community College

Attn: Justine Clegg, 950 NW. 20th St., Miami, FL 33127-4622 305-237-4234 305-237-4278 or 305-237-4116 www.mdcc.edu

The Miami-Dade Community College Midwifery Program values all forms of midwifery education and acknowledges the ongoing wisdom of apprenticeship as the original model for training midwives. To this end also, the program will utilize direct-entry midwives licensed under Chapter 467, Florida Statutes, as faculty for the primary midwifery courses. Financial aid available. Graduates of midwifery programs are eligible to apply to the Florida Council of Licensed Midwifery to take the Florida state licensure exam to become a Florida licensed midwife. Graduates of the accelerated prelicensure course must have their transcripts from their original educational program approved by the Council of Licensed Midwifery Credentialing Committee. Florida licensed midwives may qualify to practice in all other states in which direct-entry midwifery is legal, with the exception of New York state. Contact MANA or individual states' professional organizations for more information. Accelerated program for midwives certified in other states.

The Michigan School of Traditional Midwifery

P.O. Box 162, Mikado, MI 48745-0162 517-736-6583,
http://www.oscoda.net/mstm, mstm@i-star.com

Our goal is to offer both education and outlet for those who seek to pursue their midwifery calling as traditional practitioners. We wish to empower women who choose to become midwives and instill in them a sense of confidence to reach their destination. We believe those who are newly interested should be nurtured and encouraged to achieve their midwifery goals. MSTM is a positive first step toward answering your calling! MSTM conducts annual midwifery skills weekend workshops which are free for MSTM students (including room and board) and open to the public. MSTM offers two scholarships for the traditional midwifery program and also publishes a quarterly newsletter. Catalog and sample issue of *The Calling* $5.50. Midwife assistant certification.

Midwifery Institute of California

3739 Balboa St. Suite 179, San Francisco, CA 94121-2605 415-248-1671
www.birth-sex.com

We support community-based learning and apprenticeship. We support women-centered birth and value the tradition of midwifery learning as self-motivated. It is our purpose to enable students to train with qualified preceptors in both the US and abroad. Students may complete their academic preparation via at-a-distance modules (computerized) or on-site in San Francisco. Preceptors are paid by the program for training students. Linked to Heart and Hands. Students who have taken Heart and Hands may receive credit when enrolling in the Institute.

National College of Midwifery

P.O. Drawer SSS, Taos, NM 87571 505-758-1216, fax: 505-758-2683,
carla@newmex.com

Committed to training knowledgable entry-level midwives who meet NARM requirements, and supporting valid research by already certified midwives. Utilizes apprenticeship model. Offers associate of arts, BS, MS and PhD degrees in midwifery with an at-distance component available.

New Life Birth Service

2311 W. 9th St., Austin, TX 78703-4326 512-477-5452, fax: 512-477-5716

Oregon School of Midwifery

342 E. 12th Ave., Eugene, OR 97401-3244 541-338-9778, fax: 541-338-9783
www.efn.org/~osm

The goal of OSM is to improve maternal/child health and strengthen family bonds. In order to achieve these goals we offer accessible and comprehensive midwifery and doula education. We provide a structured program in the physiological and clinical aspects of childbearing while maintaining respect for the spiritual, emotional and natural process of birth. Our philosophy is centered on the midwifery model of care in which midwives support the normalcy of birth, respect family choices in childbearing, foster individualized client care, promote education and informed decision making. Two years didactic/academic; third year focused on clinical/hands on training. Doula work during first two years encouraged. Third year generally apprenticeship in homebirth or birth center practice either in US or overseas. Distance learning program pilot project beginning soon. Contact school for details.

Renaissance Woman Midwifery Institute

3106 Arizona St., Oakland, CA 94602-3950 510-530-4339

Is midwifery your calling? Honor the possibility. Ally with dynamic women pursuing education grounded in woman's ways of knowing. All paths to clinical competence are paved with both compassion and skill. There are many paths. Share laughter and tears with midwives, apprentices, mothers-to-be. Gain insight, knowledge, hands-on skill through passionate discussion, demanding didactics and practical experience. Guest speakers, special workshops, opportunities to offer doula services to homebirth families upon completion of course.

Resourcing Birth

P.O. Box 3146, Boulder, CO 80307-3146 303-499-3050, Resourcing@yahoo.com

Ongoing classes, limited apprenticeship opportunities in this direct-entry program. Terra Richardson is preceptor. Cost varies, based on classes taken. Birth Overview class available by correspondence, 10 modules cost $500.

The School of Natural Healing Midwifery Program

P.O. Box 412, Springville, UT 84663-0412 800-372-8255, fax: 801-489-8341, snh@avpro.com

Seattle Midwifery School

2524 16th Ave. S. Ste 300, Seattle, WA 98144 206-322-8834, fax: 206-328-2840, sms06@sprynet.com, Home.sprynet.com

We envision a world in which women and their families have access to the resources, information and services necessary to develop and maintain good health. Further, we envision a world in which the historically important role of women as healthcare providers, particularly as midwives, is affirmed and upheld. We intend to change the nature of healthcare, specifically maternity care and women's healthcare, by challenging the assumptions, structures, knowledge and skills upon which the current systems rest. The Seattle Midwifery School will provide information and educational services that support women's acquisition of knowledge and skills to improve and sustain their health and well-being. The school will provide training for women's healthcare providers, particularly midwives and doulas, that honors women's ways of knowing, respects the needs of adult learners, and promotes personal and professional development. We strive for quality, diversity, equity, opportunity, choice, women-centeredness, and empowerment in all our services and relationships. Seattle Midwifery School provides comprehensive theoretical and clinical education in midwifery, in a woman-centered environs that supports and honors adult learners. Students learn from a variety of teachers and clinical instructors, with range of styles and opinions about issues relevant to perinatal care. Emphasis on out-of-hospital birthing, but students have opportunity to observe and work with nurse-midwives and doctors in institutional settings. Goal is to present the range of styles and sites for midwifery practice so that students can find their own niche. Nationally accredited by the Accrediting Council for Continuing Education and Training (ACCET); recognized by the INS as an approved school for foreign students. Staff, faculty and preceptors share a heartfelt commitment to women's empowerment, midwifery, out-of-hospital birth and education that is flexible, individualized and integrated with the realities of life.

South Florida School of Midwifery

P.O. Box 557342, Miami, FL 33255-7342

State University of New York (SUNY) Health Sciences Center at Brooklyn

450 Clarkson Ave., Box 1227, Brooklyn, NY 11203 718-270-7740, chrish02@hscbklyn.edu

These one-year programs are designed to prepare qualified non-nurses and nurses to become certified midwives and nurse-midwives who are professionally prepared in full compliance with the standards established by the American College of Nurse-Midwives. Graduates from CM program will be eligible to sit for the ACNM's national certifying examination and to apply for licensure to practice midwifery within the state of New York. New York licensure does not guarantee reciprocity by any other state. CM and CNM students are integrated within the program. CNM graduates will be eligible to practice in all 50 states. ACNM approved direct-entry midwifery program. At printing, the only one of its kind in the US.

The Tennessee Birth Place

420 S. Water Ave., Gallatin, TN 37066-3311 615-452-1008 or 888-on-birth, lilyharvey@webtv.net

Seeks to give the best information about midwifery practice to aspiring and practicing midwives from all walks of life. Housing included in class fees. Taught by CPM.

Utah School of Midwifery

190 S. Canyon Ave., Springville, UT 84663-2186 801-489-1238, 888-489-1238

The purpose of the Utah College of Midwifery (UCM) is to educate and train direct-entry midwives to provide safe, high quality, low cost and personable maternity care. UCM offers a curriculum that adheres to traditional midwifery practice and current national guidelines. The midwifery coursework includes antepartum, intrapartum and postpartum care, as well as other midwifery topics. The program also emphasizes a working understanding of body systems and principles of holistic health so that the midwife can better serve the health needs of women and their families. UCM core courses are available through assisted studies (correspondence). Catalogs are available for $5 plus shipping and handling.

Nurse-Midwifery Programs

This list is not comprehensive and reflects only our current database. If you know of schools not listed here, please let us know. We have included a form on page 331 for schools and programs to send us so that we can keep our directory current.

Austin Area Birthing Center, Inc.

8500 N. Mopac Suite 502, Austin, TX 78759-8347 512-346-3224, fax: 512-345-6637

The Austin Area Birth Center is a beautiful facility dedicated to providing moms and families with a healthy birth in a nurturing environment. Apprentices get plenty of firsthand experience, live on-site, and get ample training and supervision one-on-one with an experienced midwife. Call for an application packet. Primarily intended for students who have completed didactic and academic training and taken part in a number of births. This is an opportunity for the student midwife to "primary" at births and gain the experience needed for independent practice.

Baylor College of Medicine Nurse Midwifery Program

6550 Fannin St. Ste 901 Houston, TX 77030-2720   713-798-7573

Baystate Medical Center Nurse-Midwifery Education Program

689 Chestnut St., Springfield, MA 01199-1620 413-794-4448, 413-794-8770

The program is based on a modified mastery learning curriculum that adheres to the principles of adult learning. All theoretical and clinical objectives, sub-objectives and skills are specified and organized into logical units of study (modules). The program is twelve full months in length (January through December), during which time the student develops the knowledge and skills to deliver comprehensive healthcare services to women, newborns and their families within the totality of their community. RN, BA/BS degrees conferred in any major. Three-year maternal-child health nursing, one in labor and delivery; college level course in physical assessment with clinical component within last five years.

Boston University School of Public Health Nurse-Midwifery Education Program

715 Albany St. TWS Boston, MA 02118 617-638-5012

This is the only US nurse-midwifery education program in a school of public health. First year, obtain public health degree, second year, obtain nurse-midwifery certification. Students must have commitment to underserved, rural or other needy population. Public health preparation is unique among nurse-midwifery programs.

Capitol University School of Nursing

2199 E. Main St., Columbus, OH 43209-2394 614-236-6343

Case Western Reserve University, Frances Payne Bolton School of Nursing Nurse-Midwifery Program

10900 Euclid Ave., Cleveland, OH 44106-4904 800-825-2540 ext. 2529, fax: 216-368-3542

Individualized study program; scientific and humanistic approach to academic excellence; unique ND program; can also get RN on way to CNM/MSN. Nurse-midwifery programming is very creative and flexible: multiple entry points including non-nursing and nursing with non-degree backgrounds; opportunities for those with varied and rich backgrounds to enter and move through the program; courses may be taught in intensive format (one week with preparation time before, assignment time after) to allow students to take courses for multiple reasons. Multiple exit points allow graduates to exit with nurse-midwifery credentials, credible academic degrees; also permit some master clinicians in clinical practice to obtain a doctoral degree by taking courses with intensive format scheduling so as not to disrupt practice or families. Connected to CNEP program.

Charles R. Drew University of Medicine & Science Nurse-Midwifery Program

1730 E. 120th St., Los Angeles, CA 90059-3025 213-563-4951, fax: 213-563-4923

Columbia Univ. School of Nursing Graduate Program in Nurse-Midwifery

617 W. 168th St., New York, NY 10032-3702 212-305-5236,
http://cpmcnet.columbia.edu/dept/nursing/

Contact program director Jennifer Dohrn for more information.

Community-Based Nurse-Midwifery Education Program (CNEP)

P.O. Box 528, Hyden, KY 41749 606-672-2312, CNEP@midwives.org
Program Director: Susan Stone, CNM, MSN

East Carolina University, School of Nursing (MSN)

Greenville, NC 27858 919-328-4298

Program Director: Nancy Moss, CNM, PhD

Emory University School of Nursing

531 Asbury Circle, Atlanta, GA 30322-0001 404-727-6918, fax: 404-727-0536,
http://www.emory.edu/WHSC/NURSING/PROGRAMS/MSN/midwife.html

Frontier School of Midwifery & Family Nursing, Community Nursing Educational Program (CNEP)

P.O. Box 528, Hyden, KY 41749-0528 606-672-2312, fax: 606-672-3776,
www.midwives.org

The CNEP seeks to meet the needs of prospective nurse-midwives who cannot leave their communities to obtain education in nurse-midwifery. Travel to Hyden, KY five days for midwifery-bound orientation. Levels I and II consists of courses completed in your home community. Level III is two weeks of nurse-midwifery workshops in Hyden, KY. Level IV is completed with an expert nurse-midwife, in most cases in or near your community.

Georgetown University School of Nursing Nurse-Midwifery

Box 571107 3700 Reservoir Rd. N.W., Washington, DC 20057-1107 202-687-4772, 202-687-5553, http://www.dml.georgetown.edu/schnurs/midwife1.html

The nurse-midwifery program is designed to prepare the graduate to manage a woman's normal obstetrical and gynecological needs during the childbearing years, to handle the care of the normal newborn, and to promote optimal healthcare. Upon completion of degree requirements, students are eligible to take the certification examination of the American College of Nurse-Midwives Certification Council. Located in Washington, DC, Georgetown University Nurse-Midwifery Program offers an excellent opportunity to students to get involved in health policy issues and legislation. Georgetown University is a member of the Consortium of Universities of the Washington Metropolitan Area.

Interdepartmental Nurse-Midwifery Education Program SFGH

Ward 6D, Rm. 21, 1001 Potrero Ave., San Francisco, CA 94110 415-206-5106
Program Director: Linda Ennis, CNM, MS

Institute of Midwifery, Women & Health: Philadelphia College of Textiles & Science

Rm 222 Hayward Hall, School House Lane and Henry Ave, Philadelphia, PA 19144-5444   215-843-5775, fax: 215-951-2526, imwah@bbs.acnm.org

The mission of the Institute is to advance the profession of midwifery for the betterment of women's health. The purpose of the nurse-midwifery education program is to educate nurses to become certified nurse-midwives using an economical, community-based, distance learning approach. This full-time graduate level distance learning program is based on the concept of a "school without walls." By weaving technology with tradition, we hope to provide a superb midwifery education experience. Graduates of the program can finish a master's degree through an affiliated college. Contact Jerrilyn Hobdy for more information.

Marquette University Nurse-Midwifery Program

P.O. Box 1881, Milwaukee, WI 53201-1881   414-288-3842

Med University of SC Nurse-Midwifery Program

99 Jonathan Lucas St., Charleston, SC 29401   843-792-2521

Registered nurses entering program prepare for advanced clinical practice in variety of settings as nurse-midwives; focus on the woman throughout reproductive cycle within the context of family.

Midwifery Education Program Associates, Inc.

1 West Campbell Ave., Campbell, CA 95008   408-374-3720

Program Director: Catherine A. Carr

National Association of Childbearing Centers

3123 Gottschall Rd., Perk, PA 18074-9801   215-234-8068

Contact program for details.

New York University (MA), Graduate Program in Nurse-Midwifery, School of Education, Division of Nursing

50 W. 4th St., 429 Shimkin Hall, New York, NY 10012   212-998-5895,
http://www.nyu.edu/pagea/nursing
Program Director: Patricia Burkhardt, CNM, PhD

Nurse-Midwifery Education Program, College of Allied Health Sciences

1621 East 120th St., Los Angeles, CA 90059,   213-563-4951

Program Director: Gwendolyn Spears, CNM, MSN, FACNM

Ohio State University (MA), Nurse-Midwifery Program, College of Nursing

1585 Neil Ave., Columbus, OH 43210-1289   614-292-4041, evans.27@osu.edu
Program Director: Nancy K. Lowe, CNM, PhD

Oregon Health Sciences University School of Nursing Nurse-Midwifery Program

3181 SW. Sam Jackson Park Rd., Portland, OR 97201-3098   503-494-7725
http://www.ohsu.edu/son/mp_whcn.html

Parkland School of Nurse-Midwifery

5201 Harry Hines Blvd St. 6017A, Dallas, TX 75235-7708   214-590-2580, fax: 214-590-0436,
http://www.swmed.edu/home_pages/parkland/midwifery/midwifehome.html

Based on modified modular curriculum; affiliation exists to facilitate students obtaining MS in nursing. Clinical experience in high volume setting, well-established program;

nationally known course in pharmacology; separate courses in cultural diversity, breast-feeding and gynecology. Preference given to BS and nursing students who provide evidence of commitment to care for women who are in medically underserved populations.

Pathways to Midwifery School of Nurse Health Sciences Ctr at SUNY-Stony Brook

Stony Brook, NY 11794-8240   516-444-2879,
Program Director is Ronnie Lichtman, linda.sacino@sunysb.edu

Full-time graduate program for registered nurses. Three paths for completion, for RNs with or without bachelors or as post-master's. Course work on CD-ROM, communicate by email.

Ryerson Polytechnic University School of Midwifery

Toronto, ON Canada 416-979-5104

Shenandoah Univ Division of Nursing Nurse-Midwifery Program

1775 N. Sector Ct., Winchester, VA 22601-2859   540-678-4382, 540-678-4374
540-665-5519 http://www.su.edu

Designed to prepare specialized, scholarly nurses who practice as professional nurse-midwives according to established standards and who, through scientific inquiry and continued professional growth, contribute to their discipline and profession. Nurse-midwifery graduates are prepared for their discipline and profession. Nurse-midwifery graduates are prepared to synthesize and apply knowledge, skills, values, and meanings necessary for safe, independent management and coordination of care for diverse well women, newborns and their families during the antepartum, intrapartum, postpartum and neonatal periods. In addition, they manage and promote gynecologic health of diverse well women throughout the life span. Nurse midwifery graduates support active participation of clients and families and collaborative and collegial interdisciplinary practice in diverse healthcare systems. It is intended that graduates will become leaders and positively impact those factors influencing the discipline of nurse-midwifery and the profession of nursing. Our program is user-friendly, one day a week with concentrated clinical time. Contact program for schedule information

State University of New York (SUNY) Health Sciences Center at Brooklyn

450 Clarkson Ave. Box 1227, Brooklyn, NY 11203-2098   718-270-7740,
chrish0z@hscbklyn.edu

These one-year programs are designed to prepare qualified non-nurses and nurses to become certified midwives and nurse midwives who are professionally prepared in full compliance with the standards established by the American College of Nurse-Midwives. Graduates from CM program will be eligible to sit for the ACNM's national certifying examination and to apply for licensure to practice midwifery within the state of New York. New York licensure does not guarantee reciprocity by any other state. CM and CNM students are integrated within the program. CNM graduates will be eligible to practice in all 50 states. ACNM approved direct-entry midwifery program. At printing, the only of its kind in the US.

Univerity of California Los Angeles School of Nursing, Nurse-Midwifery Ed.

P.O. Box 951702 Los Angeles, CA 90095-1702   310-825-5654

Univerity of California San Diego, Division Graduate Nursing Education

9500 Gilman Dr. Dept 809, La Jolla, CA 92093   619-543-3614, 619-543-7757

Unique program based on adult learning concepts, encourages BSNs with diverse advanced level (MSN) degrees to return to nursing via the 12 month post-masters program that offers individual bridge programs for L&D experience; two campus ed. for master's program. Heavy emphasis on primary care, involves didactic and clinical experience with FNPs and CNMs in strong, diverse clinical sites. The master's (intercampus) program is unique in that it utilizes two campuses.

UCSD Nurse-Midwifery Program, UCSF/UCSD Intercampus Graduate Program

4080 Front St. Ste. 8219, San Diego, CA 92103-2014 619-543-3614

UCSF/SFGH Interdepartmental Nurse Midwifery Education Program

6D21 San Francisco General Hospital, 1001 Potrero Ave., San Francisco, CA 94110 415-206-5106, fax: 415-206-3112

We provide excellent education toward CNM practice in an exceptional university setting. All faculty in active practice. This program has a mission to educate CNMs who will work in underserved areas. Upon graduation also receive a certificate as women's health nurse practitioner.

University of Cincinnati (MSN), Nurse-Midwifery Education Program

3110 Vine St., ML 0038, Cincinnati, OH 45221 513-558-5380, http://www.uc.edu/www/nursing

University of Colorado Health Science Center, Nurse-Midwifery Program

4200 E. 9th Ave. Box C-288, Denver, CO 80262 303-315-8654

Strength of program is 16 experienced faculty who teach and practice in three nurse-midwifery practices: sites for majority of students' clinical experience occur in first three semesters of program. Option for non-nurse, nurse with or without BS/ BA, to become nurse-midwife, for post-masters nurse or nurse-practice to return for midwifery education. All students have successfully completed the certification examination.

University of Florida College of Nursing Nurse-Midwifery Program

653 W. 8th St. Bldg 1 Fl 2, Jacksonville, FL 32209-6511 904-549-3245, 904-549-3246

This integrated master's level program prepares nurse-midwives for full-scope nurse midwifery practice which includes but is not limited to primary care, women's health, antepartum, intrapartum, newborn, postpartum and family planning. Clinical experiences include both traditional- and community-based options. Graduates have expertise in research, health policy, ethics and finance and organizational management in addition to advanced practice skills.

University of Illinois College of Nursing Nurse-Midwifery Program

m/c 802 845 S. Damen Ave. Rm 824, Chicago, IL 60612-7350 312-996-7937, fax: 312-996-8871

University of Kentucky College of Nursing Health Science Learning Center

Rm 315 760 Rose St., Lexington, KY 40536-0232 606-323-6253

Enter any semester; wide cultural clinical experiences; 1:2 faculty-student ratio in clinical. Focuses on normal changes during life cycles of woman, holistic view of contemporary family. Clinical rotation sites provide wide range of cultural diversity: from Appalachia, rural to urban, international climates. Excellence in mentorship and state-of-the-art educational tools. Classes small and taught using seminars, case presentations, experiential exp., problem-based learning.

University of Medicine and Dentistry of New Jersey, School of Health Related Professions, Nurse-Midwifery Program

65 Bergen St., Newark, NJ 07107-3001 201-982-4249, 4298, iegmaek@umdnj.edu
Program Director: Elaine Diegmann, CNM, MEd

University of Miami School of Nursing

5801 SW. 57th Ave., P.O. Box 248153 Miami, FL 33124-8153 305-247-1601
http://www.miami.edu/nur/net20/graduate/midwife.htm

University of Michigan School of Nursing Nurse-Midwifery Program

400 N. Ingalls St. Rm. 3320, Ann Arbor, MI 48109-2003 734-763-3710
734-647-0351 http://www-personal.umich.edu/~dswalker/umhome.html

Purpose of program: To prepare safe, scholarly, clinically competent nurse-midwives whose knowledge and skills reflect the core competencies defined by the ACNM. Contact program for more information.

UMDNJ Nurse Midwifery Program

65 Bergen St., Newark, NJ 07107-3001 973-972-4249

University of Missouri – Columbia Sinclair School of Nursing, Nurse-Midwifery Program

Columbia, MO 65211-5068 573-882-0277

University of Minnesota School of Nursing

6-101 Weaver-Densford Hall, 308 Harvard St. SE, Minneapolis, MN 55455-0353
612-624-6494, fax: 612-626-2359

Variety of clinical sites within the metro area, rural sites upon request. Program combines academic preparation with clinical skills for independent management and care of women and newborns. Nurse-midwives assist women and families to promote and maintain health, facilitate optimal individual and family integrity.

University of New Mexico, Nurse-Midwifery Program, College of Nursing

University of New Mexico, Albuquerque, NM 87131-1061 505-272-1184, fax: 505-272-8901, Sheilar@unm.edu

The UNM Nurse-Midwifery Educational program is organizationally within the primary care concentration of the master's in nursing program of the University of New Mexico College of Nursing, Health Sciences Center. The mission statement of the College of Nursing and the philosophy of the graduate nursing program provide the philosophical context for the educational program. In one additional year, student may become qualified as an FNP.

University of Pennsylvania Nurse-Midwifery Program

420 Guardian Dr., Philadelphia, PA 19104-4210 215-898-4335, fax: 215-573-7291
http://www.upenn.edu/nursing/courses/midwifery/midwiferyhome.html

University of Rhode Island, College of Nurse Graduate Program Nurse-Midwifery

Kingston, RI 02881-0814 401-874-5303

University of Rochester (MS), School of Nursing

601 Elmood Ave., Box SON, Rochester, NY 14642 716-275-2375

University of Southern California, Nurse-Midwifery Education Program, Department of Nursing

1540 Alcazar St., CHP 222, Los Angeles, CA 90033 213-226-3386
Program Director: Anita Bralock, CNM, MSN

University of Texas El Paso Nurse-Midwifery Program

4800 Alberta Ave., El Paso, TX 79905-2709 915-545-6490
http://www.nurse.utep.edu/nurse/midwife.htm

The curriculum prepares graduates to enter nurse-midwifery practice and function collaboratively in the healthcare system to manage the care of essentially healthy women and their infants. The border location of this program provides unique opportunities for a multicultural and international experience.

University of Utah College of Nursing Graduate Program Nurse-Midwifery

105 2000 E. Front, Salt Lake City, UT 84112-5880 801-581-8274

University of Washington School of Nursing Nurse-Midwifery Program Family & Child Nursing

Box 357262 4000 15th Ave., N.E., Seattle, WA 98195-7262 206-543-8736, fax: 206-543-6656, midwife@u.washingtonedu, http://www.son.washington.edu/~midwife/

Features availability of University of Washington faculty expertise; solid preparation in research; excellent community-based clinical sites. Program qualifies the student to sit for certification as a certified nurse-midwife. Program prepares nurses to provide comprehensive care to women throughout their life span in both ambulatory and intrapartum settings. A primary goal is to educate nurse-midwives who will work in underserved areas and communities.

USC Nurse-Midwifery Program Women's Hospital

Rm 5K40 1240 N. Mission Rd., Los Angeles, CA 90033-1019 213-226-3386, fax: 213-226-2710

Clinical experience in successful nurse-midwifery settings, faculty with extensive clinical experience, working with underserved populations. Program based at busy, renowned Los Angeles County and USC Medical Center; features exposure to a variety of perinatal settings under the direction of accomplished nurse-midwives. Twelve-year record of students' successful completion of study and pass rates of national certification exams is remarkable.

University of Texas MB School of Nursing Collaborative Nurse-Midwifery Education Program

1100 Mechanic St., Galveston, TX 77555-1029 409-772-8347, fax: 409-772-3770
www.utmb.edu

Whether caring for families during pregnancy and birth, the infant's growth and development, or throughout the woman's life span, nurse-midwives emphasize health promotion and non-intervention in normal processes.

Vanderbilt University School of Nursing Nurse-Midwifery Program

101 Godchaux Hall, 461 21, Ave. S Nashville, TN 37240-1119
615-322-3800 http://www.mc.vanderbilt.edu/nursing/level3/nursmidw.htm

Yale University Nurse-Midwifery Program

100 Church St., S New Haven, CT 06519-1703 203-785-2389
http://info.med.yale.edu/nursing/

Yeshiva University Medical School

500 W. 185th St., New York, NY 10033-3299   212-960-5400

PRE-CERTIFICATION NURSE-MIDWIFERY PROGRAMS

Ramsey Clinic

640 Jackson St., Suite 5, St. Paul, MN 55101   612-221-3820,
simonpi@mis3.sprmc.healthpartners.com

University of Miami/Jackson Memorial

1611 N.W. 12th Ave., East Tower, 3003, Miami, FL 33136   305-585-6628

CHILDBIRTH EDUCATION PROGRAMS

The following are organizations that train, certify or provide continuing education for childbirth educators. Some direct-entry schools offer training for childbirth educators as well. Please see the chart on page 299 for more details.This list is not comprehensive and reflects only our current database. If you know of schools not listed here, please let us know. We have included a form on page 331 for schools and programs to send us so that we can keep our directory current.

ALACE Childbirth Education Program

P.O. Box 382724, Cambridge, MA 02238-2724   617-441-6244

ALACE offers the only nationally recognized program developed by women and midwives. We encourage mind-body integration and prevention of unnecessary interventions. Our instructors teach families planning home, birth center, and hospital births.

American Academy of Husband-Coached Childbirth (The Bradley Method)

P.O. Box 5224, Sherman Oaks, CA 91413-5224   818-788-6662, 800-4A-Birth
www.bradleybirth.com

Strives for spontaneous, unmedicated birth for 90 percent of pregnancies. Program offers training for parenthood and also for teaching NCB. Not a school for midwifery. Trainings for teachers held 12 to 16 times per year nationally.

Birth Works, Inc.

P.O. Box 2045, Medford, NJ 08055-7045   609-953-9380 or 888 to-birth, 609-953-9380, http://members.aol.com/birthwkscd/bw.html

Birth Works because it's ancient. The art of giving birth hasn't changed; it's instinctive. However, the current medical environment presents women with an educational need. Our unique, experiential learning process gives women the tools to discover their choices, their inner voice, and ultimately, their own best way to give birth. Reading, write, evaluate research, attend three-day workshop, complete teaching manual, then teach 10-week Birth Works class for certification. Has self-study course.

ICEA Teacher Certification

P.O. Box 20048, Minneapolis, MN 55420-0048   612-854-8660, fax: 612-854-8772, www.icea.org

The International Childbirth Education Association (ICEA) is a professional organization that supports educators and other healthcare providers who believe in freedom of choice based on knowledge of alternatives in family-centered maternity and newborn care. ICEA teacher certification is not a teacher training program. However, ICEA does offer basic teacher training in its childbirth education workshops. ICEA certification recognizes professional educators who have met standards of competency in knowledge and skills. To enable candidates to meet these standards, the teacher certification program provides independent study that draws from many disciplines, including education, sociology, anthropology, physiology, psychology, midwifery, nursing and medicine. Candidates enter the program by paying the application fee. After entering the program, candidates are provided study guides. The two programs differ in the prerequisites, the study required and costs to complete. Contact ICEA for details and more information. ICEA is primarily a certifying organization, but has certain workshops and module programs to assist in the certification process.

DOULA AND LABOR ASSISTANT TRAINING
PROGRAMS AND CERTIFYING ORGANIZATIONS

This list is not comprehensive and reflects only our current database. If you know of schools not listed here, please let us know. We have included a form on page 331 for schools and programs to send us so that we can keep our directory current.

ALACE (Association of Labor Assistants and Childbirth Educators) Labor Assistant Program

P.O. Box 382724, Cambridge, MA 02238-2724 617-441-2500, fax: 617-441-3167

ALACE offers the most experienced training program for labor support providers, with an emphasis on emotional support and an introduction to physical assessments. This program is an excellent first step for aspiring midwives.

American Academy of Husband-Coached Childbirth (The Bradley Method)

P.O. Box 5224, Sherman Oaks, CA 91413-5224 818-788-6662, 800-4A Birth
www.bradleybirth.com

Strives for spontaneous, unmedicated birth for 90 percent of pregnancies. Program offers training for parenthood and also for teaching NCB. Not a school for midwifery. Trainings for teachers held 12 to 16 times per year nationally.

Birth Source

P.O. Box 29874, Los Angeles, CA 90029 323-667-2366, fax: 323-667-2212,
kelliway@loop.com

Our goal is to provide practical and accurate training opportunities for doulas and childbirth educators.

Birth Works, Inc.

P.O. Box 2045, Medford, NJ 08055-7045 609-953-9380 or 888 to-birth,
609-953-9380, http://members.aol.com/birthwkscd/bw.html

Birth Works because it's ancient. The art of giving birth hasn't changed; it's instinctive. However, the current medical environment presents women with an educational need. Our unique, experiential learning process gives women the tools to discover their choices, their inner voice, and ultimately, their own best way to give birth. Reading, write, evaluate research, attend three-day workshop, complete teaching manual, then teach 10-week Birth Works class for certification. Has self-study course.

ICEA Certified Doula Program

P.O. Box 20048, Minneapolis, MN 55420-0048   612-854-8660, www.icea.org

POSTPARTUM EDUCATOR & DOULA PROGRAMS

Birth Source

P.O. Box 29874, Los Angeles, CA 90029   323-667-2366, fax: 323-667-2212, kelliway@loop.com

Our goal is to provide practical and accurate training opportunities for doulas and childbirth educators.

ICEA Postpartum Educator Program

P.O. Box 20048, Minneapolis, MN 55420-0048 612-854-8660, www.icea.org

For more information, please see the resource section dedicated to the International Childbirth Educators Association.

LACTATION EDUCATOR
& CONSULTANT TRAINING PROGRAMS

BSC Center for Lactation Education

228 Park Ln., Chalfont, PA 18914-3135

UCLA Extension Lactation Educator Training

10995 Le Conte Ave. Ste. 711, Los Angeles, CA 90024-2883 310-825-9187, 310-825-6906, hlthsci@unex.ucla.edu, http://www.unex.ucla.edu/healthsci/directry.htm

Lactation education course is intended to prepare health professionals and other interested people to be lactation educators either in private practice or as part of their clinical employment. Emphasis is placed on maximizing professional use of scientific data and understanding problems of clinical management. It also provides them with practical information for assisting individual mothers and infants. With increasing emphasis on breastfeeding, there is a greater demand for skilled professionals to be lactation consultants either in private practice or as part of their clinical employment. The focus of this program is on maximizing professional use of scientific data and understanding problems in clinical management.

This course of study, which builds on the Lactation Educator Training Program, prepares health professionals to be lactation consultants. The didactic portion of the program includes four three-day sessions spaced over nine months which are held in Los Angeles. Additional requirements are an apprenticeship with a faculty member in Los Angeles, and a preceptorship and community observation in the student local area lactation educator (LE) and lactation consultant (LC) training.

HOMEOPATHY & NATUROPATHY SCHOOLS

American College of Naturopathic Obstetricians

44444 S.W. Corbett Ave., Portland, OR 97201-4207 503-224-4003,
wnhc@aol.com, wwwacno.org

Please contact Susan Roberts for details on their program.

Bastyr University

14500 Juanita Dr. NE, Bothell, WA 98011-4966 425-823-1300, 425-823-6222.
www.bastyr.edu

Certificate program offered for naturopathic physicians or enrolled naturopathic medical students. Grants a certificate of specialization in midwifery; graduates eligible for licensure as midwives in state of Washington. Clinical training through preceptorships with licensed birth attendants arranged by students.

Notes:

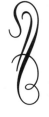

MIDWIFERY EDUCATION PROGRAMS

— Legend —

Use this list of acronyms when examining the following charts.
They are not meant to be comprehensive.
Contact schools for more information.

ADN	Associate Degree in Nursing	FNP	Family Nurse Midwifery
ADV	Advanced Training	HM	Home Study
APP	Apprenticeship Program	ICCE	ICEA Certified Childbirth Educator
BC	Birth Center	ICD	Doula
CBA	Certified Birth Attendant	INT	Intensives
CBE	Childbirth Education	LAC	Lactation and Breastfeeding Support
CCE	Certified Childbirth Educator	LS	Labor Support
CD	Certified Doula	LSP	Doula, Labor Support Program
CLIN	Clinical Site	MSN	Masters of Science, Nursing
CMM	Certified Master Midwife	MW	Midwifery
CPEI	Certified Postpartum Educator	ND	Nursing Doctorate
CTM	Certified Traditional Midwife	NM	Nurse-Midwifery
DLP	Distance Learning Program	PPD	Postpartum Doula

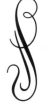

Direct-Entry Program Chart

School Name	NARM	MEAC	DLP	APP	INT	ADV	CLIN	CBE	PPD	LSP	LAC
Ancient Art Midwifery Institute		x	x		x		x				
Artemis College					x						
Association of Texas Midwives	x	x	x								
Austin Area Birthing Center, Inc.	x	x	x		x	x					
Birthingway Midwifery School		x pre								x	
Birth Rite Education Center	x	x pre		x		x		x	x	x	
Birthwise Midwifery School		x pend.			x	x				x	
Casa de Nacimiento			x		x	x					
Delphi Center for Midwifery Studies	x			x		x	x		x		
Family Birth Services Midwifery Course			x								
Florida School of Traditional Midwifery	x						x	x	x		
Hands-On Midwifery Workshops				x							
Heart & Hands Midwifery Intensives		x		x							
Hygieia College & Home Study Course			x		x		x	x	x	x	
Institute of Maternal & Child Health	x					x	x				
International School of Midwifery					x	x					
IXMUCANE					x	x					
Massachusetts Midwives' Alliance			x								
Maternidad La Luz	x	x	x		x	x					
Miami-Dade Community College					x			x			
Michigan Midwives Association				x							
Midwifery Institute of California	x	x	x	x	x						
National College of Midwifery	x	x pend.	x	x			x	x	x	x	x
New Life Birth Service	x					x	x	x	x		
Oregon School of Midwifery	x	x pre	x	x		x	x	x	x		
Renaissance Woman Midwifery Institute									x		
Resourcing Birth		x	x								
Sage Femme Midwifery School	x										
Seattle Midwifery School	x	x								x	
The Birth Center	x				x						
The Farm	x				x	x					
The Holistic Midwifery Institute			x	x	x		x	x	x	x	
The Michigan School of Traditional Midwifery		x	x	x					x		
The Tennessee Birth Place			x	x							
Utah College of Midwifery	x	x	x	x	x		x		x		

Legal Status of Direct-Entry Midwives: State by State Analysis

State	Legal By: Licensure (L) Certificate (C) Registration (R)	Legal By: Judicial Interpretation or Statutory Inference	Legal By: Not Legally Defined, but not Prohibited	Legal By: Statute, but Licensure Unavailable	Prohibited By Statute or Judicial Interpretation	CPM	MEAC Accredited Programs (Accredited, Preaccredited or Pending)	Medicaid Reimbursement
AK	L					e		x
AL				x				
AR	L					e		
AZ	L					e		x
CA	L					e	1	
CO	R					p		
CT			x			ae		
DE				x				
DC					x			
FL	L					e	2	x
GA				x				
HI				x				
ID		x				ae		
IL		x						
IN					x			
IA					x			
KS		x						
KY					x			
LA	L					e	1	
ME		x					1	
MD					x			
MA		x						
MI		x				ae		
MN				x		ae		
MS		x						
MO					x	ae		
MT	L					e		
NE			x					
NV		x						
NH	Voluntary L					e		
NJ				x				
NM	L					e	1	x
NY				x				
NC					x			
ND		x						
OH					x			
OK		x						
OR	Voluntary L					p	2	x
PA		x						
RI				x			1	
SC	L					e		x
SD			x					
TN		x				ae	2	
TX	R					p	2	
UT		x				ae	1	
VT			x			ae	1	x
VA					x			
WA	L					p	1	x
WV			x			ae		
WI			x			ae		
WY		x						

— LEGEND —

e State uses NARM Exam as part of licensure process.

ae State midwifery association uses NARM exam for certification.

p Approval of NARM exam as part of the licensure process is pending.

— School Information —

School Name	Years in Business	Program Type	Program Length	Program Size	Prerequisites	Degree/Cert.	Tuition	Email
ACHI Inst. for Midwifery Studies (AIMS) Ass. for Childbirth at Home Int. (ACHI)		DEM	min 2 yr					
Ancient Art Midwifery Institute	18	DEM, APP	3, 4 years or 6 mo(intro)	N/A			$1,600	AnctArtmi@aol.com
Arkansas Midwives School & Services		DEM	3 years		class size limited, HS diploma English prof., coursework Chemistry, A&P and nutrition		$3,500 per yr	
Artemis College		DEM	1 weekend	varies	Experienced midwives only			
Association of Texas Midwives		DEM H.S.	3 years		HM, Cert., docum. as TX midwife		$1,500	
Austin Area Birthing Center, Inc.	many	DEM, CNM	3 months	varies	Participate in 25 births, know vitals	N/A	$1,500	
Birth Rite Education Center	15	DEM, CBE, LS	2-5 years	6-18				Barefootmd@aol.com
Birthingway Midwifery School	5	DEM	3 years	9-10	20 yrs. old, HS diploma, A&P		$12,000 Aid available	
Birthwise Midwifery School	4	DEM	3 acad. sem. 2-3 yr APP	12 max	HS diploma/certificate		$4,600	birthwise@ime.net
Casa de Nacimiento		DEM- Clinical	3 months	4-5	some experience	Certificate	$2,000	
Delphi Center, Inc.		DEM	3 years		HS diploma, contact school	Assoc. deg. MW	$15,050/ 3 yrs	DelphiCntr@aol.com
Family Birth Services Midwifery Course		DEM, APP	1-3 years	8	8-10 births, accepted by preceptor	Document. TX	$500	
Florida School of Traditional Midwifery	3	DEM	3 years	10-15	3 credits English & Math	Spec. associ.	$17,942	FSTM@Juno.com
Hands-On Midwifery Workshops	5	Intensive	1 wk or 5 Sat.'s	10 max	none, basics helpful	Certificate	$475	
Heart & Hands Midwifery Intensives		DEM Intensive	10 weeks	10-20	none	Credit with MW Inst. of CA	$675 beginner $295 advanced	
Holistic Midwifery Training		DEM	1yr				$550/beg. $480 adv.	
Hygieia College & Home Study Course	17	DEM	varies		Self-healing	Diploma	$801	freestone@hubwest.com
Institute of Maternal & Child Health	16	DEM 3rd World	15 mo. min.	18-24	HS dip. or GED	Assoc. deg. MW	$2,500/quarter incl. rm/board	vsm@flash.net
Interenational School of Midwifery		DEM						
IXMUCANE		DEM, APP	3 months min.	5 max.	Prev. MW training, DEM/CNM	None	$100/week room/board	Houston@conexion.com.gt
Massachusetts Midwives' Alliance		DEM						
Maternidad La Luz	10 years	DEM, Clinical	1 year	20 max	HS Diploma, 18 yrs old, CPR, Neg TB test, & some Spanish	Certificate	$4,500 per yr	

301

School Name	Years in Business	Program Type	Program Length	Program Size	Prerequisites	Degree/Cert.	Tuition	Email
Miami-Dade Community College	37	DEM, CBE	DEM: 3 yr. Accel: 4 mo CBE: 16 wks	15-20	GED. Varies w/ different programs	AS in MW, Certificate	In St $41.25 Out St $145 per class	Cleggj@mdcc.edu
Michigan Midwives Association		Organization						
Midwifery Institute of California	3	DEM, APP Clinical/Dist.	3 years	10-20	HS diploma, exam for LM		$7,100 on site $7,400 distance	samidwife@aol.com
National College of Midwifery	4	DEM, Dist.	2-3 years	N/A	HS diploma/GED	Degree NCM NARM Cert	variable	carla@newmex.com
New Life Birth Service	18	DEM, APP	10 months	N/A	none	none	varies	
Oregon School of Midwifery	6	DEM, Dist. DONA course	3 years	max 15	Commitment to DEM. HS dipl, Pr. for CPM exam, OR licensure English prof. A&P, Neg. TB.	Certificate	$6,750 3 yrs.	daphnetree@aol.com
Renaissance Woman Midwifery Institute								
Resourcing Birth		DEM	3 years	10 max		$500 CO MWs Assoc.		
Seattle Midwifery School	20+	DEM	27 months	12-15	Coll. English, A&P, microbiology, basic nutrition, social science. Coll/2yr HS math and biology	Dipl. in Midwifery	$22,755	
South Florida School of Midwifery		DEM						
State University of New York (SUNY)	67	DEM, (CM)	1 year		BA, w/ course requirmts, Engl. prof. Experience related to MW, nursing. Contact school for full list of prereq.		$2,550/sem res $4,208/no res	
The Birth Center	8	Internship	1-4 months		Ready for hands-on experience	NARM skills	$800 per mo	
The Farm	26	DEM	varies	varies				
The Holistic Midwifery Institute	1	DEM, Intensives	varies: wkends-15 wks	20 for most	none	Certificate, CEUs	$35-$560	gbrennan@umich.edu
Michigan School of Traditional Midwifery	3	DEM Dist, MA LA, Herbology	1-2 years	N/A	none	LA, MA Cert.	$300-$975	mstm@i-star.com
The School of Natural Healing	DEM	DEM						snh@Q3.com
The Tennessee Birth Place	3	Intensives, APP	3 or 7 day, 6 mo	13	none	Certificate	$250-495.00	
Utah College of Midwifery	17	DEM	4 levels, 4 yrs	6-30	HS diploma, English prof., 2 letters of recommendation, AS in MW, BSM, MSM $25 admissions fee	OCE, CD, CBA, CTM, CMM	$55 cr. under- $75 cr. grad.	ksink@utw.com

— Nursing Schools —

School Name	Years in Business	Program Type	Program Length	Program Size	Prerequisites	Degree/Cert.	Tuition	Email
Austin Area Birthing Center, Inc.	many	CNM/DEM Clinical	3 mo	varies	Partic. in 25 births, know vitals	N/A	$1,500	swente@bcm.tmc.edu
Baylor Coll. of Med., Nurse-Midwifery Prog.	3	CNM			MSN			
Baystate Medical Center	6	CNM		1 yr.	8 students per year 3 prof. refs, current CPR cert.	RN, BA/BS Nurse-MW Cert	$12,000	
Boston University School of Public Health		CNM	2 yr	10-14	BSN, RN, GRE	MPH	$26,250	
Case Western Reserve University		CNM/CNEP	2 yr or 4 yr	16	Physical assessment	RN, CNM, MSN, ND	$650/cred. hr	
Charles R. Drew Univ. of Med. & Sci.		CNM						
Columbia Univ. School of Nursing	106	CNM						rsl@columbia.edu
Emory University School of Nursing		CNM	4 semesters		MSN, eligible to sit ACNM exam			
Frontier Sch. of MW & Fam. Nrs (CNEP)	59	CNM, Dist.	up to 5 yrs		RN w/ BA, min. 1000 on GRE, or 45 MAT. 3.0 GPA. Health exam	MSN or ND	$8,100 per yr	
Georgetown University School of Nursing	16	CNM Masters	16-27 months	13-16	BS in nursing, GPA 3+, TOEFL, acceptable score on GRE, MAT, RN license	MS in nursing; Post-master's Cert	$707 per cr	midwife@gunet.georgetown.edu
Inst. of Midwifery, Women and Health	2	CNM	21 months	15-20	RN; bachelor's in any discipline; GRE/MAT, interviews eligible to sit for CNM exam		$15,000	imwah@bbs.acnm.org
IXMUCANE		DEM, APP Clinical Site	3 - 5 mo.		Previous MW training	none	$100/wk R& B incl. Spanish $25/wk no R&B	Houston@conexion.com.gt
Marquette Univ Nurse-Midwifery Prog		CNM						
Med Univ of SC Nurse-Midwifery Prog		CNM	2 yr	9 full, 3 part	GPA 3+, GRE, 2 yr. exp. mat/child nurs., pers. interview	CNM or MSN BSN or RN	$1,210/sem res $1,330 non-res	
OR Health Sc. Univ. Sch. of Nursing		CNM			Cert., MSN, post-master's.			
Parkland School of Nurse-Midwifery		CNM	1 yr	6-12	RN; Adv. Health Asses.; GPA 3.0, 1 yr exp. in maternal/child health;	Cert. Program	$10,000 in '95	Judith.Treistman@sunysb.edu
Pathways to MW School of Nursing		CNM			good physical health			
SDSU/UCSD Nurse-Midwifery Prog		CNM						

School Name	Years in Business	Program Type	Program Length	Program Size	Prerequisites	Degree/Cert.	Tuition	Email
Shenandoah Univ Division of Nursing	2, School 103	CNM	6 semesters	10	BS in nursing, 2.8 GPA, 1 yr clinical work experience	MS in nursing, Cert. by ACNM	$400 per cr. 46 cr hrs	jfehr@su.edu
State University of New York (SUNY)	67	DEM, CM RN-based CNM	1 year		BA, w/ course requirents, Engl. pro Experience related to MW, nursing Contact school for full list of prereq		$2,550/sem res $4,208/no res	
UCSD Div Graduate Nursing Ed	4	12 mo-2 yr.	4-10		BSN, RN, Lic. in CA+1 yr L & D for post-master's, MS in any subject	NP, MS		
UCSD Nurse-Midwifery Program		MSN						
UCSF/SFGH Interdepartmental Nurse-Midwifery Education Program	21	CNM, MS	3 yr-non-nurses 15mo/2 yr/3yr	14	BA/BS, valid RN license, 3.0 GPA contact program	Certificate+MS/ RN+cert+MS		heticia@ob.ucsf.edu
UMDNJ Nurse-Midwifery Program		CNM						
University of Colorado Health Sci. Ctr Nurse-Midwifery Prog.			18mo, 28 mo	16	BSN/BS in nursing; research class; GRE, phys. asses., 1 yr exp. mat. nurs. pref. L&D	MS, ready for ACNM exam	$1,622 9 hr res $5049 nonres	
University of Florida, College of Nursing	16	Nursing MSN	4 sem. full-time	varied	BSN, client assess, statistics, add. prereq. for RN-MSN track	MSN, ready for ACNM exam.	$129./cr.hr. res $434./nonres	ahpl.umc2@mail.health.ufl.edu
University of Illinois College of Nursing		CNM	2 yr	20-30	BS/BA, RN 1 yr exp. in L&D	MS/post MS cert.	$2,033/sem res	
University of Kentucky College of Nursing		CNM	4 sem-3 yr	6-10	RN, 2 yr nurs. exp-in L&D, BC GRE -400 ea. section; phys assess	MSN/Clin. Cert N-M post-master's	$1,200 res $3,600 nonres	
University of Miami School of Nursing	20	CNM						
University of Michigan School of Nursing	8	CNM, FNP	2yr full/pt-time	14	BS in nursing, statistics, research & physical assess w/in last 5 yr, GRE	master's	$4,911 sem res $9,965 sem non	dswalker@umich.edu
University of Missouri-Columbia		CNM						
University of Minnesota School of Nursing		Nursing	6 qtr./2 yr	15 max	BS/BA, GRE, RN in US, adv.phys. phys. assess. course	Eligible for ACNM exam		
University of New Mexico	7	CNM Graduate	2 yrs.	8-10	BS, 1 yr nursing experience	MSN, post-mstrs	$2,400/yr res $8,400 nonres	ncella@unm.edu
University of Pennsylvania		CNM						
University of Rhode Island, Coll of Nrs		CNM						vmarsh@uriacc.uri.edu
University of Texas, El Paso		CNM	20 mo		MSN (completion option avail.)			
University of Utah College of Nursing		CNM						

— Childbirth Education —

School Name	Years in Business	Program Type	Program Length	Program Size	Prerequisites	Degree/Cert.	Tuition	Email
University of WA Nurse-Midwifery Prog	4	CNM	2 yrs	Max 10	BS nursing or ADN & BS other	CNM master's	$1,744 res qrtr. $4,322 non-res	midwife@u.washington.edu
Univ. of Washington School of Nursing		CNM	2yr	10	BS/BA or ACT-PEP exam; RN req. BS/BA fr. NLN accr. prog.	MSN	$1,500 per qrtr	
USC Nurse-Midwifery Program		CNM	11.5 mo	12	BS/BA, RN lic, contact prog	MW Cert, MSN	$11,800	
UTMB School of Nursing	5	Nursing, MSN	5 semesters	10-12	BSN, 1 year L&D exp.	MSN, Cert N.M.	$34/cred. res $278 non-res	jkvale@sonpo.utmb.edu
Vanderbilt University School of Nursing		CNM						
Yale Univ Nurse-Midwifery Program								
Yeshiva Univ Medical School		med	11.5 mo	12	BS/BA, phys. assmt, RN, perinatal nurs. exp., pref L&D	Cert. MW, MSN	$11,800	
ALACE-Childbirth Education program	3	CBE, LA	Approx. 6 mo.	20	none	Ntl. certification	$575 or $695	alacehq@aol.com
Am. Academy of Husband-Coached Childbirth (The Bradley Method)	32	CBE	4 day workshop plus 9 months	15	natural birth or OB experience	Cert. in the Bradley Method	$795	
Birth Source	4	Adv. CD train.	varies	varies	varies	DONA Cert.	varies	kelliway@loop.com
Birth Works, Inc.	15	CBE	18 months	6-12 wkshop	Complete teacher profile	CCE	$395 $195 Teacher Tr.	BirthWksCD@aol.com
Birth Rite Education Center	15	DEM, CBE, LS	2-5 years	6-18				Barefootmd@aol.com
The Holistic Midwifery Institute	1	DEM,Inten.	varies	20 - 35	none	Cert, CEUs	$35-$560	gbrennan@umich.edu
ICEA Teacher Certification		CBE, CD, CPE	varies	N/A	ICCE, ICCE-CPE, ICD	varies	varies	
Institute of Maternal & Child Health	16	DEM, clinical	15 mo min	18-24	HS dip. or GED or equiv.	AS Midwifery	$2,500/qrtr room & board	vsm@flash.net
Miami-Dade Community College		DEM Ed	DE 3yr Ad 4mo CBE: 16wks.	15-20	GED, contact college	AS in MW, Cert.	$41.cr in-st. $145cr out-st	Cleggj@mdcc.edu
New Life Birth Service	18	DEM, APP	10 mo	N/A	none	none	varies	
Utah College of Midwifery	17	DEM	4 levels, 1 yr ea	6-30	HS dipl. Engl prof. 2 letters recomm $25 admissions processing fee	AS MW, BSM, CCE, CD, CBA, CTM, MSM	$55 per cr under, $75 per cr grad.	ksink@utw.co

THE MANA STATEMENT OF VALUES AND ETHICS

We, as midwives, have a responsibility to educate ourselves and others regarding our values and ethics and to reflect them in our practices. Our exploration of ethical midwifery is a critical reflection of moral issues as they pertain to maternal/child health on every level. This statement is intended to provide guidance for professional conduct in the practice of midwifery, as well as for MANA's policy making, thereby promoting quality care for childbearing families. MANA recognizes this document as an open, ongoing articulation of our evolution regarding values and ethics.

First, we recognize that values often go unstated and yet our ethics (how we act), proceed directly from a foundation of values. Since what we hold precious, that is, what we value, infuses and informs our ethical decisions and actions, the Midwives Alliance of North America wishes to explicitly affirm our values as follows:

I. WOMAN AS AN INDIVIDUAL WITH UNIQUE VALUE AND WORTH:

A. We value women and their creative, life-affirming and life-giving powers which find expression in a diversity of ways.

B. We value a woman's right to make choices regarding all aspects of her life.

II. MOTHER AND BABY AS WHOLE:

A. We value the oneness of the pregnant mother and her unborn child; an inseparable and interdependent whole.

B. We value the birth experience as a rite of passage; the sentient and sensitive nature of the newborn; and the right of each baby to be born in a caring and loving manner, without separation from mother and family.

C. We value the integrity of a woman's body and the right of each woman and baby to be totally supported in their efforts to achieve a natural, spontaneous vaginal birth.

D. We value the breastfeeding relationship as the ideal way of nourishing and nurturing the newborn.

III. THE NATURE OF BIRTH:

A. We value the essential mystery of birth.

B. We value pregnancy and birth as natural processes that technology will never supplant.

C. We value the integrity of life's experiences; the physical, emotional, mental, psychological and spiritual components of a process are inseparable.

D. We value pregnancy and birth as personal, intimate, internal, sexual and social events to be shared in the environment and with the attendants a woman chooses.

E. We value the learning experiences of life and birth.

F. We value pregnancy and birth as processes which have lifelong impact on a woman's self esteem, her health, her ability to nurture and her personal growth.

IV. THE ART OF MIDWIFERY:

A. We value our right to practice the art of midwifery. We value our work as an ancient vocation of women which has existed as long as humans have lived on earth.

B. We value expertise which incorporates academic knowledge, clinical skill, intuitive judgement and spiritual awareness.

C. We value all forms of midwifery education and acknowledge the ongoing wisdom of apprenticeship as the original model for training midwives.

D. We value the art of nurturing the intrinsic normalcy of birth and recognize that each woman and baby have parameters of well-being unique unto themselves.

E. We value the empowerment of women in all aspects of life and particularly as that strength is realized during pregnancy, birth and thereafter. We value the art of encouraging the open expression of that strength so women can birth unhindered and confident in their abilities and in our support.

F. We value skills which support a complicated pregnancy or birth to move toward a state of greater well-being or to be brought to the most healing conclusion possible. We value the art of letting go.

G. We value the acceptance of death as a possible outcome of birth. We value our focus as supporting life rather than avoiding death.

H. We value standing for what we believe in the face of social and political oppression.

V. WOMAN AS MOTHER:

A. We value a mother's intuitive knowledge of herself and her baby before, during and after birth.

B. We value a woman's innate ability to nurture her pregnancy and birth her baby; the power and beauty of her body as it grows and the awesome strength summoned in labor.

C. We value the mother as the only direct care provider for her unborn child.

D. We value supporting women in a non-judgmental way, whatever their state of physical, emotional, social or spiritual health. We value the broadening of available resources whenever possible so that the desired goals of health, happiness and personal growth are realized according to their needs and perceptions.

E. We value the right of each woman to choose a care giver appropriate to her needs and compatible with her belief systems.

F. We value pregnancy and birth as rites of passage integral to a woman's evolution into mothering.

G. We value the potential of partners, family and community to support women in all aspects of birth and mothering.

VI. THE NATURE OF RELATIONSHIP:

A. We value relationship. The quality, integrity, equality and uniqueness of our interactions inform and critique our choices and decisions.

B. We value honesty in relationship.

C. We value caring for women to the best of our ability without prejudice against their age, race, religion, culture, sexual orientation, physical abilities or socioeconomic background.

D. We value the concept of personal responsibility and the right of individuals to make choices regarding what they deem best for themselves. We value the right to true informed choice, not merely informed consent to what we think is best.

E. We value our relationship to a process larger than ourselves, recognizing that birth is something we can seek to learn from and know, but never control.

F. We value humility in our work.

G. We value the recognition of our own limits and limitations.

H. We value direct access to information readily understood by all.

I. We value sharing information and our understanding about birth experiences, skills and knowledge.

J. We value the midwifery community as a support system and an essential place of learning and sisterhood.

K. We value diversity among midwives; recognizing that it broadens our collective resources and challenges us to work for greater understanding of birth and each other.

L. We value mutual trust and respect, which grows from a realization of all of the above.

These values reflect our feelings regarding how we frame midwifery in our hearts and minds. However, due to the broad range of geographic, religious, cultural, political, educational and personal backgrounds among our membership, how we act based on these values will be very individual. Acting ethically is a complex merging of our values and these background influences combined with the relationship we have to others who may be involved in the process taking place. We call upon all these resources when deciding how to respond in the moment to each situation.

We acknowledge the limitations of ethical codes which present a list of rules which must be followed, recognizing that such a code may interfere with, rather than enhance, our ability to make choices. To apply such rules we must have moral integrity, an ability to make judgments, and we must have adequate information; with all of these an appeal to a code becomes superfluous. Furthermore, when we set up rigid ethical codes we may begin to cease considering the transformations we go through as a result of our choices as well as negate our wish to foster truly diversified practice. Rules are not something we can appeal to when all else fails. However, this is the illusion fostered by traditional codes of ethics. MANA's support of the individual's moral integrity grows out of an understanding that there cannot possibly be one right answer for all situations.

We acknowledge the following basic concepts and believe that ethical judgements can be made with these thoughts in mind:

• Moral agency and integrity are born within the heart of each individual.

• Judgments are fundamentally based on awareness and understanding of ourselves and others and are primarily derived from ones own sense of moral integrity with reference to clearly articulated values. Becoming aware and increasing our understanding are on-going processes facilitated by our efforts at personal growth on every level. The wisdom gained by this process cannot be taught or dictated but one can learn to realize, experience and evaluate it.

• The choices we can or will actually make may be limited by the oppressive nature of the medical, legal or cultural framework in which we live. The more our values conflict with those of the dominant culture, the more risky it becomes to act truly in accord with our values.

• The pregnant woman and midwife are both individual moral agents unique unto themselves, having independent value and worth.

• We support ourselves and the women and families we serve to follow and make known the dictates of our own conscience as our relationship begins, evolves and especially when decisions must be made which impact us or the care being provided. It is up to all of us to work out a mutually satisfactory relationship when and if that is possible.

It is useful to understand the two basic theories upon which moral judgments and decision making processes are based. These processes become particularly important when one considers that in our profession, a given woman's rights may not be absolute in all cases, or in certain situations the woman may not be considered autonomous or competent to make her own decisions.

One of the main theories of ethics states that one should look to the consequences of the act (i.e. the outcome) and not the act itself to determine if it is appropriate care. This point of view looks for the greatest good for the greatest number. The other primary ethical theory states that one should look to the act itself (i.e. type of care provided) and if it is right, then this could override the net outcome. This is a more process oriented, feminist perspective. As midwives we weave these two perspectives in the process of making decisions in our practices. Since the outcome of pregnancy is ultimately an unknown and is always unknowable, it is inevitable that in certain circumstances our best decisions in the moment will lead to consequences we could not foresee. In summary, acting ethically is facilitated by:

• Carefully defining our values.

• Weighing the values in consideration with those of the community of midwives, families and culture in which we find ourselves.

• Acting in accord with our values to the best of our ability as the situation demands.

• Engaging in on-going self-examination and evaluation.

There are both individual and social implications to any decision-making process. The actual rules and oppressive aspects of a society are never exact, and therefore conflicts may arise and we must weigh which choices or obligations take precedence over others. There are inevitably times when resolution does not occur and we will be unable to make peace with any course of action or may feel conflicted about a choice already made. The community of women, both midwives and those we serve, will provide a fruitful resource for continued moral support and guidance.

BIBLIOGRAPHY:

Cross, Star. 1989. MANA Ethics Chair. Unpublished draft of MANA Ethics code.

Daly, Mary. 1978. *Gyn Ecology: The Metaethics of Radical Feminism*. Beacon Press: Boston, MA.

Hoagland, Sarah Lucia. 1988. *Lesbian Ethics: Toward New Value*. Institute of Lesbian Studies: Palo Alto, CA.

Johnson, Sonia. 1987. *Going Out of Our Minds: The Metaphysics of Liberation*. Crossing Press: Freedom, CA.

CODE OF ETHICS FOR CERTIFIED NURSE-MIDWIVES

A certified nurse-midwife has professional moral obligations. The purpose of this code is to identify obligations which guide the nurse-midwife in the practice of nurse-midwifery. This code further serves to clarify the expectations of the profession to consumers, the public, other professionals and to potential practitioners.

1. Nurse-midwifery exists for the good of women and their families. This good is safeguarded by practice in accordance with the ACNM Philosophy and ACNM Standards for the Practice of Nurse-Midwifery.

2. Nurse-midwives uphold the belief that childbearing and maturation are normal life processes. When intervention is indicated, it is integrated into care in a way that preserves the dignity of the woman and her family.

3. Decisions regarding nurse-midwifery care require client participation in an ongoing negotiation process in order to develop a safe plan of care. This process considers cultural diversity, individual autonomy and legal responsibilities.

4. Nurse-midwives share professional information with their clients that leads to informed participation and consent. This sharing is done without coercion or deception.

5. Nurse-midwives practice competently. They consult and refer when indicated by their professional scope of practice and/or personal limitations.

6. Nurse-midwives provide care without discrimination based on race, religion, life-style, sexual orientation, socioeconomic status or nature of health problem.

7. Nurse-midwives maintain confidentiality except when there is a clear, serious and immediate danger or when mandated by law.

8. Nurse-midwives take appropriate action to protect clients from harm when endangered by incompetent or unethical practices.

9. Nurse-midwives interact respectfully with the people with whom they work and practice.

10. Nurse-midwives participate in developing and improving the care of women and families through supporting the profession of nurse-midwifery, research, and the education of nurse-midwifery students and nurse-midwives.

11. Nurse-midwives promote community, state and national efforts such as public education and legislation, to ensure access to quality care and to meet the health needs of women and their families.

Source: Ad Hoc Committee on Code of Ethics Approved by Board of Directors May 18, 1990

MIDWIVES ALLIANCE OF NORTH AMERICA (MANA)
MANA CORE COMPETENCIES FOR BASIC MIDWIFERY PRACTICE

The Midwives Alliance of North America was created to organize midwives and to develop educational standards, practice guidelines and support systems for all midwives.

Our core competencies are the basis for standard entry-level preparation of a midwife. Curricula for learning midwifery skills are based on the core competencies. Individual schools or programs are responsible to develop their own curricula based on the core competencies that have been identified. The core competencies are:

MANA CORE COMPETENCIES

GUIDING PRINCIPLES OF PRACTICE

I. The midwife provides care according to the following principles:

A. Midwives work in partnership with women and their chosen support community throughout the caregiving relationship.

B. Midwives respect the dignity, rights and the ability of the women they serve to act responsibly throughout the caregiving relationship.

C. Midwives work as autonomous practitioners, collaborating with other health and social service providers when necessary.

D. Midwives understand that physical, emotional, psycho-social and spiritual factors synergistically comprise the health of individuals and affect the childbearing process.

E. Midwives understand that female physiology and childbearing are normal processes, and work to optimize the well-being of mothers and their developing babies as the foundation of caregiving.

F. Midwives understand that the childbearing experience is primarily a personal, social and community event.

G. Midwives recognize that a woman is the only direct care provider for herself and her unborn baby; thus the most important determinant of a healthy pregnancy is the mother herself.

H. Midwives recognize the empowerment inherent in the childbearing experience and strive to support women to make informed decisions and take responsibility for their own well-being.

I. Midwives strive to insure vaginal birth and provide guidance and support when appropriate to facilitate the spontaneous process of pregnancy, labor, and birth, utilizing medical intervention only as necessary.

J. Midwives synthesize clinical observations, theoretical knowledge, intuitive assessment and spiritual awareness as components of a competent decision making process.

K. Midwives value continuity of care throughout the childbearing cycle and strive to maintain continuous care within realistic limits.

L. Midwives understand that the parameters of "normal" vary widely and recognize that each pregnancy and birth are unique.

GENERAL KNOWLEDGE AND SKILLS

II. The midwife provides care incorporating certain concepts, skills and knowledge from a variety of health and social sciences, including, but not limited to:

A. Communication, counseling, and teaching skills.

B. Human anatomy and physiology relevant to childbearing.

C. Community standards of care for women and their developing infants during the child-bearing cycle, including midwifery and bio-technical medical standards and the rationale for and limitations of such standards.

D. Health and social resources in her community.

E. Significance of and methods for documentation of care through the childbearing cycle.

F. Informed decision making.

G. The principles and appropriate application of clean and aseptic technique and universal precautions.

H. The selection, use and care of the tools and other equipment employed in the provision of midwifery care.

I. Human sexuality, including indications of common problems and indications for counseling.

J. Ethical considerations relevant to reproductive health.

K. The grieving process.

L. Knowledge of cultural variations.

M. Knowledge of common medical terms.

N. The ability to develop, implement and evaluate an individualized plan for midwifery care.

O. Woman-centered care, including the relationship between the mother, infant and their larger support community.

P. Knowledge of various health care modalities as they apply to the childbearing cycle.

CARE DURING PREGNANCY:

III. The midwife provides healthcare, support and information to women throughout pregnancy. She determines the need for consultation or referral as appropriate. The midwife uses a foundation of knowledge and/or skill which includes the following:

A. Identification, evaluation and support of maternal and fetal well-being throughout the process of pregnancy.

B. Education and counseling for the childbearing cycle.

C. Pre-existing conditions in a woman's health history which are likely to influence her well-being when she becomes pregnant.

D. Nutritional requirements of pregnant women and methods of nutritional assessment and counseling.

E. Changes in emotional, psycho-social and sexual variations that may occur during pregnancy.

F. Environmental and occupational hazards for pregnant women.

G. Methods of diagnosing pregnancy.

H. Basic understanding of genetic factors which may indicate the need for counseling, testing or referral.

I. Basic understanding of the growth and development of the unborn baby.

J. Indications for, risks and benefits of bio-technical screening methods and diagnostic tests used during pregnancy.

K. Anatomy, physiology and evaluation of the soft and bony structures of the pelvis.

L. Palpation skills for evaluation of the fetus and uterus.

M. The causes, assessment and treatment of the common discomforts of pregnancy.

N. Identification of, implications of, and appropriate treatment for various infections, disease conditions and other problems which may affect pregnancy.

O. Special needs of the Rh- woman.

CARE DURING LABOR, BIRTH AND IMMEDIATELY THEREAFTER:

IV. *The midwife provides healthcare, support and information to women throughout labor, birth, and the hours immediately thereafter. She determines the need for consultation or referral as appropriate. The midwife uses a foundation of knowledge and/or skill which includes the following:*

A. The normal process of labor and birth.

B. Parameters and methods for evaluating maternal and fetal well-being during labor, birth and immediately thereafter, including relevant historical data.

C. Assessment of the birthing environment, assuring that it is clean, safe and supportive, and that appropriate equipment and supplies are on hand.

D. Emotional responses and their impact during labor, birth and immediately thereafter.

E. Comfort and support measures during labor, birth and immediately thereafter.

F. Fetal and maternal anatomy and their interactions as relevant to assessing fetal position and the progress of labor.

G. Techniques to assist and support the spontaneous vaginal birth of the baby and placenta.

H. Fluid and nutritional requirements during labor, birth and immediately thereafter.

I. Assessment of and support for maternal rest and sleep as appropriate during the process of labor, birth and immediately thereafter.

J. Causes of, evaluation of, and appropriate treatment for variations which occur during the course of labor, birth and immediately thereafter.

K. Emergency measures and transport for critical problems arising during labor, birth or immediately thereafter.

L. Understanding of and appropriate support for the newborn's transition during the first minutes and hours following birth.

M. Familiarity with current bio-technical interventions and technologies which may be commonly used in a medical setting.

N. Evaluation and care of the perineum and surrounding tissues.

POSTPARTUM CARE:

V. *The midwife provides healthcare, support and information to women throughout the postpartum period. She determines the need for consultation or referral as appropriate. The midwife uses a foundation of knowledge and/or skill which includes but is not limited to the following:*

A. Anatomy and physiology of the mother during the postpartum period.

B. Lactation support and appropriate breast care including evaluation of, identification of, and treatments for problems with nursing.

C. Parameters and methods for evaluating and promoting maternal well-being during the postpartum period.

D. Causes of, evaluation of and treatment for maternal discomforts during the postpartum period.

E. Emotional, psycho-social and sexual variations during the postpartum period.

F. Maternal nutritional requirements during the postpartum period including methods of nutritional evaluation and counseling.

G. Causes of, evaluation of, and treatments for problems arising during the postpartum period.

H. Support, information and referral for family planning methods as the individual woman desires.

NEWBORN CARE:

The entry-level midwife provides healthcare to the newborn during the postpartum period and support and information to parents regarding newborn care. She determines the need for consultation or referral as appropriate. The midwife uses a foundation of knowledge and/or skill which includes the following:

A. Anatomy, physiology and support of the newborn's adjustment during the first days and weeks of life.

B. Parameters and methods for evaluating newborn wellness including relevant historical data and gestational age.

C. Nutritional needs of the newborn.

D. Community standards and state laws regarding indications for, administration of, and the risks and benefits of prophylactic bio-technical treatments and screening tests commonly used during the neonatal period.

E. Causes of, assessment of, appropriate treatment and emergency measures for neonatal problems and abnormalities.

PROFESSIONAL, LEGAL AND OTHER ASPECTS:

VII. The entry-level midwife assumes responsibility for practicing in accord with the principles outlined in this document. The midwife uses a foundation of knowledge and/or skill which includes the following:

A. MANA's documents concerning the art and practice of midwifery.

B. The purpose and goal of MANA and local (state or provincial) midwifery associations.

C. The principles of data collection as relevant to midwifery practice.

D. Laws governing the practice of midwifery in her local jurisdiction.

E. Various sites, styles, and modes of practice within the larger midwifery community.

F. A basic understanding of maternal/child healthcare delivery systems in her local jurisdiction.

G. Awareness of the need for midwives to share their knowledge and experience.

WELL-WOMAN CARE & FAMILY PLANNING:

VIII. Depending upon education and training, the entry-level midwife may provide family planning and well-woman care. The practicing midwife may also choose to meet the following core competencies with additional training. In either case, the midwife provides care, support and information to women regarding their overall reproductive health, using a foundation of knowledge and/or skill which includes the following:

A. Understanding of the normal life cycle of women.

B. Evaluation of the woman's well-being including relevant historical data.

C. Causes of, evaluation of, and treatments for problems associated with the female reproductive system and breasts.

D. Information on, provision of or referral for various methods on contraception.

E. Issues involved in decision-making regarding unwanted pregnancies and resources for counseling and referral.

ACNM: THE CORE COMPETENCIES
FOR BASIC MIDWIFERY PRACTICE

May 1997

The core competencies for basic midwifery practice represent the delineation of the fundamental knowledge, skills and behaviors expected of a new practitioner; as such, they serve as guidelines for educators, students, healthcare professionals, consumers, employers and policymakers and constitute the basic requisites for graduates of all nurse-midwifery and midwifery education programs accredited by the American College of Nurse-Midwives (ACNM)*.

Midwifery practice is based on the Core Competencies for Basic Midwifery Practice, The Standards for the Practice of Nurse-Midwifery and the Code of Ethics promulgated by the American College of Nurse-Midwives. Midwives who have been certified by the ACNM or the ACNM Certification Council, Inc. (ACC) assume responsibility and accountability for their practice as primary care providers.

Midwifery education is based on a theoretical foundation in the health sciences as well as clinical preparation which focuses on the knowledge, judgment and skills deemed necessary to provide primary care and independent management of women and newborns within a healthcare system that provides for medical consultation, collaborative management, or referral as appropriate. Recognizing that creativity, innovation and individuality are essential to the vitality of the profession, each education program may develop its own unique identity and may choose to extend beyond the core competencies into other areas of healthcare. In addition, each graduate is responsible for complying with the laws of the jurisdiction where the practice of midwifery is conducted.

The ACNM defines the midwife's role in primary care based on the Institute of Medicine's definition (1994), the ACNM's Philosophy (1989), and the ACNM Board of Directors' Position Statement on Primary Care by Nurse-Midwives (1992). Primary care is the provision of integrated, accessible healthcare services by clinicians who are accountable for addressing the large majority of personal healthcare needs, developing a sustained partnership with patients, and practicing within the context of family and community. Certified nurse-midwives (CNMs) and certified midwives (CMs) are often the initial contact for providing healthcare to women and they provide such care on a continuous and comprehensive basis. As a primary provider, the CNM or CM assumes responsibility for provision of and referral for appropriate services within a defined scope of practice.

The concepts and skills identified below and the midwifery management process outlined in the sections that follow apply to all components of midwifery care and comprise the foundation upon which practice guidelines and curriculum content must be built. This document is reviewed and revised at least every five years to reflect changing trends and new developments in midwifery practice and must be adhered to in its entirety.

HALLMARKS OF MIDWIFERY

The art and science of midwifery are characterized by these hallmarks: recognition of pregnancy and birth as a normal physiologic and developmental process and advocacy of nonintervention in the absence of complications; recognition of menses and menopause as a normal physiologic and developmental process; promotion of family-centered care; empowerment of women as partners in healthcare; facilitation of healthy family and interpersonal relationships; promotion of continuity of care; health promotion, disease prevention and health education; advocacy for informed choice, participatory decision-making, and the right to self-determination; cultural competency and proficiency; skillful communication, guidance and counseling; therapeutic value of human presence; value of and respect for differing paths toward knowledge and growth; effective communication and collaboration with other members of the healthcare team; promotion of a public healthcare perspective; care to vulnerable populations.

COMPONENTS OF MIDWIFERY CARE: PROFESSIONAL RESPONSIBILITIES OF CNMs AND CMs

The professional responsibilities of CNMS and CMS include, but are not limited to, these components:

Knowledge of the history of midwifery; knowledge of the legal basis for practice; knowledge of national and international issues and trends in women's health and maternal/newborn care; support of legislation and initiatives to promote high quality healthcare services; knowledge of issues and trends in healthcare policy and systems; commitment to the ACNM's Philosophy, Standards and Code of Ethics; participation in midwifery education; systematic collection of practice data to document midwifery care outcomes; ability to evaluate, apply, interpret and collaborate in research; participation in self-evaluation, peer review, continuing education, and other activities that ensure and validate quality practice; development of leadership skills.

COMPONENTS OF MIDWIFERY CARE: MIDWIFERY MANAGEMENT PROCESS

The midwifery management process includes:

Systematically compiling and updating a complete and relevant database for the comprehensive assessment of each client's health, including a thorough health history and physical examination; identifying problems and formulating diagnoses based upon interpretation of the database; identifying healthcare needs/problems and establishing healthcare goals in collaboration with the client; providing information and support to enable women to make informed decisions and to assume primary responsibility for their own health; developing a comprehensive plan of care with the client; assuming primary responsibility for the implementation of individualized plans; obtaining consultation, planning and implementing collaborative management, and referral or transferring the care of the client as appropriate; Initiating management of specific complications, emergencies and deviations from normal; evaluating, with the client, the achievement of healthcare goals and modifying the plan of care as appropriate.

COMPONENTS OF MIDWIFERY CARE: THE CHILDBEARING FAMILY

I. PRE-CONCEPTION CARE

A. Independently manages care of the woman who is preparing for pregnancy

B. Applies knowledge of midwifery practice that includes, but is not limited to, the following:

1. Reproductive anatomy and physiology related to conception

2. Impact of health, family and genetic history on pregnancy outcomes

3. Health and laboratory screening to evaluate the potential for a healthy pregnancy

4. Assessment of readiness for pregnancy of the woman and her family including emotional, psychosocial and sexual factors

5. Nutritional assessment and counseling

6. Influence of environmental and occupational factors, health habits and behavior on pregnancy planning

II. CARE OF THE CHILDBEARING WOMAN

A. Independently manages care of the woman during pregnancy, childbirth and the postpartum period

B. Applies knowledge of midwifery practice in the antepartum period that includes, but is not limited to, the following:

1. Anatomy and physiology of conception, pregnancy and lactation

2. Diagnosis of pregnancy

3. Genetics, placental physiology, embryology and fetal development

4. Epidemiology of maternal and perinatal morbidity and mortality

5. Influence of environmental and occupational factors, health habits and maternal behaviors on pregnancy outcomes

6. Emotional and psychosexual change during pregnancy

7. Health risks including domestic violence, sexually transmitted diseases, substance, alcohol and tobacco use

8. Effect of maternal nutrition on pregnancy outcomes

9. Indicators of normal pregnancy and deviations from normal

10. Assessment of the progress of pregnancy and fetal well-being

11. Etiology and management of common discomforts of pregnancy

12. Management techniques and therapeutics, including complementary therapies** to facilitate healthy pregnancy and outcome

13. Anticipatory guidance related to birth, lactation, parenthood and change in the family constellation

14. Pharmacokinetics and pharmacotherapeutics of medications commonly used during pregnancy

15. Principles of group education

C. Applies knowledge of midwifery practice in the intrapartum period that includes, but is not limited to, the following:

1. Anatomy and physiology of the structures and processes of labor

2. Anatomy and physiology of the fetus

3. Diagnosis and assessment of labor and its progress through the four stages

4. Assessment of maternal and fetal status during labor

5. Indicators of deviations from normal including complications and emergencies

6. Measures to support psychosocial needs during labor and delivery

7. Management techniques and therapeutics, including complementary therapies, to facilitate normal labor progress

8. Techniques for (i) administration of local anesthesia, including pudendal blocks, (ii) spontaneous vaginal delivery, (iii) third stage management, and (iv) performance and repair of episiotomy and repair of lacerations

9. Techniques for management of emergency complications and abnormal birth events

10. Pharmacokinetics and pharmacotherapeutics of medications commonly used during labor and birth

D. Applies knowledge of midwifery practice in the postpartum period that includes, but is not limited to, the following:

1. Anatomy and physiology of the puerperium

2. Emotional, psychosocial and sexual changes of the puerperium

3. Postpartum self-care, infant care, contraception and family relationships

4. Management techniques and therapeutics, including complementary therapies, to facilitate a healthy puerperium

5. Methods of facilitation or suppression of lactation

6. Deviations from normal and appropriate interventions including management of complications and emergencies

7. Management of discomforts of the puerperium

8. Pharmacokinetics and pharmacotherapeutics of medications commonly used during the puerperium

III. Newborn Care

A. Independently manages the care of the newborn

B. Applies knowledge of midwifery practice that includes, but is not limited to, the following:

1. Effect of maternal/fetal risk factors on the newborn

2. Anatomy and physiology of the newborn

3. Nutritional needs of the newborn

4. Bonding and attachment theory

5. Evaluation of neonatal status: (i) physical and behavioral assessment, (ii) gestational age assessment, and (iii) common screening and diagnostic tests per formed on the neonate

6. Methods to facilitate adaptation to extrauterine life: (i) stabilization at birth, (ii) resuscitation, and (iii) emergency management

7. Promotion and management of breast-feeding

8. Indications of deviation from normal and appropriate interventions

9. Management techniques to facilitate integration of the newborn into the family

10. Pharmacokinetics and pharmacotherapeutics of common medications used in the neonatal period

Components of Midwifery Care: The Primary Care of Women

I. Health Promotion and Disease Prevention

A. Independently manages primary health screening of women through the life cycle

B. Applies knowledge of midwifery practice that includes, but is not limited to, the following:

1. Anatomy and physiology

2. Growth and development patterns for the woman across the life span

3. Basic principles of clinical epidemiology as they affect women's health

4. National defined goals and objectives for health promotion and disease prevention

5. Parameters for assessment of physical and mental health

6. Utilization of nationally defined screening recommendations to promote health and detect/prevent disease

7. Management techniques and therapeutics, including complementary therapies, to facilitate health

8. Pharmacokinetics and pharmacotherapeutics of immunizations

II. Management of Common Health Problems

A. Assumes responsibility for the triage of common health problems presented by women and for management, collaboration, co-management and/or referral to appropriate levels of healthcare services within the CNM's or CM's defined scope of practice

B. Applies the knowledge of midwifery practice that includes, but is not limited to, the following:

1. Anatomy and pathophysiology related to frequently occurring conditions

2. Etiology of common health problems of essentially healthy women

3. Parameters for differential diagnosis of common presenting health problems

4. Management techniques and therapeutics, including complementary therapies, for the treatment of common health problems of essentially healthy women

5. Pharmacokinetics and pharmacotherapeutics of frequently prescribed medications for common health problems

6. Skills in healthcare team leadership and management to ensure that presenting healthcare concerns are addressed completely by a multi-disciplinary healthcare team and community services

III. FAMILY PLANNING/GYNECOLOGIC CARE

A. Independently manages the care of women seeking family planning and/or gynecologic services

B. Applies knowledge of midwifery practice that includes, but is not limited to, the following:

1. Anatomy and physiology of the reproductive systems, including the breast, through the life cycle

2. Human sexuality

3. Common screening and diagnostic tests

4. Parameters for differential diagnosis of common gynecologic problems including sexually transmitted diseases

5. Essentials of barrier, hormonal, mechanical, chemical, physiologic and surgical conception control methods

6. Management techniques and therapeutics, including complementary therapies, for common gynecologic problems and family planning needs

7. Counseling for sexual behaviors that promote health and prevent disease

8. Resources for counseling and referral for unplanned or undesired pregnancies, sexual concerns, infertility, and other gynecologic problems

9. Pharmacokinetics and pharmacotherapeutics of frequently prescribed medications for family planning and gynecologic care

IV. PERIMENOPAUSE AND POST-MENOPAUSE

A. Independently manages the care of women during the perimenopause and post-menopause

B. Applies knowledge of midwifery practice that includes, but is not limited to, the following:

1. Anatomy and physiology of the systems as affected by the aging process

2. The effects of the menopause of physical and mental health

3. Nutritional needs of the aging woman

4. Common screening and diagnostic tests pertinent to the evaluation of the health of women with advancing age

5. Identification of deviations from normal and appropriate interventions

6. Counseling and education for health maintenance and health promotion in the aging woman

7. Management techniques and therapeutics, including complementary therapies, for alleviating the common discomforts that accompany aging

8. Pharmacokinetics and pharmacotherapeutics of frequently prescribed medications and treatments for the perimenopausal and menopausal woman

* Midwifery as used throughout this document refers to the education and practice of certified nurse-midwives (CNMs) and certified midwives (CMs) who have been certified by the American College of Nurse-Midwives (ACNM) or ACNM Certification Council, Inc (ACC).

** Complementary therapies as used throughout this document refer to those therapeutic measures for which there is some evidence of safety and effectiveness.

MANA STANDARDS AND QUALIFICATIONS
FOR THE ART AND PRACTICE OF MIDWIFERY

revised January, 1997

The midwife recognizes that childbearing is a woman's experience and encourages the active involvement of family members in her care.

1. Skills: Necessary skills of a practicing midwife include the ability to:

   • Provide continuity of care for the woman and her family during the maternity cycle,

   • Assess and provide care for healthy women during pregnancy, birth and the postpartum period and for newborns during the first six weeks of life;

   • Identify and assess deviations from normal;

   • Maintain proficiency in life-saving measures by regular review and practice;

   • Deal with emergency situations appropriately.

   • In addition, a midwife may choose to provide well-woman care.

   It is affirmed that judgement and intuition play a role in competent assessment and response.

2. Appropriate equipment: Midwives are equipped to assess maternal, fetal newborn well-being; to maintain a clean and/or aseptic technique; to treat maternal hemorrhage; and to resuscitate mother or infant.

3. Records: Midwives keep accurate records of care provided for each woman such as are acceptable in current midwifery practice. Records shall be held confidential and provided to the woman on request.

4. Data collection: Midwives collect data for their practice on a regular basis. It is highly recommended that this be done prospectively, following the guidelines and using the data form developed by the MANA Statistics and Research Committee.

5. Compliance: Midwives will inform and assist parents regarding the public health requirements of the jurisdiction in which the midwifery practice will occur.

6. Medical consultation and referral: All midwives recognize that there are certain conditions when medical consultations are advisable. The midwife shall make a reasonable attempt to assure that her client has access to consultation and/or referral to a medical care system when indicated.

7. Screening: Midwives respect the woman's right to self-determination within the boundaries of responsible care. Midwives continually assess each woman regarding her health and well-being relevant to the appropriateness of midwifery services. Women will be informed of this assessment. It is the right and responsibility of the midwife to refuse or discontinue services in certain circumstances. Appropriate referrals are made in the interest of the mother or baby's well-being or when the required or requested care is outside the midwife's legal or personal scope of practice as described in her protocols.

8. Informed choice: Each midwife will present accurate information about herself and her services, including but not limited to:

   • Her education in midwifery

   • Her experience level in midwifery

   • Her protocols and standards

   • Her financial charges for services

   • The services she does and does not provide

   • The responsibilities of the pregnant woman and her family

9. Continuing education: Midwives will update their knowledge and skills on a regular basis.

10. Peer review: Midwifery practice includes an on-going process of case review with peers.

11. Protocols: Each midwife will develop protocols for her services that are in agreement with

the basic philosophy of MANA and in keeping with her level of understanding. Each midwife is encouraged to put her protocols in writing.

REFERENCES:

American College of Nurse-Midwives documents.

ICM membership and joint study on maternity, FIGO, WHO, etc. Revised 1972.

New Mexico regulations for the practice of lay midwifery. Revised 1982.

North West Coalition of Midwives. *Standards for Safety and Competency in Midwifery.*

Varney, Helen. *Nurse-Midwifery.* Blackwell Scientific Pub., Boston, MA 1980.

GOALS OF MANA

To expand communication and support among North American midwives.

To form an indentifiable and cohesive organization representing the profession of midwifery on a regional, national and international basis.

To promote guidelines for the education of midwives and to assist in the development of midwifery education programs.

To promote research in the field of midwifery as a quality healthcare option.

To promote and support a woman's right to choose her care provider and place of birth.

To promote public education and midwifery advocacy.

CATEGORIES OF PROFESSIONAL MIDWIVES

DIRECT-ENTRY MIDWIVES

"Direct-entry" midwives, who are licensed in some states, are not required to become nurses before training to be midwives. The Midwifery Education and Accreditation Council (MEAC) is currently accrediting direct-entry midwifery educational programs and apprenticeships in the United States. Direct-entry midwives' legal status varies according to state, and they practice most often in birth centers and in homes.

CERTIFIED PROFESSIONAL MIDWIVES

Certified professional midwives (CPMs) may gain their midwifery education through a variety of routes. They must have their midwifery skills and experience evaluated through the North American Registry of Midwives (NARM) and pass the NARM Written Examination and Skills Assessment. The legal status of these nationally credentialed direct-entry midwives varies from state to state (see page 300). In some of the states where they are also individually licensed, midwives' services are reimbursable through Medicaid and private insurance carriers.

CERTIFIED NURSE-MIDWIVES

Certified nurse-midwives (CNMs) are educated in both nursing and midwifery. After attending an educational program accredited by the American College of Nurse Midwives Certification Council (ACC), they must pass the ACC examination and can be licensed in the individual states in which they practice, most often in hospitals and birth centers.

— Approved by MANA Board 10/3/94

This information was taken from the MANA homepage.

STANDARDS FOR THE PRACTICE
OF NURSE-MIDWIFERY

Nurse-midwifery practice is the independent management of women's healthcare, focusing particularly on pregnancy, childbirth, the postpartum period, care of the newborn, and the family planning and gynecological needs of women. The certified nurse-midwife (CNM) practices within a healthcare system that provides for consultation, collaborative management or referral as indicated by the health status of the client. Certified nurse-midwives practice in accord with the Standards for the Practice of Nurse-Midwifery, as defined by the American College of Nurse-Midwives (ACNM). The nurse-midwife is committed to maintaining a high standard of professional care, to participating in the education of nurse-midwives, and to promoting the concepts of nurse-midwifery practice in the community.

STANDARD I

Nurse-midwifery care is provided by qualified practitioners

The practitioner: Is certified by the ACNM-approved certifying agent. Shows evidence of continuing competency as required by the American College of Nurse-Midwives. Is in compliance with the legal requirements of the jurisdiction where the nurse-midwifery practice occurs.

STANDARD II

Nurse-midwifery care supports individual rights and self-determination within boundaries of safety

The certified nurse-midwife: Practices in accord with the Philosophy and the Code of Ethics of the American College of Nurse-Midwives. Provides clients with a description of the scope of nurse-midwifery services and information regarding the client's rights and responsibilities. Provides clients with information on other providers and services when requested or when care required is not within the scope of practice of the individual nurse-midwife. Promotes involvement of support persons in the practice setting.

STANDARD III

Nurse-midwifery care is comprised of knowledge, skills and judgments that foster the delivery of safe and satisfying care

The certified nurse-midwife: Collects and assesses client care data, develops and implements a plan of management and evaluates the outcome of care. Demonstrates the clinical skills and judgments described in the ACNM Core Competencies for Basic Nurse-Midwifery Practice. Practices in accord with the ACNM Standards for the Practice of Nurse-Midwifery. Practices in accord with the policies of the nurse-midwifery service/practice that meet the requirements of the particular institution or practice setting. Expands clinical practice in accordance with ACNM Guidelines for the Incorporation of New Procedures into Nurse-Midwifery Practice.

STANDARD IV

Nurse-midwifery care is based upon knowledge, skills and judgments which are reflected in written policies/practice guidelines

The certified nurse-midwife: Describes the parameters for the service/practice for nurse-midwifery management, physician management and collaborative management. Establishes practice guidelines for each specialty area, which include but are not limited to:

Antepartum

Criteria for admission to the nurse-midwife service, parameters and methods for assessing the progress of pregnancy, parameters and methods for assessing fetal well-being, indicators of risk in pregnancy and appropriate intervention, parameters for medications prescribed/used during pregnancy.

Intrapartum

Parameters and methods for assessing progress of labor and birth, parameters and methods for assessing maternal and fetal status, parameters for medications and solutions prescribed/used during labor and birth, management of birth and the immediate postpartum period, methods to facilitate the newborn's adaptation to extrauterine life.

Significant Deviations from Normal and Appropriate Interventions

Parameters and methods for assessing the immediate well-being of the newborn

Postpartum/Newborn

Parameters and methods for assessing the postpartum status of the mother, parameters and methods for assessing the well-being of the newborn, parameters for medications prescribed/used in the puerperium, significant deviations from normal and appropriate interventions.

Family Planning/Gynecology

Parameters and methods for assessing general physical and emotional status of the client, parameters for medications and devices prescribed/used, significant deviations from normal and appropriate interventions.

Standard V

Nurse-midwifery care is provided in a safe environment

The certified nurse-midwife: Demonstrates knowledge of and utilizes federal and state regulations that apply to practice environment and infection control. Promotes adequate staffing in the clinical setting where the nurse-midwife practices. Demonstrates appropriate techniques for emergency management including arrangements for emergency transportation.

Standard VI

Nurse-midwifery care occurs within the healthcare system of the community using appropriate resources for referrals to meet medical, psychosocial, economic and cultural or family needs

The certified nurse-midwife: Demonstrates a safe mechanism for obtaining medical consultation, collaboration and referral. Uses community services. Demonstrates knowledge of medical, psychosocial, economic, cultural and family factors that may affect care.

Standard VII

Nurse-midwifery care is documented in legible, complete health records

The certified nurse-midwife: Uses records that facilitate communication of information to consultants and institutions. Facilitates clients' access to their records. Provides written documentation of risk assessment, course of management and outcome of care. Provides for prompt entry on the health record of laboratory tests, treatments and consultations. Provides a mechanism for sending a copy of the health record on referral or transfer to other levels of care. Treats records as confidential documents.

Standard VIII

Nurse midwifery care is evaluated according to an established program for quality assessment that includes a plan to identify and resolve problems

The certified nurse-midwife: Participates in a program of quality assurance/ improvement for the evaluation of nurse-midwifery practice within the setting in which it occurs and within legal requirements. Collects client care data systematically and is involved in analysis of that data for the evaluation of the process and outcome of care. Seeks consultation to review problems identified by the quality assurance/improvement program. Acts to resolve problems that are identified. Participates in peer review.

Midwifery
Ancient Art of Touching the Future

Ancient Art Midwifery Institute

The standard of excellence in academic midwifery education since 1981

We offer the original midwifery home study course developed by Carla Hartley
Self-paced program • Comprehensive curriculum
Individual assistance • On-line Study Group
Affordable Tuition • 0% Interest Payment Plans

Student Options:

Documented Apprenticeship • Advanced Academics • Philomath Option
Abbreviated Academics • Childbirth Educator Certification Option

We also offer:

Introduction to Midwifery • All My Babies Video
Helping Hands, The Apprentice Workbook by Carla Hartley

P.O. Box 788 Claremore, OK 74018-0788
Telephone 918-342-2926 • 818-902-0449
FAX 818-902-0449 • e-mail AnctArtMi@aol.com
Visit our website: http://members.aol.com/anctartmi/index.html

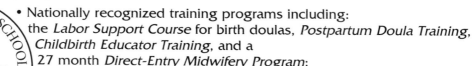
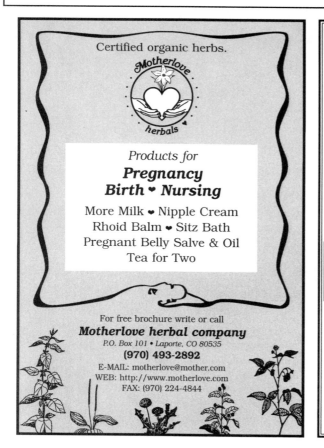
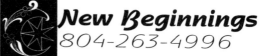
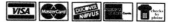

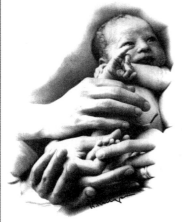
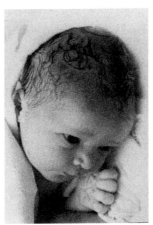
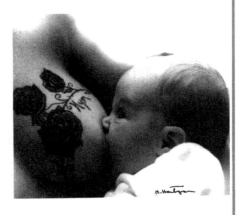

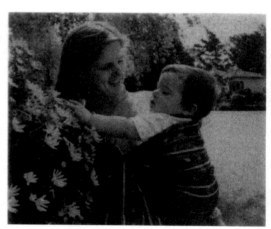
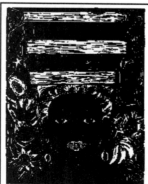

MIDWIFERY TODAY CONFERENCE TAPES

Various speakers, 1992 – 98. (Midwifery Today, P.O. Box 2672, Eugene, OR 97402, $9.00 single cassettes, $16.00 double cassettes, request a complete list.)

Two years ago I was all set to attend the annual Midwifery Today conference in Eugene. I had saved money and was about to reserve plane tickets, when last-minute changes of plans had to be made. So I did the next best thing in the following years: I acquired some of the conference tapes.

Admittedly, there were a few lumps in my throat as I listened to the taped sessions; the atmosphere of sharing and caring during the conference sessions is palpable, and this can make you acutely aware of what you've missed by not being there in person. My favorite tape that expresses this feeling of sisterhood is Jill Cohen's "Philosophy of Midwifery" tape. The lecture and group participation is excellent, inspiring and thought-provoking.

If you can't save enough for air fare, lodging and other expenses, do the next best thing with your money: spend a sizable amount of your savings on some of the conference tapes. Or, if you have attended any of the conferences, relive your favorite classes or attend the ones you missed—on tape. You will learn a lot and feel more connected to your worldwide network of colleagues.

Reviewer Sue LaLeike lives in Florida with her family. She is a contributing editor at Midwifery Today.

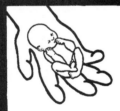

The Midwifery Today Homepage

http://www.midwiferytoday.com

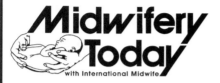 # Online

Updated Weekly!

New Features include:

- Online specials for Web customers. Come see our new special product discounts every two weeks!
- Tip of the week. Coming soon, a weekly midwifery trick to add to your birth bag!
- Jan's Musings. Don't miss the wisdom of our editor, Jan Tritten, in her weekly commentary, coming soon!
- News updates and new articles will be posted frequently.

Don't miss the latest!

Your online resource for birth and midwifery.

<u>Conferences</u> <u>Products</u> <u>Midwifery Today</u> <u>Magazine</u> <u>The Birthkit</u>

<u>Related Sites</u> <u>Books</u> <u>Directory of Midwives</u> <u>Email</u>

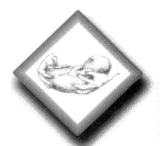

Send us email!
Subscriptions/orders: Midwifery@aol.com
Editorial: Mtedit@aol.com

If you love birth, you'll love Midwifery Today

Learn about birth and midwifery with the news, reviews, birth stories and information you'll receive four times a year.

When you open our pages, you'll...

▶ Learn from articles written by midwives & other birth practitioners from around the world

▶ Discover techniques that work in Tricks of the Trade

▶ Keep informed about the latest publications with Media Reviews and Journal Abstracts

▶ Learn new insights from a homebirth, birth center and hospital CNM with Marion's Message

▶ Stay aware of midwifery worldwide with the International Midwife (IM) section

▶ Each issue is thematically oriented, such as:

- Prolonged Labor
- Keeping Birth Normal
- Hemorrhage
- Bridging the Gap
- Homebirth
- Birth Center

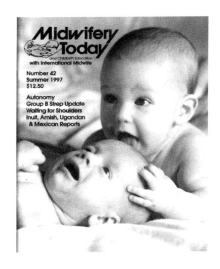

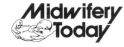

Midwifery Today, Inc.
PO Box 2672-857, Eugene OR 97402
(800) 743-0974, (541) 344-7438,
fax (541) 344-1422
http://www.midwiferytoday.com
Midwifery@aol.com

Want healthier babies and easier births?
Learn tricks expert midwives use!

These unique collections of life-saving tips, suggestions and remedies used by experienced midwives and birth practitioners around the world are perfect for birth practitioners of any kind and make wonderful gifts for midwives, doulas and any birth practitioner.

Life of a Midwife: A Celebration of Midwifery

This is the companion guide to *Paths to Becoming a Midwife*. With these two books you will understand what it is like to be a midwife.

Practicing and aspiring midwives can:

• Learn from ideas, experiences, joys and tribulations of many birth practitioners

• Read about character, roles, realities and ways of practice

Aspiring midwives will:

• Discover what it takes to be a midwife

• See if the profession is for you. Know what midwifery involves before you invest your life in it

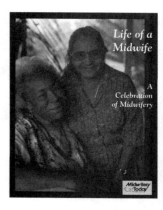

$25

Tricks of the Trade

You will learn about:
• Prenatal Care • Organizing Your Practice • Postpartum
• First, Second and Third Stage • Educating Parents
• Taking Care of the Babies • Special Features include:
• Tear Prevention and Nutrition • Herbal Formulary

Wisdom of the Midwives:
Tricks of the Trade II

$20

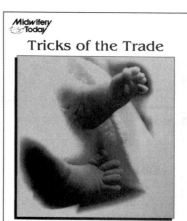

This volume is full of ideas and techniques to help babies and mothers at births you attend.

Learn about:
• Counseling as a Tool in Your Birth Kit
• Nutrition and Healthy Birth Ideas
• Herbs / Homeopathy / Chinese Medicine
• Pregnancy
• Premature Rupture of Membranes
• More First Stage Help and much more!

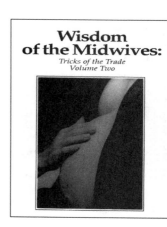

$25

If you are a school or birth resource and wish to update or add your school information, please fill out this form as completely as possible:

School Name:

Years in Business:

Address:

Phone: **Fax:**

Email: **Homepage:**

Program Type:

Program Length:

Class Size:

Prerequisites:

Degree/Certification:

Tuition:

Mission Statement/Philosophy:

Additional information:

Please check the appropriate boxes describing your organization:

☐ **Apprenticeship**

☐ **Certified Nurse-Midwifery**   ☐ **Advanced Training**

☐ **Childbirth Education**   ☐ **NARM**

☐ **Direct-Entry or Lay Midwifery**   ☐ **MEAC Accredited**

☐ **Doula/Labor Support training**   ☐ **ACNM**

☐ **Other Programs**   ☐ **Lactation**

☐ **Postpartum**   ☐ **Distance Learning/Correspondence**

ORDER FORM

Please send me the following books:

___ copies of Life of a Midwife at $25 each $_____
(the feel for a midwife's life in story, articles and photos)

___ copies of Tricks of the Trade, Vol. 1, at $20 each $_____
(midwives' techniques and tricks)

___ copies of Wisdom of the Midwives (Tricks...Vol. 2), at $25 each $_____
(midwives' techniques and tricks, insights)

___ copies of Paths to Becoming a Midwife, at $29.^{95} ea. $_____
See box for great discounts on bulk orders.

Subtotal for books:	$_____
Shipping and handling:	$_____
Subtotal:	$_____

US: up to $10.00=$2.50; $10.01–$25=$4.00; $25.01–$65=$7.50; $65.01–$100=$10; over $100=$12
• Additional Speed Shipping: UPS 2nd day air: $8; overnight – $22 US Only
Canada/Mexico: up to $10.00=$3; $10.01–$25=$5; $25.01–$65=$9; $65.01–$100=$12; over $100=$15
Other International (ground): up to $10.00=$3.25; $10.01 $25=$5.75; $25.01–$65=$10.25; $65.01– $100=$13.25; over $100=$15.50

BULK DISCOUNT RATES*:	
5–15	30%
16–25	40%
26+	50%

*Per title
Other discounts don't apply

Name _____

Street Address_____

City, State, Zip & Country_____

Phone _____

Profession_____

❏ Check   ❏ MasterCard   ❏ Visa   ❏ Card No. _____
Exp. _____

Name on credit card _____

Signature _____

❏ *Midwifery Today* magazine!

2 years: ❏ U.S. $95   ❏ Mexico/Canada $113   ❏ All other countries $143
1 year: ❏ U.S. $50   ❏ Mexico/Canada $60   ❏ All other countries $75

Please start my subscription with: ❏ Current issue   ❏ Other ___

Midwifery Today, Inc.
P.O. Box 2672-857 • Eugene, OR, 97402 USA
(541) 344-7438 • (800) 743-0974 • fax (541) 344-1422
Midwifery@aol.com • http://www.midwiferytoday.com